MODERN PERSPECTIVES IN PSYCHIATRY
Edited by John G. Howells

11

MODERN PERSPECTIVES IN PSYCHOSOCIAL PATHOLOGY

MODERN PERSPECTIVES IN PSYCHIATRY

Edited by John G. Howells

Modern Perspectives in Psychosocial Pathology

Edited by

JOHN G. HOWELLS
M.D., F.R.C.Psych., D.P.M.

BRUNNER/MAZEL, *Publishers* • New York

Library of Congress Cataloging-in-Publication Data

Modern perspectives in psychosocial pathology.

   (Modern perspectives in psychiatry ; 11)
   Includes bibliographies and indexes.
   1. Mental illness.   2. Psychology, Pathological.
I. Howells, John G.   II. Series. [DNLM: 1. Mental
Disorders.   2. Social Problems. W1 MO167P v.11 / WM 100
M6883]
RC454.M58   1988   616.89   88-2873
ISBN 0-87630-511-7

Copyright © 1988 by John G. Howells

Published by
BRUNNER/MAZEL, INC.
19 Union Square
New York, New York 10003

MANUFACTURED IN THE UNITED STATES OF AMERICA

10 9 8 7 6 5 4 3 2 1

EDITOR'S PREFACE

The Modern Perspectives Series is an international encyclopedia of psychiatry. The ten volumes already published cover the psychiatry of all age periods — infancy, childhood, adolescence, adulthood, middle age, and old age — together with explorations into world psychiatry, into the special fields of psycho-obstetrics, into the psychiatric aspects of surgery, and a special volume on general clinical psychiatry.

The Series now continues with this volume on psychosocial pathology, to be followed by two volumes devoted to main nosological entities — the neuroses and the affective disorders.

Modern Perspectives in Psychosocial Pathology, focuses on how psychopathology in individuals and families impinges on society, creating social psychopathology, or arises in society itself as a social group expression of psychopathology. Social psychopathology becomes a matter for social concern, social action, and social treatment. The first chapters describe social pathology arising through children and are followed by chapters showing the expression of social pathology through adults. The volume concludes with chapters demonstrating social pathology arising as a social group phenomenon.

The aim of each volume in the Series has remained as stated in the first volume of the Series. *Modern Perspectives in Psychosocial Pathology* is thus planned to bring the facts from the growing points of psychiatry, and pertinent related fields, to the attention of the clinician at as early a stage as possible. A complete coverage of the field is not attempted. A single volume is not a textbook. To give an international flavor to the Series the Editor feels free to wander over the world, inviting acknowledged experts to present a topic to the readership. Each contributor has the task of selecting, appraising, and explaining the available knowledge on his subject for the benefit of colleagues who may be less acquainted with that field. Special consideration is given to the requirements of psychiatrists in training.

The Editor eschews any interests or biases of his own. Thus ranging over

v

the possible topics, it becomes apparent that those to be covered select themselves. Together, they speak of eclecticism. Although leaning toward the clinical, applied and basic sciences, clinical and biobehavioral sciences, dynamic and biological psychiatry stand comfortably together.

In this volume, as in all previous volumes in the Series, the Editor has profited by the zeal and flair of his Assistant Editor, Mrs. Livia Osborn. This he gratefully acknowledges.

CONTENTS

vii

MODERN PERSPECTIVES IN PSYCHIATRY
Edited by John G. Howells

11

MODERN PERSPECTIVES IN PSYCHOSOCIAL PATHOLOGY

1

CHILD ABUSE: WILL WE EVER FIND A "VACCINE" OR "CURE"?

Marilyn Heins, M.D.

Vice Dean, Professor of Pediatrics,
University of Arizona College of Medicine,
Health Sciences Center,
Tucson, Arizona

Child abuse is not a new problem; it has become increasingly more visible, it affects large numbers of children, and — to date — is difficult both to treat and to prevent. All professionals who deal with children — physicians, nurses, counselors, teachers — need a special awareness of child abuse because appropriate intervention can be lifesaving. Also, society as a whole must pay attention to this potentially fatal and often crippling "disease," which carries a costly price tag. Although we use the term "child abuse," the locus of the "pathology" lies in the parents or caretakers. The child is the victim of this pathology. Yet, if the condition were more accurately called "inadequate parenting syndrome," less attention might be paid to it. Thus, Kempe, in 1962, did a great service to children when he coined the term "battered child" (25).

A WORD OF HISTORY

There have been several excellent reviews of the history of child abuse (36, 38, 43). I summarized the history of child abuse in a Landmark Perspective article that accompanied the republication of Kempe's landmark article in the *Journal of the American Medical Association* (19).*

---

*Reprinted with permission. Copyright 1984, American Medical Association.

Violence against infants and children is at least as old as recorded history. Infanticide was an accepted practice for dealing with unwanted children in prehistoric and ancient cultures in the face of scarce resources. Darwin actually postulated that one could correlate the beginning of human civilization with infanticide. "Our early semi-human progenitors would not have practiced infanticide. . . . For the instincts of the lower animals are never so perverted as to lead them regularly to destroy their own offspring."

We know from the Bible that ritual sacrifice of children — or near-misses in the case of Isaac and Moses — was common. In the Judeo-Christian tradition of counteracting infanticide, the customs of circumcision and baptism serve as symbols substituting for the sacrifice of children. After these rituals, infants are provided with both a given name and a family name, which bonds the child to the protecting family that has allowed him life. Early Roman law gave the father the absolute right of life or death over his child, but the Christian church began to preach against infanticide in the fourth century, and Roman laws making infanticide a capital offense followed. These laws were the beginning of the notion of parens patriae, which defines the right of the state to intervene in the family on behalf of the child. Yet, infanticide, especially of illegitimate children, continued through the 19th century. Abandonment rather than frank murder became the method most often used to get rid of unwanted children. The first foundling home to save the lives of abandoned children was not established until 787 A.D.

Concomitant with the Protestant Reformation arose the belief that children should be educated and disciplined in order to create a godly society on earth. Discipline became a sacred duty of families; the Puritans even established the death penalty for disobedient children, although there is no documentation of its use. Calvinist doctrine dictated that children should be whipped regularly to help rid them of innate depravity. Through the 17th century, flogging of children was common; most of these children today would be considered victims of physical abuse.

The 18th century brought enlightenment in the care of children. Locke and Rousseau both held that children were shaped by their experience and were innocent before being corrupted by society. Corporal punishment was no longer considered necessary to ensure salvation. By the 19th century children came to be relatively well treated unless they were poor and forced to work at an early age. In this country, one of the earliest social reforms was directed against the widespread use of child labor, and, when the Children's Bureau was established in 1912 to oversee the health and welfare of children, it was housed in the Department of Labor.

The first recorded case of child abuse in this country occurred in New York in 1874. A church worker calling on an elderly lady in a tenement learned that an eight-year-old child by the name of Mary Ellen, who was in the care of foster parents, was being starved and beaten. The church worker tried to remove Mary Ellen from her home, but appeals to the police and the Department of Charities were futile. She then appealed to Henry Bergh (who had founded the American Society for the Prevention of Cruelty to Animals in 1866). He persuaded the court to accept the case, and Mary Ellen was subsequently removed from the home and placed in an orphanage called "The Sheltering Arms." The foster mother was found guilty of assault and battery and sentenced to prison for a year. Mary Ellen died in 1961 at the age of 96 years after marrying and raising four children. In 1875, the American Society for Prevention of Cruelty to Children was founded, and the establishment of child welfare agencies followed.

With the onset of better economic conditions in our country, children became better cared for. They were clean and well fed; parents had more leisure time to devote to the children. The American childhood seemed idyllic when compared with earlier times and with childhood in other nations. This likely led to a mind-set that held that parental abuse of children was not possible. In such a milieu, how did physicians recognize that children were being abused?

We now know that the first medical article on child abuse was written in Paris in 1860 by Ambroise Tardieu, a professor of legal medicine. He reported on autopsies of 32 children who had died violently, mainly at the hands of their parents. Tardieu's article described the same medical lesions (multiple injuries and traumatic lesions of skin, bone, and brain) and the same demographic and social factors (the perpetrators were generally the parents who had discrepant explanations for the injuries) as Kempe et al. described more than 100 years later.

In 1946, the father of pediatric radiology, John Caffey, described six cases of multiple fractures in the long bones of infants who had chronic subdural hematomas — signs classic for physical abuse. At one time he postulated that a clotting defect as yet unrecognized was responsible for this entity. Caffey noted that there was no roentgeno-graphic evidence of any underlying pathological bone condition in these children, that subdural hematomas were best explained by trauma, and that the bone lesions were traumatic in nature, adding, "The injuries which caused the fractures in the long bones of these patients were either not observed or were denied when observed. The motive for denial has not been established." According to Dr. Frederic Silverman, Dr. Caffey believed that these children were victims of inflicted injury but was concerned about legal repercus-sions. In 1953, Silverman was the first to say that caretakers "may permit trauma and be unaware of it, may recognize trauma but forget or be reluctant to admit it, or may deliberately injure the child and deny it."

In 1956, Caffey further solidified our thinking about child abuse in a speech before the Congress of the British Institute of Radiology urging early diagnosis to save abused children from further injury: "The correct early diagnosis of injury may be the only means by which the abused youngsters can be removed from their traumatic environment and their wrongdoers punished."

Woolley and Evans in 1955 noted the chronic nature of parentally inflicted trauma as well as "instability" in the parents of these chil-dren. Subsequently, several articles on what is now called child abuse were published in pediatric, orthopedic, and social work journals. Although we can only speculate on how widely these articles were read, it is clear that child abuse was considered a minor aberration of parenting that rarely was seen and that was likely to be found in children of disadvantaged families. Indeed, a paper on child abuse submitted by Kempe to the Society of Pediatric Research in 1959 was read by title, as it was not considered important enough to be put on the program.

In a letter dated October 29, 1983, Dr. Kempe wrote:

My involvement in child abuse was at first far from humane; it was, candidly, intellectual, at least at part. Day after day, while making rounds at the University of Colorado Medical School whose Depart-ment of Pediatrics I headed since 1956, I was shown children with diagnoses by residents and by consultants and attending physicians which simply were examples of either ignorance or denial. I thought very much of the latter. I was shown children who had thrived for seven months and then developed "spontaneous subdural hematoma." "Multiple bruises of unknown etiology" in whom all tests were normal, who had no bleeding disorders and who did not bruise on the ward even when they fell. "Osteogenesis imperfecta tarda" . . . in kids who had normal bones by x-ray except that they showed on whole body x-ray many healing fractures which could be dated. "Impetigo" in kids with skin lesions which were clearly cigarette burns. "Accidental burns of buttocks" in symmetrical form which could only occur from dunking a child who had soiled into a bucket of hot water to punish soiling. In these cases and many others we did often learn from one or both parents, in time and with patient and kindly approaches, that these were all inflicted accidents or injuries.

In the fall of 1959, William Droegemueller, M.D., currently professor and chairman of obstetrics-gynecology at the University of North Carolina, was a senior medical student at the University of Colorado. He remembers that both Kempe and his colleague, Henry Silver, were young and dynamic role models who inspired a large number of the graduating students to enter pediatrics. Dr. Droegemueller wanted to do a research project in this stimulating department but was not interested in the available research possibilities. Dr. Silver suggested seeing Dr. Kempe, who wanted to determine how widespread was the phenomenon of inflicted injuries in childhood. Together the medical student and Dr. Kempe surveyed hospital directors and district attorneys about the incidence of abuse; 71 hospitals and 77 district attorneys responded. When Dr. Droegemueller graduated in 1960, he left the data behind in two shoeboxes. Dr. Kempe retrieved and collated the information.

Dr. Kempe continued,

I have always had a visceral dislike for sloppy thinking in diagnosis and treatment, and I did not sit still for this fairly uniform cover-up which was based for the most part on denial or fear of what the physician's next step should be in getting it all laid out and making a treatment plan. I had seen "battered children" as a student at San Francisco County Hospital and so had everyone, but not in the private or middle class setting. . . . My teachers said, these terrible events were caused by drunk fathers or inadequate mothers and referred them to Social Services. I was able to enlist Brandt Steele to see these folks as a psychiatrist can. . . . Our social workers and I formed a "team" to discuss all cases for the week, go over all fractures in the x-ray department in children under two as a case finding tool. We finally figured out that 10% of all our ER (emergency room) trauma visits in children were due to child abuse. My own field of smallpox research remained very much an active matter but I wanted a chance to get to all pediatricians. This came when after being a member of the Program Committee of the American Academy of Pediatrics for five years, by rotation I became its Chairman for the 1961 meeting in Chicago. One prerogative of that job was the planning of a morning plenary session and on a day when most attended in the ballroom of the Old Palmer House. I wanted a title that would get their attention and named this the "Battered Child Syndrome." The presentation went all morning and the room with well over a thousand people was totally quiet. Nobody seemed to leave and after we were done a great many doctors came up and for the next two hours talked of cases in their private practice which they had missed. . . . The press and radio picked it up from there.

DEFINITION

In Kempe's original article the "battered child syndrome" was defined as "a clinical condition in young children who have received serious physical abuse, generally from a parent or foster parent." In 1970 the working definition of physical abuse of children was "the intentional, non-accidental, use of physical force or intentional, non-accidental acts of omission, on the part of a parent or other caretaker interacting with a child in his care, aimed at hurting, injuring, or destroying that child" (15). The Federal Child Abuse Prevention and Treatment Act of 1974 (Public Law 93-247) has a more global definition, which includes: "physical or mental injury, sexual abuse, negligible treatment or maltreatment of a child under the age of 18 by a person who is responsible for the child's welfare under circumstances which indicate that the child's health or welfare is harmed or threatened thereby" (33). Thus, emotional abuse, sexual abuse, and neglect have been added to physical abuse, which not only broadens the definition of child abuse, but also has increased the number of reported cases.

INCIDENCE

The number of reported cases and the rate of reports per 1,000 children have both risen in the United States. According to data obtained from the National Study on Child Neglect and Abuse Reporting, an estimated

1,726,649 children were reported to child protective service agencies in 1984, an increase of nearly 17% since the previous year and 158% since 1976 (2). The estimated rate of reporting has gone from 10.1 per 1,000 in 1976 to 27.3 per 1,000 in 1984, a nearly threefold increase. Physical injury was reported in 25% of all cases, with major physical injury in 3.3%.

Although this represents the most comprehensive reporting data currently available, it is important to remember that for all but five states, duplicate reports are included; i.e., a child or family member may be listed more than once in the total. There is also a wide variation in reporting rates from the jurisdictions, ranging from 6.9 to 55.1 per 1,000 child population. The only conclusion one can draw concerning this variation is that more children are reported in the high-rate states, not that more children are maltreated.

Cases Reported

About 42% of the reported cases were substantiated by child protective service agencies. Substantiation varies among the jurisdictions, and cases that are not substantiated could represent true child maltreatment. Also, economic conditions can cause variations in the ability of an agency to respond to reported cases.

Slightly less than half of all reported cases were reported by professionals, 11% by physicians, with the remainder about equally divided between school personnel or child-care providers, law enforcement, and social service workers. The largest single group of reports, 36%, came from nonprofessionals such as friends, neighbors, relatives, or self.

A higher percent of cases reported by professionals were substantiated, but this could reflect both greater case severity and the likelihood that the fact a professional did the reporting is taken into account in making substantiation decisions. Nearly half the cases reported were opened for protective services. About 10% of the cases with identified maltreatment were closed after investigation; 18% resulted in foster care or out-of-home placement.

Families Involved

Forty-eight percent of the reported families involved were receiving public assistance compared to 12% of all U.S. families. The reported families had a larger average number of children in the household (2.1) than in the United States as a whole (1.9). Thirty-seven percent of the reported families had a single female caretaker, in contrast to 23% of all U.S. families with children under 18. A recent retrospective study revealed that abusive punishment is twice as common in single-parent households as in two-parent families (41).

The data reported above from the National Study on Child Neglect and Abuse Reporting include reported cases of abuse and neglect, nearly half of which are not substantiated. Yet common sense tells us that the number and rate of reported cases fall far short of the actual number of cases — and there is good evidence to support this. Based on the Gelles and Strauss survey, an estimated 1.5 million children from two-parent families were subjected to severe violence in 1985 (2). If one adds the large numbers of cases that can be expected to occur in single-parent households, the number is probably much larger. Putting the two data sets together, only one injured child out of seven is reported, and this extrapolation does not take neglect or sexual abuse into account.

Gelles and Strauss, who obtained their data by asking parents about violence toward their children, found that there was a substantial *decrease* in parental reports of violence against children between 1975 and 1985 (37). Possible explanations for this include differences in data collection techniques, a greater public awareness of child abuse and its consequences leading to a reluctance to self-report, or a true decline in violence against children. These authors do not see a conflict between their data and the national reporting data. Rather they interpret that the increase in reporting — nearly half of which comes from more nonprofessionals such as self or friends — means more parents are seeking help.

Reporting by Professionals

In the National Study of Incidence and Severity of Child Abuse, tabulated reports made by hospitals between May 3, 1979 and April 30, 1980, over 77,000 cases of abuse were recognized by hospitals. These reports, as could be expected, involved severe injuries and were more likely to be reported in black children from urban areas. Hospitals did not report almost half the cases that met the criteria for reporting when analyzed by the study staff (17).

With regard to reporting, one further study should be called to the reader's attention. When data from the National Study on Child Neglect and Abuse Reporting between 1976 and 1982 were analyzed, the methodology permitted a comparison between cases of maltreatment known to professionals but not reported and those cases reported. Two-thirds of cases were *not* reported despite legislative mandate that professionals report. There was remarkable consistency in the source of the reports through the years. Trend data from this study point out the great demand on child protective services and corroborate the fact that reported cases represented only a fraction of all maltreated children (1).

Physicians in all states are required by statute to report suspected cases of child abuse. However, compliance is far from universal. Physicians interviewed to ascertain what influenced whether or not they reported child abuse indicated that abuse is rare in the private practice setting, that they are concerned about losing patients if they report, and that they lack confidence in community agencies that handle reported cases of child abuse (29). Although 98% of physicians felt bruising a child with a belt is not appropriate punishment, only 48% said they would report this as abuse. Older physicians were less likely than younger physicians to report. We know that physicians are more likely to report cases from minority homes and from low-income homes than they are to report cases from white, middle-class homes. Yet child abuse can and does occur in families from all social classes.

Reluctance of physicians to report is puzzling, especially as every statute mandating reporting provides immunity from civil or criminal liability for the person reporting. In addition, the physician may be liable for failing to report, and in one case in California, the physician and hospital were sued for failing to report a severely injured child who became permanently brain damaged (33).

DIAGNOSIS

Diagnosis starts with the physician's awareness of the possibility that the patient could have the disease, which, in turn, is based on the physician's fundamental knowledge of the disease and its clinical features. The clinician takes a careful history, which includes appropriate questions, looks for specific signs in the physical examination, and confirms suspicions with diagnostic tests such as x-ray and laboratory.

History Taking

Table 1 summarizes key information the physician can elicit when obtaining a focused history. It is not usually helpful to ask, "Were you abused as a child?" However, asking the parent about his or her attitudes toward child discipline and following up with a question about discipline in the

Table 1
Factors That Should Be Covered in Taking History
of Suspected Child Abuse Cases

Parental Factors
    Young parents
    Abused in own childhood
    History of abuse in patient or sibling
    Alcohol
    Drugs
    Poor impulse control
    Marked dependency
    Social isolation
    Spouse violence
    Mental illness
    Limited intelligence and/or illiteracy
    Belief in physical punishment
    Ignorance about child development or nurturance needs
    Marital stress
    Expectations inconsistent with child development

Situational Factors
    Social stress
    Economic stress
    Emotional stress
    Unemployment
    Single parenting
    Divorce
    Inadequate child spacing
    Inadequate help in child care

Child Factors
    Considered abortion of child
    Disappointed over sex of child
    Prematurity
    Neonatal complications requiring hospitalization
    Retardation
    "Difficult child"
    Colic
    Excessive crying
    Unexplained trauma
    Accident history inconsistent with trauma
    Accident history inconsistent with developmental age
    History of frequent trauma
    History of previous abuse

parent's own childhood may elicit valuable information. "Tell me about your parents" and "What was the worst thing you remember about your childhood?" are two additional useful questions. It is important to elicit from all parents, whether or not abuse is suspected, information about household status (divorce, single parenting, degree of economic sufficiency, recent move, parental employment, child care arrangements, etc.) and support systems (to whom does the parent turn in times of stress? what is the availability of friends and family?).

If possible, an assessment of the parent's functional status as both a person and a parent should be ascertained. "How are *you* feeling?" "On a scale of 1 to 10, with the highest possible happiness, where would you place yourself now? Why?" "Would you say, compared to your friends, you have more, the same, or fewer worries? What are they?"

Although denial may prevent the clinician from learning the truth, questions about drugs and alcohol should always be asked. Such questions show your concern for both the child and the parent.

Because there is a correlation between abuse and deficient attachment, it is important for the clinician to know whether the child was premature or had other neonatal complications necessitating separation from the parents. The child's developmental status, as well as the parent's perception of this status, should both be ascertained. The clinician should also ask what temperament the child has and whether or not the parent perceives the child as excessively demanding or difficult.

It is also wise to question parents about siblings and other children currently in the home (for example, the mother might have the care of a divorced sister's baby) and to inquire about their health, developmental status, and disposition.

It is crucial for the clinician to understand clearly the "pathophysiology" of accidents in order to understand the probability that an accident occurred in the child and that it caused the injury. For example, "He blacked his eyes when he fell off his tricycle" is unlikely in a 15-month-old who cannot pedal a tricycle and especially unlikely if both eyes are black and the forehead is not bruised. Similarly, "Tommy turned on the hot water in the tub" is an implausible explanation for second-degree burns of the buttocks, which are more likely to have been caused when the parent dipped the child into very hot water to clean the diaper area or to punish the child.

Parents often say that the child injured himself or herself or that an older sibling caused the injury. The physician must carefully weigh the probability of a sibling being responsible for the injury, taking into account the sibling's age, developmental status, and personality factors. As today's parents are worried about being thought of as abusive, a nonaccusatory, supportive tone during questioning is important.

If the child is old enough to question, it is suggested that parents not be present when the clinician does so. Taping the interview both provides an accurate record and prevents the child from having to repeat the story. It goes without saying that the language used should be appropriate to the child's developmental level and that rapport should be established before questioning starts. It is important to avoid suggesting answers to the child or forcing the child into statements the child does not wish to make. When a child voluntarily says that an adult caused his or her injury, this is usually the case. Similarly when one parent attributes the injury to the other parent, this is usually correct unless a custody battle is taking place.

When the clinician is confronted with evidence of physical injury, the questioning about that injury must be fairly detailed. It is important to find out when the injury occurred (accidents between midnight and 6:00 A.M. are suspect, as are injuries that occurred considerably earlier than the time of seeking medical attention), what the sequence of events was, and who was with the child at the time of injury.

Findings on Physical Examination

Table 2 lists possible findings likely to be found on physical examination.

Skin manifestations. The most important thing the clinician can do to avoid missing a case of child abuse is to have a clear understanding of the etiology of visible marks on the child. More than 90% of child abuse cases will have skin manifestations (34). The location of the bruise is one of the best ways to differentiate between inflicted and accidental injury. Buttocks and lower-back bruises are likely to be due to abusive punishment. Bruises on a child's inner thighs, buttocks, or upper or lower back do not usually result from a fall, which generally causes bruising over a bony prominence (elbow, knee, forehead, or chin). Face and ear bruises as well as mouth lesions are common in abuse. Bruises on the neck are usually caused by finger or rope marks. Abrasions radiating out from each corner of the mouth may be due to a gag put in place to prevent or stop screaming. Pinch marks or crescent-shaped nail marks may be seen on the penis.

The age of a bruise can be estimated from the color. A swollen and tender bruise that is red, blue, or purple is less than two days old. The change in color to green as heme pigment is broken down occurs in about

Table 2
Evidence of Abuse on Physical Examination

General
Young child – usually under three
Appearance ranges from normal, healthy looking, well dressed to malnourished, dirty, inadequately clothed

Behavior
Negative
Unhappy
Isolated
Abusive toward others
Excessive or absent anxiety when separated from parents
Constantly seeking attention
Developmental delay

Skin and Mucosal Surfaces
Bruises of different ages, especially on back, inner thighs, buttocks, side of head or face
Outline of fingertips or thumbs, belt buckle, cord, or other objects
Crescent marks of fingernails
Lacerations
Unusual rash
Patterned burns
Punctate burns from cigarettes or cigars
Immersion burns on buttocks, hands, or feet
Rope burns on wrist or ankles
Mouth and lip injuries

Head
Subdural hematoma
Cephalohematoma
Intracranial bleeding

Eyes
Subconjunctival hemorrhage
Retinal hemorrhage
Papilledema
Traumatic cataract

Extremities
Evidence of fractures
Evidence of dislocation

Abdomen
Bruises
Masses (hematomas)
Evidence of intraabdominal injury or rupture
Evidence of renal bleeding

Genitalia and Rectum
Severe diaper rash and/or hyperpigmentation
Thickening of labia
Horizontal diameter of vaginal opening greater than 4 mm in prepubertal child
Bruises
Bleeding
Tears
Condyloma acuminatum
Evidence of trauma or infection on pelvic or rectal examination
Lax rectal tone

five days. By the seventh day, the green has changed to yellow, and finally, the bruise becomes brownish. Bruises of varying age, bruises on multiple parts of the body, and bruises on soft parts of the body, such as the cheek or abdominal wall, should always be suspect.

Bruises that have a shape are likely to be caused by an object such as a belt buckle or a cord used in beating. The so-called "two and eight" bruises are seen after a severe shaking and result from two thumb bruises on the neck, chest, or arms, and eight finger bruises on the back. A bite mark is likely to have been made by an adult—not a young sibling—if there is more than 3 cm between the two canine impressions.

Similarly, burns due to inflicted abuse have distinctive patterns. Round, punctate burns which are usually multiple are caused by a cigarette, cigar, match, or incense stick. Immersion burns are stocking/glove in nature or doughnut shaped on the buttocks. Such burns have distinct margins. Patterned burns can resemble the iron or stovetop burner that inflicted them (3). Location of the burn can suggest a nonaccidental cause. For example, a burn on the back of the hand is likely to be due to abuse; accidental burns tend to occur on the palm or the inside of the fingers (35).

Lacerations or abrasions, especially on the mouth, gums, eyes, or genitalia, can be due to inflicted injuries. A laceration of the lip mucosa from the alveolar margin of the gum can result from a blow on the mouth.

Although all children bruise themselves repeatedly, especially on the bony prominences, the presence of bruises *not* on bony prominences and of bruises of different ages indicates the repetitive and chronic nature of abusive actions against children.

Bone injuries. According to Kessler, 20% of physically abused children exhibit some roentgenographic evidence of bone trauma (26). Chip fractures and evidence of subperiosteal hematomas, as well as frank fractures in various stages of healing, can be visualized on x-ray. However, it takes 10 to 14 days for a subperiosteal hematoma to calcify, so a repeat x-ray is needed in the child who may not be brought back for follow-up. Early signs of bone trauma can be diagnosed by a bone scan, which can show evidence of subperiosteal reaction in five to seven days. Increased uptake in occult fractures of ribs and hairline fractures of long bones can sometimes be seen within 24 hours.

Other injuries. Inflicted abdominal trauma can cause injury to, or rupture of, abdominal organs. Such children may present with shock or a rigid abdomen—and may have little or no evidence of bruising on the abdomen. Any unexplained or poorly explained abdominal injury is suspect of abuse. Head injury can cause unconsciousness, evidence of increased intracranial pressure, or seizures. These signs, in the absence of another explanation, could indicate abuse.

Observations. Observing parent-child interactions can be useful. Fontana and his colleagues quantitatively analyzed videotaped interaction between abusive and nonabusive mothers and their children. Compared to nonabusive mothers, abusive mothers spent less time looking at their children, had less focused attention for the child, were more likely to fire words and actions at the child without noticing the child's response, issued more directives, and were more physically coercive (12). Abuse can be viewed as a "lack of mutual attunement between caretaker and child, of which acts of physical violence are dramatic exemplars."

Helfer points out that there are three components to the sequence of events we call child abuse: the potential to abuse in the parent, the special characteristics of the child, and the precipitating stress (20). Both the potential for abuse and some of the characteristics of the child could have the same root cause: an abusive parent who suffered from inadequate parenting in his or her own childhood. This, in turn, can result in lack of attunement between the parent and child, which can lead, for example, to excessive crying in an infant or negativism or apathy in a toddler. Other special characteristics of a child that can predispose to abuse include illness, developmental delay, or difficult temperament.

Mistaken "evidence." There are two possible diagnostic errors physicians can make in child abuse. A type 1 error is failing to diagnose a case of abuse; a type 2 error is falsely labeling a case as abuse which is not (14). We know that doctors can be wrong in diagnosing suspected child abuse. Autopsies performed on 10 children, who died suddenly and who were suspected of being abused, revealed that there was a nonabuse cause for the suspicious presenting findings (27). These ranged from meningitis with disseminated intravenous coagulation to sudden infant death syndrome with postmortem lividity. Mongolian spots in Caucasian children can look like bruises. A direct hit with a hard ball can cause a round bruise, as can a suction cup toy pressed against the forehead by a young child. Home remedies practiced by certain cultural groups, such as coin rubbing, can leave bruises. A case of Schönlein-Henoch purpura was recently misdiagnosed as child abuse (6).

PROGNOSIS

Child abuse can be fatal. A survey tabulating newspaper stories of abuse in 1962 reported a 22% fatality rate (11). The overall mortality in Gil's series was 3.4%, and an additional 5% of the children suffered permanent damage (15). Long-term follow-up of child abuse cases revealed a high incidence of physical or developmental deviation from normal, although some of these children may have been so affected before the abuse. Homicide is the only leading cause of death in children under 15 that has increased in incidence and now is one of the five leading causes of death in childhood. The majority of young homicide victims are killed by parents, caretakers, or relatives (7).

Recidivism is high. In a dysfunctional family that has not received treatment, the same conditions for abuse (the parent, the child, and the stress) are still present. As many as 20% of children are reabused (22).

There are other long-range effects. We know that abusive parents were likely to have been abused themselves. Steele feels that it is rare *not* to elicit a history of maltreatment in an abusive parent's childhood (45). Sometimes true amnesia of childhood events has occurred; more frequently there is denial of abuse. Careful questioning can reveal a history of beatings not thought of as abuse because it was considered punishment for bad behavior. Without intervention, it is likely that the abused children of today will become the abusing parents of tomorrow. It is frightening to think that the pool of potentially dysfunctional parents increases as the number of abused children increases. There is also evidence that criminality and other forms of violence are associated with abuse as a child (4, 10).

TREATMENT

Treatment of the child includes removal from the abusive parent (or removal of the abusive parent as, for example, jailing a criminally abusive father). Treatment of the problem of child abuse requires lengthy rehabilitative programs for the parent and family.

There have been four stages in our approach to the treatment of abused children (18). The first stage, denial, prevailed until the early articles associating intentional infliction of injuries with physical and roentgenographic lesions of abuse were published in the 1950s. At that time "attempts to consider parental love invincible became futile" (28). The next stage was punitive; child abusers were treated as criminals. Next came a "pseudopunitive" approach. The abuser was not sent to jail, but the child was taken away from the abuser.

The rehabilitative approach is relatively recent, and reviews are mixed. Rehabilitation of child abusers is costly, requiring both a team approach and long-term treatment. Psychotherapy of the abusive parent alone is not enough and can even precipitate further abuse (31). Further, abusive parents are characterized by suspicion and isolation, so they are likely to both break appointments and change their residence, making follow-up difficult. The abusive parent needs education and support — the former to lower unrealistic expectations of the child, the latter to increase the parent's own self-esteem.

The First National Child Abuse and Neglect Program Evaluation was a study of over 1,700 adults who abused or neglected their children. Thirty percent reabused or neglected their children during treatment. The variables most likely to predict recidivism were the "seriousness" of the original maltreatment as well as the magnitude of family dysfunction and stress. The variables associated with success (no further abuse) were supplementation of case management with lay counseling or participation in Parents Anonymous. Overall, however, only 42% of parents were less likely to abuse or neglect after the treatment period ended (8).

Currently 150,000 children are in foster care because of child maltreatment (40). Foster care is likely to be the disposition in cases of children from poor families who had physical injuries (23). The impact of foster care has not been systematically evaluated. However, one study looked at school attendance and performance in a group of maltreated children in foster care and matched maltreated children left in their home. Attendance had improved for both groups, but both groups were doing poor work in school, so that there was no evidence for any rehabilitative effect of foster care in this parameter.

It is apparent that we have no sure "cure" for child abuse. It is true that removal of the child from a dangerous, abusive environment can be lifesaving. However, removal of children from their families is fraught with difficulties. Foster care is not a permanent solution; only rarely can relatives provide a stable home. Rehabilitation of the family offers the most promise, but to date, costs have prevented large-scale treatment or evaluative studies.

PREVENTION

What about a "vaccine" to prevent child abuse? Identification and intervention are the twin hopes for prevention of abuse.

If parents likely to abuse their children could be identified, perhaps those scarce resources now used to protect the child after the abuse has occurred could be utilized to prevent abuse in the first place. A study comparing abusive and nonabusive mothers showed that abusers were characterized by lower self-concept and greater ignorance about what they thought of themselves and what they would like to be (39). Prebirth prediction of how the mother and infant would interact was studied. When both mother and father were assessed prebirth as above average on adaptation, competence, and relationship capacity and held a positive view of marriage, mother-baby interaction was more likely to be positive (30).

There is some evidence that intervention, usually in the form of home visits, can prevent abuse. Such intervention has been shown to reduce the incidence of injuries. In one study there were significantly fewer incidents of abuse and neglect during the first two years in homes visited by a nurse. In addition, children in visited homes were punished less and were provided with more play material (32).

Because inadequate parenting is the problem, efforts to improve parenting skills and to enhance positive parent-child interaction should help prevent abuse. Perinatal coaching, home care training, techniques to improve interpersonal skills, and crash "courses in childhood" for adults who were inadequately parented themselves, all have potential value (24). The lay health visitor program to provide home support for new mothers is an effective methodology (16).

Early skin-to-skin contact with newborns enhances bonding and attachment for mothers — and fathers. Birthing rooms, rooming in, and coaching new parents in newborn behavior can all help the process of attachment. Dr. Ann Wilson teaches new parents four important aspects of new babies: newborns have different states of consciousness affecting how they react to stimulation, newborns are sociable, newborns are selective in how much and what kind of stimulation they can process, and each baby is unique in ways that affect interaction with the parent (47). Incorporating this knowledge and coaching into all postpartum care should enhance parenting.

Screening to identify future abusers, if perfected, could pinpoint the parents for whom intervention is indicated. Methods used for screening include questionnaires, interviews, and observations of interactions. Areas studied are early childhood experiences, interaction skills, perception about children, and presence or absence of family dysfunction and stress. Unfortunately, there is a 20% misidentification error in the best of research studies (42). Dangers lie in both directions: failing to identify a potential abuser, and incorrectly labeling a parent as a potential abuser.

WHERE DO WE GO FROM HERE?

Two major directions emerge. First, we must find a way to diminish violence in our homes, in our society, and between nations. Second, we must provide resources to prevent and treat child abuse.

Violence has always been part of our mammalian heritage. One physician who cared for many cases of child abuse recognized that some failures of parenting could be attributed to what he called an "evolutionary" mechanism that enables parents themselves to survive, given their limited actual and emotional resources. This is a mechanism shared by other species that kill their own kind, such as lions, hippos, and wolves (9).

There are "costs" of parenting. Each parent must sacrifice for the child's well-being, growth, and survival. The parent's energy and resources are finite; devoting these to the child means the energy and resources are not available for the parent. Human parenting is a lengthy process and, in the case of limited resources, may produce overwhelming pressures on the parent (5). Limited resources are common in families with children born in quick succession. Infanticide and cannibalism of babies is seen in some cultures at times of stress or famine.

Family violence is a response to structural stress in the family. A precondition for its occurrence is the socialization family members received themselves as children. Exposure to violence as a child creates a role model for violence and provides "basic training for violence" (13, 46). We all get angry; most of us are socialized to learn that violent acts against people or property are not tolerated by our society. Unfortunately, many persons are socialized in homes where violence is frequent and condoned. As it occurs behind closed doors, societal sanctions do not apply unless the degree of violence precludes its continuing secrecy.

Tacit condoning of violence occurs every day on TV screens. It has been estimated that the average American child will watch 13,000 murders on TV before reaching adulthood (44). Violence in the news is depicted graphically and repeatedly.

Recognition of the degree of violence in the public and private sectors of society is the first step. Realization that interpersonal skills, communicative techniques, and tolerance of frustration can be taught — and learned — is the next step. Schools should incorporate these "subjects" into the curricula. Parent education, encompassing not only parenting skills but also how to deal with feelings such as anger and frustration, should be a mandatory part of education for all children.

A society that does not protect its children is making a very poor investment in its own future. Funds for adequate child protective services must be found; research dollars to seek the "cure" and "vaccine" for child abuse must also be provided in amounts large enough to be meaningful.

There has been little involvement of medical specialties other than pediatrics in the area of child abuse. Helfer notes that psychiatry, both adult and child, has, for the most part, avoided the issues of abuse and neglect. Also, family practitioners need more training and involvement in child abuse — a hallmark of family violence. Helfer advocates that all medical specialties incorporate the subject of child abuse and neglect into residency training and board certification (21). Professionals who work in child abuse need more interdisciplinary training.

As I noted elsewhere (19), 100 years went by between the year Mary Ellen's abuse came to the attention of the nation and the passage of the Federal Child Abuse Prevention and Treatment Act of 1974. Physicians have an obligation to lead the way toward both a cure and a vaccine. Another century must not elapse before child abuse and neglect become as rare as polio and smallpox.

REFERENCES

1. American Humane Association (1984). *Trends in child abuse and neglect: A national perspective.* Denver, CO: The American Humane Association.
2. American Humane Association (1986). *Highlights of official child neglect and abuse reporting, 1984.* Denver, CO: The American Humane Association.
3. American Medical Association Council on Scientific Affairs (1985). AMA diagnostic and treatment guidelines concerning child abuse and neglect. *JAMA, 254,* 796.
4. BAIN, I. (1963). The physically abused child. *Pediatrics, 31,* 895.
5. BOLTON, F. G. (1983). *When bonding fails.* Beverly Hills, CA: Sage Publications.
6. BROWN, J., & MELINKOVICH, P. (1986). Schönlein-Henoch purpura misdiagnosed as suspected child abuse. *JAMA, 256,* 617.
7. CHRISTOFFEL, K. K. (1984). Homicide in childhood: A public health problem in need of attention. *Am. J. Public Health, 74,* 68.
8. COHN, A. H. (1982). Organization and administration of programs to treat child abuse and neglect. In E. H. Newberger (Ed.), *Child abuse.* Boston: Little, Brown.
9. COMERCI, G. D. (1983). Foreword. In F. G. Bolton, *When bonding fails.* Beverly Hills, CA: Sage Publications.
10. DUNCAN, G. M., FRAZIER, S. H., et al. (1958). Etiological factors in first-degree murder. *JAMA, 168,* 1755.
11. FONTANA, V. J. (1964). *The maltreated child: The maltreatment syndrome in children.* Springfield, IL: Charles C Thomas.
12. FONTANA, V. J. & ROBISON, E. (1984). Observing child abuse. *J. Pediatr., 105,* 655.
13. GELLES, R. J. (1972). *The violent home: A study of physical aggression between husbands and wives.* Beverly Hills, CA: Sage Publications.
14. GELLES, R. J. (1982). Child abuse and family violence: Implications for medical professionals. In E. H. Newberger (Ed.), *Child abuse.* Boston: Little, Brown.

15. GIL, D. G. (1970). *Violence against children: Physical child abuse in the United States.* Cambridge, MA: Harvard University Press.
16. GRAY, J. & KAPLAN, B. (1980). The lay health visitor program: An eighteen-month experience. In C. H. Kempe & R. E. Helfer (Eds.) *The battered child* (3rd ed.) Chicago: University of Chicago Press.
17. HAMPTON, R. L. & NEWBERGER, E. H. (1985). Child abuse incidence and reporting by hospitals: Significance of severity, class, and race. *Am. J. Public Health, 75,* 56.
18. HEINS, M. (1983). The necessity for reporting child abuse. In D. Ganos, R. E. Lipson, et al. (Eds.), *Difficult decisions in medical ethics.* New York: Alan R. Liss.
19. HEINS, M. (1984). The "battered child" revisited. *JAMA, 251,* 3295.
20. HELFER, R. E. (1984). The epidemiology of child abuse and neglect. *Pediatr. Ann., 13,* 745.
21. HELFER, R. E. (1985). Where to now, Henry? A commentary on the battered child syndrome. *Pediatrics, 76,* 993.
22. JOHNSON, B. & MORSE, H. (1968). Injured children and their parents. *Children, 15,* 147.
23. KATZ, M. H., HAMPTON, R. L., et al. (1986). Returning children home: Clinical decision making in cases of child abuse and neglect. *Am. J. Ortho., 56,* 253.
24. KEMPE, C. H. & HELFER, R. E. (Eds.) (1980). *The battered child* (3rd ed.) Chicago: University of Chicago Press.
25. KEMPE, C. H., SILVERMAN, F. N., et al. (1962). The battered-child syndrome. *JAMA, 181,* 17.
26. KESSLER, D. B. (1985). Pediatric assessment and differential diagnosis of child abuse. In E. H. Newberger & R. Bourne (Eds.), *Unhappy families: Clinical and research perspectives on family violence.* Littleton, Massachusetts: PSG Publishing Company.
27. KIRSCHNER, R. H. & STEIN, R. J. (1985). The mistaken diagnosis of child abuse. *Am. J. Dis. Child. 139,* 873.
28. KOMISARUK, R. & SCHORNSTEIN, H. (1965). *Clinical observations of the abused child syndrome.* Report of the Conference on Child Abuse. Detroit, Michigan: Wayne State University.
29. MORRIS, J. L., JOHNSON, C. F., et al. (1985). To report or not to report. *Am. J. Dis. Child., 139,* 194.
30. OATES, D. S. & HEINICKE, C. M. (1985). Prebirth prediction of the quality of the mother-infant interaction: The first year of life. *J. Fam. Issues, 6,* 523.
31. OATES, K. (1986). *Child abuse and neglect: What happens eventually?* New York: Brunner/Mazel.
32. OLDS, D. L., HENDERSON, C. R., et al. (1986). Preventing child abuse and neglect: A randomized trial of nurse home visitation. *Pediatrics, 78,* 65.
33. PAGE, S. L. (1982). The law, the lawyer, and medical aspects of child abuse. In E. H. Newberger (Ed.), *Child abuse.* Boston: Little, Brown.
34. *Pediatric News* (May 1986). Suspect abuse when site, shape, color of a child's bruises or burns inconsistent with parent's account. *Pediatr. News, 20,* 58.
35. *Pediatric News* (August 1986). Pattern, site, history identify nonaccidental burn. *Pediatr. News, 20,* 56.
36. RADBILL, S. X. (1968). A history of child abuse and infanticide. In R. E. Helfer and C. H. Kempe (Eds.), *The battered child.* Chicago: University of Chicago Press.
37. RIESENBERG, D. E. (1986). Child mistreatment remains an ugly problem. *JAMA, 255,* 2723.
38. ROBIN, M. (1982). Sheltering arms: The roots of child protection. In E. H. Newberger (Ed.), *Child abuse.* Boston: Little, Brown.
39. ROSEN, B. & STEIN, M. T. (1980). Women who abuse their children *Am. J. Dis. Child., 134,* 947.
40. RUNYAN, D. K. & GOULD, C. L. (1985). Foster care for child maltreatment, II. Impact on school performance. *Pediatrics, 76,* 841.

41. SACK, W. H., MASON, R., et al. (1985). The single-parent family and abusive child punishment. *Am. J. Ortho.*, *55*, 252.
42. SCHNEIDER, C., HELFER, R. E., et al. (1980). Screening for the potential to abuse: A review. In C. H. Kempe and R. E. Helfer (Eds.), *The battered child* (3rd ed.) Chicago: University of Chicago Press.
43. SMITH, S. M. & PAGAN, D. (1979). The battered young child. In J. G. Howells (Ed.), *Modern perspectives in the psychiatry of infancy.* New York: Brunner/Mazel.
44. SOMERS, A. R. (1976). Violence, television and the health of American youth. *N. Engl. J. Med.*, *294*, 811.
45. STEELE, B. F. (1985). Generational repetition of the maltreatment of children. In E. J. Anthony & G. H. Pollock (Eds.), *Parental influences in health and disease.* Boston: Little, Brown.
46. STRAUS, M. A., GELLES, R. J., et al. (1980). *Behind closed doors: Violence in the American family.* New York: Anchor Press/Doubleday.
47. WILSON, A. L. (1980). Promoting a positive parent-baby relationship. In C. H. Kempe and R. E. Helfer (Eds.), *The battered child* (3rd ed.) Chicago: University of Chicago Press.

2

CHILD MOLESTERS

GEORGE W. BARNARD, M.D.

Professor and Chief,
Consultation-Liaison Service

A. KENNETH FULLER, M.D.

Resident Psychiatrist

and

LYNN ROBBINS, B.S.

Research Associate,
Department of Psychiatry,
University of Florida,
Gainesville, Florida

During the last decade public and scientific awareness of the problem of child molestation has increased dramatically. Clinicians are increasingly confronted with this complex, contemporary issue that crosses clinical, legal, and social boundaries. The purpose of this chapter is to provide the clinician with a basic understanding of the physiological and psychosocial characteristics of the child molester, discuss diagnostic assessment techniques, and explain selected treatment modalities.

No uniform definition of the child molester exists. Pedophilia is defined in the *International Classification of Diseases* (86) as sexual deviations in

The authors wish to acknowledge the contribution of the staff of the sex offender treatment unit at North Florida Evaluation and Treatment Center for their valuable suggestions in the preparation of this manuscript. In particular, we thank Dennis Gies, Administrator; Gustave Newman, M.D., Clinical Director; and Theodore Shaw, Director of Sex Offender Treatment Unit.

which an adult engages in sexual activity with a child of the same or opposite sex. Lanyon (55) defines child molesters as "older persons whose conscious sexual desires and responses are directed, at least in part, toward dependent, developmentally immature children and adolescents who do not fully comprehend these actions and are unable to give informed consent" (p. 176). The Council on Scientific Affairs of the American Medical Association (22) broadens the definition to the sexual exploitation of a child for the gratification or profit of an adult.

Reliable figures on the incidence of child molestation are not available. In 1984 there were 100,000 reported cases of child sexual abuse in the United States, according to the American Humane Association (7). Four of the most recent and representative studies of prevalence of child sexual abuse confirm this high incidence. Russell (76), Wyatt (87), and Finkelhor (25, 27) reported the percentage of the women who experienced sexual abuse in their childhood to be 38%, 45%, 19%, and 15%, respectively. The divergencies in response rates may be due in part to the different criteria used in defining experiences as sexual abuse (88). No one knows how many instances go unreported, although Russell (76) found only 2% of intrafamilial and 6% of extrafamilial child sexual abuse experiences had been reported to the police.

By self-report, if the child molester remains undetected in the community, he may commit hundreds of sexually abusive acts toward children (5). The enormous effect that child molesters have on young lives makes the necessity for early identification and treatment readily apparent.

ETIOLOGY

The motivation for child molesting is complex and comprised of sexual and nonsexual factors. The etiological theories of child-molesting behavior are extremely divergent, ranging from hormonal imbalance to early childhood experience to ignorance about sexuality. Finkelhor's conceptualization (8, 25) is the best available. His model has four nonexclusive factors: (1) emotional congruence, (2) sexual arousal, (3) blockage, and (4) disinhibition.

Emotional Congruence

The emotional congruence theories imply that the molester's sexual attraction to children fulfills his special emotional needs. The child molester prefers children as sexual partners because they function at his emotional level and can more easily respond to his needs. The particular needs are numerous and probably differ for different molesters. Some need mastery of prior emotional trauma. Others need to fully control their sexual partner. Arrested emotional development may cause perpetrators to express immature sexual and emotional urges toward children. Research has empirically confirmed few of these ideas. However, Langevin et al. (54) found a trend for molesters to be aroused by the idea of "dominating the fearful child," and Howells (45) documented the special emotional meaning that children's lack of dominance has for child molesters. Child molesters appear to have been sexually victimized as children more than the average. In our study of incarcerated child molesters, 56% reported they were sexually abused as children, with a mean age of first occurrence at 8.5 years (84).

Sexual Arousal

Other theories pertain to the notion that relating to a child is exceptionally arousing sexually for at least some child molesters. Investigations of incarcerated child molesters (29, 68) provide consistent empirical support for this proposition. It is suggested that sexual imprinting occurs during a critical period of life, followed by a conditioning process through which fantasies of sex with children are strengthened by repetition, masturbation, and positive reinforcement. Simply having the arousal response pattern to children, however, does not imply that an individual will act on it. Situational stress, such as the loss of a job or the discovery of his wife's adultery, may trigger the sexual acting out. Likewise, disinhibiting agents such as alcohol or drugs may allow his overt sexual behavior with the child to occur.

Blockage

Blockage theories are based on the proposition that child molesters have chronic or episodic difficulty in gaining satisfaction of emotional and sexual needs through adult partners. This obstruction or inhibition is believed by some to begin with early trauma or from dynamics in the family of origin, resulting in fear and difficulty relating to adult females. General sexual inhibition, sexual anxiety, or difficulties in current relationships also have been used to explain this blockage. Research evidence supporting these theories is scant. Howells (44) found that molesters generally are shy and passive; Goldstein and Kant (37) documented that molesters have a fairly high degree of sexual inhibition and anxiety. There is mixed evidence regarding their unusual fears of relating to adult women.

Disinhibition

Theories of disinhibition have attempted to explain why some persons are capable of overcoming the legal and moral proscriptions against sexual contact with children. Many people with a strong desire to have sexual contact with children are probably inhibited by societal taboos. Likewise, simply being sexually aroused by children is not sufficient in itself to produce molestation. Because of its disinhibiting effects and established role in 30 to 40% of molestations, alcohol has been cited as a factor in undermining these inhibitions (8). Other theories suggest a variety of disinhibiting factors such as mental retardation, organicity, social isolation, social stress, loneliness, and subcultures that find child sexual abuse condonable. The best empirical evidence on this proposition is on alcohol and social isolation (20).

DESCRIPTION AND CLASSIFICATION

Classification

The classification systems of child molesters are primarily based on clinical description and generally lack scientific evidence for classificatory validity. Despite limitations, the classifications are felt to be clinically useful provided clinicians remember that the narrow stereotypes are rarely, if ever, found in pure form in practice. Most molesters present as composites of the various types.

Preference versus situational. The sexual orientation of preference or fixated child molesters is toward children and adolescents. According to Groth (39), a *"fixated child offender* is a person who has, from adolescence, been sexually attracted primarily or exclusively to significantly younger people, and this attraction has persisted throughout his life, regardless of what other sexual experiences he has had" (p. 6).

Situational or regressed child molesters depart from their primary sexual orientation to age mates as a result of precipitating stressors. The involvement with children begins in adulthood and is usually isolated or episodic. In such cases the victim may be understood as a surrogate for a preferred but unavailable adult. The assumption is that sexual development was normal until some intervening factor produced the return to a previous developmental level and sexual object choice. Disturbances in adult sexual romantic relationships, alcohol abuse, and situational stress are suggested as factors in the origin of regressed, situational child molestation. A high association of drinking, alcoholism, and child molestation is reported (71).

Incest versus nonincest. Despite the pervasiveness of the incest taboo, the incidence of intrafamilial child sexual abuse is alarmingly high (76). Failure of the incest avoidance mechanism is supported by studies (26, 77) showing rates of sexual abuse in stepfather families to be up to seven times greater than for biological-father families. Incest is discussed further in Chapter 3, this volume.

Violent versus nonviolent. Violence occurs in 10 to 15% of sexual offenses against children (55, 62). The use of violence distinguishes the child rapist, who more closely resembles rapists of adult females, from nonviolent child molesters. Generally nonviolence offenders coax or pressure children into sexual activity; i.e., the child gives sex in exchange for attention, acceptance, recognition, and material gain; whereas child rapists use threat, intimidation, and physical force. Violent child molestations may be best understood as an intense intermingling of aggression and sexual urges.

Males versus females. Child sexual abuse is primarily perpetuated by males. Many experts in the field (40, 65), however, argue that the number of female child molesters is seriously underestimated. Victims of female abuse may be more reluctant to report the offense than victims of male abuse because of cultural attitudes that perceive sexual abuse by females as being less serious and traumatic. It has been suggested that women as primary caretakers can mask their sexual abusive acts more easily than men. The increase in the reporting of all types of child sexual abuse has been paralleled by a rise in the proportion of female offenders. Finkelhor (25) reported that sexual abuse by women occurs in roughly 20% of the cases with male victims and 5% of the cases with female victims.

Juvenile versus adult. According to the Seattle Institute for Child Advocacy Committee for Children (23), the majority of adult sex offenders committed their first offense as teenagers. The average age of first offense is estimated to be 13 to 15 years. Like their adult counterparts, a vast majority (90 to 95%) of juvenile sex offenders are male, although the reports of abuse by juvenile girls are increasing. The most common setting for abuse by juveniles is when babysitting. Early intervention is necessary to avoid lifelong patterns of sexually abusive behavior affecting the lives of many victims. Research is needed to determine factors associated with continuance of molestation into adulthood.

Endocrine and Psychosocial Characteristics

Rada et al. (72) showed that plasma testosterone levels in child molesters fall within normal limits, albeit at a lower mean level than in their normal controls or rapists. A more recent investigation by Gaffney and Berlin (32) compared endocrine studies in men with pedophilia, in nonpedophiliac paraphilias, and in normal male controls. When the subjects were infused with luteinizing hormone releasing hormone (LHRH), the pedophile group showed a much higher elevation of luteinizing hormone than did the other two groups. The authors concluded that the data were indicative of a hypothalamic-pituitary-gonadal dysfunction in some pedophiles.

Clinicians find certain cognitive distortions common to many of the child molesters seen in their practice. Abel, Becker, and Cunningham-Rathner (3) summarize these distorted beliefs as follows: a child who does not physically resist really wants sex; having sex with a child is a good way to teach the child about sex; children don't tell about sex with an adult because they really enjoy it; sometime in the future our society will realize that sex with children is really all right; an adult who feels a child's genitalia is not really being sexual with the child, so no harm is really being done; when a child asks about sex it means that the child wants to see the adult's sex organs or have sex with the adult; and a relationship with the child is enhanced by having sex with him/her.

Groth et al. (40) found no sociodemographic characteristics that differentiated child molesters from the general population: not race, religion, intelligence, education, occupation, or socioeconomic status.

The literature (16, 20, 25) as well as our investigation (84) of the childhood and adolescent characteristics of rapists and child molesters indicates antecedent factors common in the life histories of many sex offenders. Abandonment by parents, parental separation or divorce, neglect, physical or sexual abuse, familial violence, frequent arguments, and parental problem drinking were major characteristics in the family histories of our population, as was the notable absence of a close relationship with the father. The family of origin and childhood situations of many child molesters were chaotic. The absence of nurturance, physical affection, or examples of healthy sexuality has been noted. Many sex offenders share the following premorbid features: history of physical and/or sexual abuse; alcohol or substance abuse; preoccupation with sexuality; ignorance, confusion, or guilt about their sexuality; societal and peer pressure to be macho, aggressive, controlling, or violent; marital stress; interpersonal deficits; no or few friends while growing up; and the absence of moral development. They tend to have feelings of anxiety, powerlessness, fear, inadequacy, anger, and low self-esteem.

Although these characteristics are frequently found in sex offenders, they should not be seen as being exclusively associated with them. Individuals with similar life histories and psychosocial characteristics may have normal, healthy nondeviant sexual interests and behaviors throughout their life. Controlled studies comparing normal populations with child molesters are needed before one can make definitive statements pertaining to a "typical profile of the child molester." Early intervention or prevention of sexual abuse may be facilitated by clinician awareness of these descriptive characteristics. If practitioners are aware of these traits and behaviors, they can elucidate additional information during the clinical interview to determine whether the individual has committed or has the urge to commit sex offenses. Only in this way will clinicians be able to intervene before the list of victims expands.

ASSESSMENT ISSUES

Clinical Interview

Child molesters present as ordinary individuals. In the initial interview the clinician frequently will be confronted by a person who denies any type of sexual involvement with the child whether the patient is referred for paraphiliac activity or unrelated problems. In contrast with many patients, the child molester often presents as an individual without major psychopathology, and his lifestyle may appear to be average. When interviewing a child molester, the clinician may have to probe, challenge, and confront to get the essential information. A general psychiatric evaluation with specific inquiry into the sexual area is essential. Detailed information pertaining to the child molester's sexual offenses and his current social situation should be obtained. Histories — family, educational, sexual, marital, military, occupational, criminal, medical, psychiatric, and substance abuse — are required. The clinician should not rely solely on self-report. When possible, information should be secured from other sources, such as victims' statements, depositions, arrest reports, attorneys, and documents from educational, mental health, military, vocational, social service, and criminal justice agencies.

Psychological Testing

In addition to this historical information, the comprehensive assessment of the child molester includes evaluation of intelligence, reading ability, general personality factors, interests, needs, attitudes, beliefs, motivations, and interpersonal factors. Standardized psychological tests and inventories provide a quantitative means for comparison with a normal population and, in case of those standardized on a population with known paraphilias, a comparison with sexually deviant populations.

At North Florida Evaluation and Treatment Center (NFETC), a forensic treatment facility for incarcerated sex offenders in Gainesville, Florida, we have implemented a broad-based assessment program. The test battery consists of 13 tests: We obtain an estimated verbal intelligence quotient from the Shipley Institute of Living Scale (43, 81). The Wide Range Achievement Test (47) provides an estimate of grade reading level. The Personality Research Form-E (46) yields 20 different personality measures related to impulse expression and control, orientation to work and play, orientation toward autonomy and control, intellectual and aesthetic orientations, and ascendancy and interpersonal orientations. The Interpersonal Behavior Survey (61) measures the presence of aggressive and assertive behaviors and assesses their effects on interpersonal interactions. This instrument's ability to detect excesses and deficits of these behaviors has great utility in treatment planning and outcome evaluation. The Minnesota Multiphasic Personality Inventory (MMPI) (41), Thematic Apperception Test (TAT) (63), and Rorschach Test (74) give measures of psychopathology. Since so many of the child molesters abuse alcohol, we administer the Michigan Alcoholism Screening Test (79), an instrument devised to detect alcoholism. In addition to these general personality measures, specialized inventories document the resident's sexual attitudes, beliefs, and experiences. The Clarke Sex History Questionnaire (52, 78) is an instrument that investigates sexual experiences throughout the lifespan. It requires detailed responses of the nature, frequency, and diversity of sexual activity. Cognitive distortions related to pedophilia are detected through the Abel Pedophilia Cognition Scale (4). The Burt Scales (19) measure acceptance of interpersonal violence and rape myth, sex role stereotyping, sex role satisfaction, adversarial sexual beliefs, and sexual conservatism.

Abel and Becker's Sexual Interest Cardsort (2) measures the degree of sexual arousal or repulsion to scenarios describing different sexual variants. The Multiphasic Sex Inventory (64) assesses a wide range of psychosexual characteristics of the sexual offender. It measures sex knowledge, sexual deviance, interest in atypical sexual behavior, and degree of sexual dysfunction.

The Computer Assisted Psychosocial Assessment (CAPSA), an instrument we developed, provides an extremely detailed narrative history covering the subject's developmental, educational, sexual, marital, occupational, and military history. His medical history including psychiatric illnesses and problems with alcohol and drugs are documented, as well as the offender's criminal record as a juvenile and adult.

Physiological Assessment

In the past decade the measurement of sexual arousal patterns has become an important component in the assessment of sex offenders (21, 57, 75). Investigators have used different psychophysiological parameters, including electromyographic activity (EMG), galvanic skin resistance (GSR), and pupil dilation, to determine sexual arousal patterns. The preferred and most widely used technique employs the penile plethysmograph, which measures the vasocongestive engorgement of the penile corporea while the offender is exposed to sexual stimuli, by measuring either the circumference or the volume of the penis.

In the circumferential measurement technique the subject is seated alone in a room with a mercury strain gauge fitted over his penis while exposed to sexual stimuli. The stimuli may be slides of different age groups of nude male and female individuals, movies depicting different types of sexual activity, or audiotaped descriptions of sexual encounters.

Measurements of penile reactions to visual stimuli can differentiate between child molesters and normals (70). Although the researchers found that child molesters claimed to have adult sexual preferences, they registered increased arousal to children. Furthermore, they could differentiate between male- and female-oriented child molesters. Heterosexual child molesters had peak arousal toward female children; homosexual child molesters had peak arousal to male children; and bisexual child molesters responded most to female children. Avery-Clark and Laws (9) were able to differentiate pedophiles with a known history of violence from pedophiles with no violent history.

Freund, Chan, and Coulthard (30) observed that phallometry correctly identified 95% of heterosexuals and homosexuals who prefer mature sexual objects. This discriminatory power lessens somewhat when testing pedophiles, although its value is still apparent. Two-thirds of admitting pedophiles and one-third of nonadmitting were correctly identified.

Although the phallometric measurements offer the best method for discriminating between child molesters and nonmolesters, a word of caution should be offered. Some therapists are giving expert testimony in court labeling a person a child molester based solely on his arousal pattern. These professionals are overstepping the limits of the procedure and the data it yields. Likewise, at this stage of knowledge it is not appropriate to use these response data as a sole predictor of future acts or an indicator for release from prison.

There are limitations to penile plethysmography. Numerous studies (1, 30, 56, 58) indicate that phallometric responses can be faked, and not all offenders respond to stimuli in the laboratory setting. As phallometric procedures generally are unstandardized, efforts are currently underway to develop standards for sexual assessment laboratories. We believe the reliability of penile plethysmography for child molesters would be improved by using rating scales of sexual maturity as a criterion for categorization of stimulus materials (31). Currently arbitrarily established age categories that do not take into account the wide variation in growth and development among children and adolescents are used.

Integrating the Assessment Data

Child molesters, generally speaking, have high levels of denial and rationalization. Because of the high levels of denial, the clinician may wish to confront the patient with the findings from clinical observations, psychological assessment, documents, and phallometric testing. Abel, Rouleau, and Cunningham-Rathner (6) found that in 62.2% of cases where the patients had denied any deviant interests, they subsequently acknowledged them when confronted with their arousal responses to the paraphiliac stimuli.

At the conclusion of this complex assessment at our laboratory, a computerized report is printed out containing the psychosocial history and interpretative test results. The emphasis is placed on procuring extensive information because we base diagnosis and prognosis on these data. A multidisciplinary team reviews this report, formulates treatment objectives, and institutes an individualized treatment program.

TREATMENT

Goals

The general aim of treatment for child molesters, as in all forms of sexual deviancy, is to reduce, prevent, or otherwise avoid sexual victimization and sexual offenses. Langevin and Lang (53) point out the pedophiles' reluctance to give up ego syntonic behavior that they experience as positive and rewarding. When asked in one study (28), very few pedophiles indicated they wanted to lose their pedophilia. To reduce the risk of the child molester committing future offenses requires effecting changes in the internal psychological predisposition of the offender, in his external living environment, in his behavior, or some combination thereof. The offender must develop internal controls or be externally controlled to prevent his acting out such interests. We discuss four treatment modalities: (1) organic, (2) psychotherapeutic, (3) behavioral, and (4) psychosocial approaches.

Organic

Testosterone, an androgen, is the most important hormone in the maintenance of and effects on male sexual behavior. There are two organic treatments for the child molester that reduce sexual interests by lowering the androgen level: surgical castration and antiandrogen medication.

Throughout history surgical castration has been practiced on sex offenders as a preventive intervention as well as a retribution for deviant sexual behavior. Castration, the removal of testes in a man, results in a complete shutdown of androgen production from the testes, which produces 95% of the body's total testosterone. Various studies of recidivism have rates varying between 1.1% and 16.8% (15, 17, 83). Serious criticism of the methodology of the recidivism studies has been raised (42). Bradford (17), however, in a review of castration as a treatment for sexual offenders, concludes: "There is no doubt that castration, even allowing the largest margin for methodological difficulties, has a massive impact on sexual recidivism in the post castration state" (p. 368). Regardless of the efficacy of the treatment, we do not consider castration to be an acceptable treatment modality owing to the many ethical considerations involved with this irreversible procedure.

In contrast to castration, antiandrogens provide a reversible means of lowering male sexual hormones and, therefore, sexual drive. The reduction in strength of arousal is temporary, and arousal to inappropriate stimuli returns when the therapy is discontinued.

Recent studies have indicated that the use of antiandrogens, such as medroxyprogesterone acetate (MPA) and cyproterone acetate (CPA), suppresses libido and overt sexual behavior in sex offenders (10, 11, 14, 15, 33). The outcome studies evaluating the effectiveness of MPA have shown 83% effectiveness during treatment and 65% relapse with discontinuation of treatment. The recidivism rates of sexual offenders ranged from 54% to 100% prior to treatment with CPA and fell to zero with treatment (17). Relapse was associated with failure of compliance, with drug or alcohol intake, and with lack of pair-bondedness to a significant other. Numerous side effects from MPA and CPA have been documented. In most cases the side effects are not very severe or dangerous, but may affect compliance.

Standard psychopharmacological agents are generally not indicated for altering the child molester's deviant sexual arousal. When the molester suffers from severe psychopathology, treatment must be directed toward the underlying illness. For example, antipsychotic medications may be indicated in the offender with schizophrenia or other thought disorders. Major affective disorders may require lithium therapy or antidepressant medication.

Neither endocrine chemotherapy nor psychotropic medication eliminates deviant sexual interests. If nothing has been done during the period of medication to modify deviant arousal patterns, molesting behavior may reemerge when medication ceases. The period under medication provides the opportunity to develop appropriate sexual conduct through psychotherapy, behavior therapy, or psychosocial education.

Psychotherapy

Since the 1960s many psychotherapeutic approaches, both individual and group, have been tried with child molesters. The literature on individual psychotherapy for child molesters is sparse and predominantly consists of case reports (51). Group psychotherapy is particularly well suited to overcome the denial, rationalization, and repression of child molesters. In our experience, the child molester must be motivated in order to profit from psychotherapy. Treatment is intensive, demanding, and time consuming. This section is an account of the group approach implemented at NFETC by David Hutchinson, former Director of the Sex Offender Treatment Unit. For additional psychotherapeutic approaches the reader may consult Knopp (49, 50), Langevin and Lang (53), Giarretto (35, 36), Quinsey (66), Resnik and Peters (73), and Silver (82).

When the child molester enters group, the therapist first determines his emotional needs. If an emotional fixation from a traumatic event in child-hood is noted, reliving the experience with guidance from the therapist helps to master the overwhelming feelings of helplessness and fear. Many have repressed these feelings. Others have taken a course of identifying with the aggressor and seek to master anxiety or helplessness by exerting dominance over a young child. In the process, the offender isolates the affective component and loses contact with those feelings of sensitivity which would permit empathy and caring for others. In therapy the patient is assisted in recognizing the hurt, frightened child within. With the sup-port of the group and therapist he often becomes aware of his anger and rage. Experiencing an emotional catharsis permits the child molester to regain contact with the repressed affect. Many experiences of reliving the traumatic events are necessary in order to complete the intrapsychic inte-gration. This affective experiencing sets the stage for receptivity to change.

In psychotherapy the patient not only deals with traumatic events from the past, but also explores other dynamic factors. With the aid of the therapist and group members, he is given the opportunity to explore his own sexuality and to investigate the onset of his normal and deviant sexu-ality. Often previously forgotten memories or screened memories that con-ditioned the pedophilic arousal patterns are remembered as the child mo-lester reenacts his sexual experience with his child victim during role play.

Group psychotherapy permits the offender to gain insight into the origin of his psychopathology, to learn how it is manifested in everyday life, and to analyze his belief systems. The group environment encourages and facil-itates change and development of healthier styles of relating to others. For example, a patient may not know how to experience intimacy and close-ness outside a sexual encounter. In therapy he is encouraged to separate these needs by developing an intimate relationship without sex. He may find that some facets of his life have been overinhibited. During his devel-opmental years he learned not to express his frustration and appropriate anger directly, but rather to express his repressed feelings with occasional outbursts or in a passive aggressive manner. In therapy more direct and appropriate means of asserting his needs are learned. This process of cogni-tive mastery promotes self-awareness and provides a rational component for organizing and integrating change.

An offender may have sexually arousing deviant thoughts and fantasies, but only occasionally follows through with actual child molestation. In therapy he reviews the antecedent circumstances surrounding his loss of control. Commonly deviant fantasies are acted upon while intoxicated or after a self-defeating experience with an adult female. In either case becoming aware of the antecedent disinhibiting or displacement factors helps prevent recurrence of sexual abuse through management of actions and habits. Role playing is a useful technique in imparting empathy for the victim and promoting personal insight. In addition, it reinforces therapeutic learning through rehearsal, repetition, and continued practice of new behaviors.

Behavioral Approaches

Behavioral therapies are important in the treatment of child molesters. Their emphasis is on the patient's current functioning, a data-based approach to specific treatment interventions, and the use of measurable changes in cognitive, affective, physiological, or interpersonal behavior to assess treatment progress. Many behavioral interventions have been demonstrated to be effective in clinical and research settings for some offenders. The interested reader may refer to other writers (38, 48, 67, 80) for descriptions of the procedures, theoretical formulations, and empirical evidence for their effectiveness.

The focus of behavioral approaches for child molestation is twofold: (1) to decrease the strength of deviant sexual arousal and preference, and (2) to increase preference and capacity for sexual activities with age-appropriate partners.

In the present decade comprehensive behavioral treatment packages (4, 60, 69) are in vogue. Early reviews (24) are optimistic for these comprehensive behavioral models, but further evaluation and scrutiny are needed. Briefly, the strategy is to assess the strengths and weaknesses of the offender and to administer treatment only to the deficit areas. These multidimensional approaches often employ several parts that combine aversive and positive paradigms. The most common interventions designed to decrease heightened sexual arousal to children are masturbatory satiation, covert sensitization to unacceptable sexual behavior, and cognitive restructuring strategies, such as stress and anger management, thought stopping, and relapse prevention.

The masturbatory satiation technique (59) requires the subject to masturbate to ejaculation while verbalizing nondeviant sexual material and then to continue to masturbate after ejaculation for a prolonged, refractory period while verbalizing deviant sexual fantasies. Satiation sessions may be audiotaped and spot-checked by a therapist for compliance and proper procedure.

Covert sensitization (4) is based on the belief that child-molesting behaviors are usually the product of a lengthy chain of events involving fantasy and other preassaultive behaviors. The child molester is helped to recognize the sequential elements of his paraphilic arousal and to identify the most highly aversive consequences (ostracized by family, prison term, sadistic rape of himself, etc.) of his molesting children. The offender verbalizes the sequences leading to the paraphilic activity. At the moment of intense arousal he switches to the highly aversive thoughts. Subsequently, the expectation is that the child molester will recognize the antecedent thoughts and actions of his paraphilic behavior and be able to turn off his arousal by substituting the aversive thoughts for the erotic ones.

Cognitive restructuring is exemplified by a treatment manual (34) for relapse prevention with sexual offenders. This method involves six group therapy sessions followed by 52 weekly individual follow-up sessions. The technique requires motivation and cultivates a self-control perspective, with the offender taking the responsibility for his own treatment. Continued self-monitoring, improved coping skills, improved social interactions, and constructive lifestyle habits are used to promote adaptive functioning, self-efficacy, and decreased recidivism.

Masturbatory conditioning and fading are two techniques employed to develop preference arousal to age-appropriate sexual stimuli (12). Masturbatory conditioning is a technique where the offender masturbates to favorite deviant fantasies but changes to a nondeviant, age-appropriate fantasy at the moment of orgasm. Brownell et al. (18) found that the method increased the arousal to nondeviant stimuli but did not change the pattern of deviant sexual arousal. Thus the patterns may be independent.

Some sex abusers reported having difficulty switching between fantasies at the point of orgasm. This led to the suggestion of using other shaping techniques. In the fading technique (13), the subject views stimulus slides on which inappropriate and appropriate sexual objects are superimposed. The inappropriate stimuli are clearly perceptible at first but then gradually fade as the appropriate slides become visible.

Behavioral therapy appears promising but has its own inherent weaknesses. Behaviorists often downplay development of adaptive functioning for sexual and affectional drives. Interpersonal, familial, psychosocial, and general-systems issues often are not addressed.

Psychosocial Education

Psychosocial strategies can be divided into before-the-molestation and after-the-molestation interventions. Before-the-molestation strategies attempt to prevent sexual abuse by equipping children with knowledge and skills to protect themselves, keeping adolescents and adults from becoming offenders, and educating the public about the magnitude and seriousness of this problem. An outline and the rationale of an approach for primary prevention is available from the National Committee for the Prevention of Child Abuse (20). After-the-molestation intervention consists of teaching a known offender the life management skills lacking in his socialization that will allow him to function interpersonally, to cope more adaptively, and to stop his abusive behavior.

The psychosocial rehabilitation of an identified child molester involves several components (40). A basic program in human sexuality is indicated for child molesters who have limited or erroneous sexual knowledge. Sex education focuses on myths about sex, common concerns, reproduction, sexual roles, gender identity, and variations in sexual behavior, values, and attitudes. Role playing, assertiveness training, anger modulation, social-skills training, and similar techniques are directed toward improving the offender's interpersonal communication, self-control, and empathy. As many child molesters were physically, sexually, or emotionally victimized as youngsters, these offenders are helped to understand the impact of this trauma on current attitudes, values, behavior, and fantasy. Understanding the aftereffects of sexual assault from the victim's perspective helps the offender to more fully understand and empathize with the victim. The effectiveness of this approach is largely untested; however, as a technique it has several advantages. The goals are identified and approached in an organized, structured fashion; each component is time-limited, which is particularly suitable for offenders with low endurance who need instant gratification.

PROGNOSIS

The effectiveness of treatment of the child molester is dependent on a number of variables (20, 24, 53, 55, 85): (a) the greater the degree of compliance, motivation, and willingness to persist in treatment, the better the prognosis; (b) the longer the molesting behavior has been established and the earlier in life it developed, the poorer the prognosis; (c) incestuous child sexual abuse situations resolve more easily than nonrelated, preference pedophilic situations; (d) the ability to manage life crises and fiscal responsibility lessens the chances of reoffending; (e) concomitant substance abuse, psychopathology, and constrictive religious or moral beliefs do not bode well for treatment success; and (f) a cooperative and committed adult sex partner and good heterosocial skills improve the likelihood of the child molester managing his urges and modifying his preference for children.

Because of the limited treatment outcome data, we strongly advocate an extended follow-up on each offender.

REFERENCES

1. ABEL, G. G., BARLOW, D. H., BLANCHARD, E. B., & MAVISSAKALIAN, M. (1975). Measurement of sexual arousal in male homosexuals: Effects of instructions and stimulus modality. *Arch. Sex. Behav., 4*, 623.
2. ABEL, G. G., & BECKER, J. V. (1985). *Sexual interest cardsort*. Atlanta, GA: Behavioral Medicine Laboratory, Emory University.
3. ABEL, G. G., BECKER, J. V., & CUNNINGHAM-RATHNER, J. (1984). Complications, consent and cognitions in sex between children and adults. *Int. J. Law Psychiatry, 7*, 89.
4. ABEL, G. G., BECKER, J. V., CUNNINGHAM-RATHNER, J., ROULEAU, J. L., KAPLAN, M., & REICH, J. (1984). *The treatment of child molesters*. Atlanta, GA: Behavioral Medicine Laboratory, Emory University.
5. ABEL, G. G., MITTELMAN, M. S., & BECKER, J. V. (1985). Sexual offenders: Results of assessment and recommendations for treatment. In M. H. Ben-Aron, S. J. Hucker, & C. D. Webster (Eds.), *Clinical criminology: Current concepts*. Toronto: M & M Graphics.
6. ABEL, G. G., ROULEAU, J., & CUNNINGHAM-RATHNER, J. (1986). Sexually aggressive behavior. In: W. J. Curran, A. L. McGarry, and S. A. Shah (Eds.), *Forensic psychiatry and psychology: Perspectives and standards for interdisciplinary practice*. Philadelphia: Davis.
7. American Humane Association, Children's Division, 9725 E. Hampden Avenue, Denver, CO 80231, personal communication.
8. ARAJI, S., & FINKELHOR, D. (1985). Explanations of pedophilia: Review of empirical research. *Bull. Am. Acad. Psychiatry Law, 13*, 17.
9. AVERY-CLARK, C. A., & LAWS, D. R. (1984). Differential erection response patterns of sexual child abusers to stimuli describing activities with children. *Behav. Ther., 15*, 71.
10. BANCROFT, J. (1977). Hormones and sexual behaviour. *Psychol. Med., 7*, 553.
11. BANCROFT, J., TENNENT, G., LOUCAS, K., & CASS, J. (1974). The control of deviant sexual behaviour by drugs: 1. Behavioural changes following oestrogens and anti-androgens. *Br. J. Psychiatry, 125*, 310.
12. BARLOW, D. H. (1973). Increasing heterosexual responsiveness in the treatment of sexual deviation: A review of the clinical and experimental evidence. *Behav. Ther. 4*, 655.
13. BARLOW, D. H., & AGRAS, W. S. (1973). Fading to increase heterosexual responsiveness in homosexuals. *J. Appl. Behav. Anal., 6*, 355.
14. BERLIN, F. S. (1983). Sex offenders: A biomedical perspective and a status report on biomedical treatment. In J. G. Greer & I. R. Stuart (Eds.), *The sexual aggressor: Current perspectives on treatment*. New York: Van Nostrand.
15. BERLIN, F. S., & MEINECKE, C. F. (1981). Treatment of sex offenders with antiandrogenic medication: Conceptualization, review of treatment modalities, and preliminary findings. *Am. J. Psychiatry, 138*, 601.
16. BONIELLO, M. J. (1986). The family as "stage" for creating abusive children. *Connections Prev. Child Sexual Abuse, 1*, 4.
17. BRADFORD, J. M. W. (1985). Organic treatments for the male sexual offender. *Behav. Sci. Law, 3*, 355.
18. BROWNELL, K. D., HAYES, S. C., & BARLOW, D. H. (1977). Patterns of appropriate and deviant sexual arousal: The behavioral treatment of multiple sexual deviations. *J. Consult. Clin. Psychol., 45*, 1144.

19. BURT, M. R. (1980). Cultural myths and supports for rape. *J. Personality Soc. Psychol.*, *38*, 217.
20. COHN, A., FINKELHOR, D., & HOLMES, C. (1985). *Preventing adults from becoming child sexual molesters*. Working Paper Number 25. Chicago, IL: National Committee for the Prevention of Child Abuse.
21. CONTE, J. R. (1985). Clinical dimensions of adult sexual abuse of children. *Behav. Sci. Law*, *3*, 341.
22. Council on Scientific Affairs of the American Medical Association. (1985). AMA diagnostic and treatment guidelines concerning child abuse and neglect. *JAMA*, *254*, 796.
23. DOWNER, A. (1985). *Prevention of child sexual abuse: A trainer's manual*. Seattle, WA: Seattle Institute for Child Advocacy Committee for Children.
24. EARLS, C. M., & QUINSEY, V. L. (1985). What is to be done? Future research on the assessment and behavioral treatment of sex offenders. *Behav. Sci. Law*, *3*, 377.
25. FINKELHOR, D. (1984). *Child sexual abuse: New theory and research*. New York: Free Press.
26. FINKELHOR, D. (1980). Risk factors in the sexual victimization of children. *Child Abuse Neglect*, *4*, 265.
27. FINKELHOR, D. (1979). *Sexually victimized children*. New York: Free Press.
28. FREDERIC, B. (1975). An enquiry among a group of pedophiles. *J. Sex Res.*, *11*, 242.
29. FREUND, K. (1967). Diagnosing homo- or heterosexuality and erotic age-preference by means of a psychophysiological test. *Behav. Res. Ther.*, *5*, 209.
30. FREUND, K., CHAN, S., & COULTHARD, R. (1979). Phallometric diagnosis with "nonadmittors." *Behav. Res. Ther.*, *17*, 451.
31. FULLER, A. K., BARNARD, G. W., ROBBINS, L., & SPEARS, H. (in press). Sexual maturity as a criterion for classification of phallometric stimulus slides. *Arch. Sex. Behav.*
32. GAFFNEY, G. R., & BERLIN, F. S. (1984). Is there hypothalamic-pituitary-gonadal dysfunction in paedophilia? A pilot study. *Br. J. Psychiatry*, *145*, 657.
33. GAGNE, P. (1981). Treatment of sex offenders with medroxyprogesterone acetate. *Am. J. Psychiatry*, *138*, 644.
34. GEORGE, W. H., & MARLATT, G. A. (1986). *Relapse prevention with sexual offenders: A treatment manual*. Tampa, FL: Florida Mental Health Institute.
35. GIARRETTO, H. (1982). A comprehensive child sexual abuse treatment program. *Child Abuse Neglect*, *6*, 263.
36. GIARRETTO, H. (1982). *Integrated treatment of child sexual abuse: A treatment and training manual*. Palo Alto, CA: Science and Behavior Books.
37. GOLDSTEIN, M. J., & KANT, H. S. (1973). *Pornography and sexual deviance*. Berkeley, CA: University of California Press.
38. GROSSMAN, L. S. (1985). Research directions in the evaluation and treatment of sex offenders: An analysis. *Behav. Sci. Law*, *3*, 421.
39. GROTH, A. N. (1978). Patterns of sexual assault against children and adolescents. In A. W. Burgess, A. N. Groth, L. L. Holmstrom & S. M. Sgroi (Eds.), *Sexual assault of children and adolescents*. Lexington, MA: Lexington.
40. GROTH, A. N., HOBSON, W. F., & GARY, T. S. (1982). The child molester: Clinical observations. In J. Conte & D. A. Shore (Eds.), *Social work and child sexual abuse*. New York: Haworth.
41. HATHAWAY, S. R., & MCKINLEY, J. C. (1967). *The Minnesota Multiphasic Personality Inventory*. Minneapolis: University of Minnesota Press.
42. HEIM, N., & HURSCH, C. J. (1979). Castration for sex offenders: Treatment or punishment? A review and critique of recent European literature. *Arch. Sex. Behav.*, *8*, 281.
43. HEINEMANN, A. W., HARPER, R. G., FRIEDMAN, L. C., & WHITNEY, J. (1985). The relative utility of the Shipley-Hartford Scale: Prediction of Wais-R IQ. *J. Clin. Psychol.*, *41*, 547.

44. HOWELLS, K. (1981). Adult sexual interest in children: Considerations relevant to theories of aetiology. In M. Cook & K. Howells (Eds.), *Adult sexual interest in children*. New York: Academic Press.
45. HOWELLS, K. (1979). Some meanings of children for pedophiles. In M. Cook & G. Wilson (Eds.), *Love and attraction: An international conference*. Oxford: Pergamon.
46. JACKSON, D. N. (1984). *Personality Research Form Manual*. Port Huron, MI: Research Psychologist Press.
47. JASTAK, S., & WILKINSON, G. S. (1984). *The Wide Range Achievement Test – Revised*. Wilmington, DE: Jastak Associates.
48. KELLY, R. J. (1982). Behavioral reorientation of pedophiliacs: Can it be done? *Clin. Psychol. Rev., 2*, 387.
49. KNOPP, F. H. (1984). *Retraining adult sex offenders: Methods and models*. Syracuse, NY: Safer Society Press.
50. KNOPP, F. H. (1985). *The youthful sex offender: The rationale and goals of early intervention and treatment*. Syracuse, NY: Safer Society Press.
51. LANGEVIN, R. (1983). *Sexual strands: Understanding and treating sexual anomalies in men*. Hillsdale, NJ: Erlbaum.
52. LANGEVIN, R., HANDY, L., PAITICH, D., & RUSSON, A. (1985). Appendix A: A new version of the Clarke Sex History Questionnaire for Males. In R. Langevin (Ed.), *Erotic preference, gender identity, and aggression in men: New research studies*. Hillsdale, NJ: Erlbaum.
53. LANGEVIN, R., & LANG, R. A. (1985). Psychological treatment of pedophiles. *Behav. Sci. Law, 3*, 403.
54. LANGEVIN, R., HUCKER, S. J., BEN-ARON, M. H., PURINS, J. E., & HOOK, H. J. (1985). Why are pedophiles attracted to children? Further studies of erotic preference in heterosexual pedophilia. In R. Langevin (Ed.), *Erotic preference, gender identity, and aggression in men: New research studies*. Hillsdale, NJ: Erlbaum.
55. LANYON, R. I. (1986). Theory and treatment in child molestation. *J. Consult. Clin. Psychol., 54*, 176.
56. LAWS, D. R., & HOLMEN, M. L. (1978). Sexual response faking by pedophiles. *Criminal Justice Behav., 5*, 343.
57. LAWS, D. R., & OSBORN, C. A. (1983). How to build and operate a behavioral laboratory to evaluate and treat sexual deviance. In J. G. Greer & I. R. Stuart (Eds.), *The sexual aggressor: Current perspectives on treatment*. New York: Van Nostrand.
58. LAWS, D. R., & RUBIN, H. B. (1969). Instructional control of an autonomic sexual response. *J. Appl. Behav. Anal., 2*, 93.
59. MARSHALL, W. L. (1979). Satiation therapy: A procedure for reducing deviant sexual arousal. *J. Appl. Behav. Anal., 12*, 10.
60. MARSHALL, W. L., EARLS, C. M., SEGAL, Z., & DARKE, J. L. (1983). A behavioral program for the assessment and treatment of sexual aggressors. In K. Craig & R. McMahon (Eds.), *Advances in clinical behavior therapy*. New York: Brunner/Mazel.
61. MAUGER, P. A., & ADKINSON, D. R. (1980). *Interpersonal Behavior Survey (IBS) manual*. Los Angeles: Western Psychological Services.
62. MRAZEK, P. J., LYNCH, M. A., & BENTOVIM, A. (1983). Sexual abuse of children in the United Kingdom. *Child Abuse Neglect, 7*, 147.
63. MURRAY, H. A. (1943). *Thematic Apperception Test manual*. Cambridge, MA: Harvard University Press.
64. NICHOLS, H. R., & MOLINDER, I. (1984). *Multiphasic Sex Inventory manual*. Tacoma, WA: Nichols and Molinder.
65. PLUMMER, K. (1981). Pedophilia: Constructing a sociological baseline. In M. Cook & K. Howells (Eds.), *Adult sexual interest in children*. London: Academic Press.
66. QUINSEY, V. L. (1977). The assessment and treatment of child molesters: A review. *Can. Psychol. Rev., 18*, 204.

67. QUINSEY, V. L., & MARSHALL, W. L. (1983). Procedures for reducing inappropriate sexual arousal: An evaluation review. In J. G. Greer, & I. R. Stuart (Eds.), *The sexual aggressor: Current perspectives on treatment.* New York: Van Nostrand Reinhold.
68. QUINSEY, V. L., CHAPLIN, T. C., & CARRIGAN, W. F. (1979). Sexual preferences among incestuous and nonincestuous child molesters. *Behav. Ther., 10,* 562.
69. QUINSEY, V. L., CHAPLIN, T. C., MAGUIRE, A. M., & UPFOLD, D. (1988). The behavioral treatment of rapists and child molesters. In E. K. Morris, & C. J. Braukmann (Eds.), *Behavioral approaches to crime and delinquency: Application, research, and theory.* New York: Plenum Press.
70. QUINSEY, V. L., STEINMAN, C. M., BERGERSEN, S. G., & HOLMES, T. F. (1975). Penile circumference, skin conductance, and ranking responses of child molesters and "normals" to sexual and nonsexual visual stimuli. *Behav. Ther., 6,* 213.
71. RADA, R. T. (1976). Alcoholism and the child molester. *Ann. NY Acad. Sci., 273,* 492.
72. RADA, R. T., LAWS, D. R., & KELLNER, R. (1976). Plasma testosterone levels in the rapist. *Psychosom. Med., 38,* 257.
73. RESNIK, H. L. P., & PETERS, J. J. (1967). Outpatient group therapy with convicted pedophiles. *Int. J. Group Psychother., 17,* 151.
74. RORSCHACH, H. (1942). *Psychodiagnostics, a diagnostic test based on perception.* New York: Grune & Stratton.
75. ROSEN, R. C., & KEEFE, F. J. (1978). The measurement of human penile tumescence. *Psychophysiology, 15,* 366.
76. RUSSELL, D. E. H. (1983). The incidence and prevalence of intrafamilial and extrafamilial sexual abuse of female children. *Child Abuse Neglect, 7,* 133.
77. RUSSELL, D. E. H. (1984). The prevalence and seriousness of incestuous abuse: Stepfathers vs. biological fathers. *Child Abuse Neglect, 8,* 15.
78. RUSSON, A. E. (1985). Appendix B: Sex History Questionnaires scoring manual. In R. Langevin (Ed.), *Erotic preference, gender identity, and aggression in men: New research studies.* Hillsdale, NJ: Erlbaum.
79. SELZER, M. L. (1971). The Michigan Alcoholism Screening Test: The quest for a new diagnostic instrument. *Am. J. Psychiatry, 127,* 1653.
80. SERBER, M., & WOLPE, J. (1971). Treatment of the sex offender: Behavioral therapy techniques. *Int. Psychiatr. Clin., 8,* 53.
81. SHIPLEY, W. C. (1939). *Shipley Institute of Living Scale for Measuring Intellectual Impairment: Manual of directions and scoring key.* Hartford, CT: The Institute of Living.
82. SILVER, S. N. (1976). Outpatient treatment for sex offenders. *Social Work, 21,* 134.
83. STURUP, G. K. (1972). Castration: The total treatment. In H. L. P. Resnik & M. E. Wolfgang (Eds.), *Sexual behaviors: Social, clinical, and legal aspects.* Boston: Little, Brown.
84. TINGLE, D., BARNARD, G. W., ROBBINS, L., NEWMAN, G., & HUTCHINSON, D. (1986). Childhood and adolescent characteristics of pedophiles and rapists. *Int. J. Law Psychiatry, 9,* 108.
85. WHEELER, J. R. (1986). Should behavioral interventions be used with adolescent sexual offenders? *Connections Prev. Child Sexual Abuse, 1,* 6.
86. World Health Organization. (1977). *International statistical classification of diseases, injuries, and causes of death* (9th rev.), Section V—Mental disorders. Geneva: WHO.
87. WYATT, G. E. (1985). The sexual abuse of Afro-American and white-American women in childhood. *Child Abuse Neglect, 9,* 507.
88. WYATT, G. E., & PETERS, S. D. (1986). Issues in the definition of child sexual abuse in prevalence research. *Child Abuse Neglect, 10,* 231.

3

EVALUATION AND TREATMENT FOR INCEST VICTIMS AND THEIR FAMILIES: A PROBLEM-ORIENTED APPROACH

JEAN M. GOODWIN, M.D., M.P.H.

Professor of Psychiatry and Director, Joint Academic Programs,
Medical College of Wisconsin and
Milwaukee County Mental Health Complex,
Milwaukee, Wisconsin

Surveys indicate that 16% of women in the general population have experienced sexual contact with a relative and 1 to 4% have experienced father-daughter incest (1, 2). In psychiatric populations the prevalence is higher, with 35% of female psychiatric inpatients reporting incest experiences in childhood with fathers, stepfathers, mothers, grandparents, older brothers, or uncles (3). Males in the general population are less well studied. There is considerable anecdotal evidence that in the most severely disturbed families all children — both male and female — are sexually and/or otherwise abused, often by multiple family members — both male and female (4). One survey shows that over half of therapists — psychiatrists, psychologists, and family counselors — have treated at least one child or adult incest victim in the past year (5).

In the past 10 years certain evaluation and treatment strategies have become routine for child incest victims (6). In the initial phase this routine includes: (1) a complete *physical examination*, (2) *investigation* to document abuse and to detect *other victims*, (3) *legally mandated reporting* to protective services and in some jurisdictions to law enforcement, (4) interview and evaluation of *the alleged abuser* and other family members, and (5) assessment of the child for *post-traumatic symptoms*. Treatment of child victims tends to be similarly organized around the same five axes: (1) structuring adequate *physical care*, which sometimes requires placement of the child away from the abuser or both parents, (2) individual and group treatment of abused and/or neglected *siblings*, (3) guidance and support for family members as they progress through various *legal interventions*, (4) individual, group, behavioral, couples', and family therapy to rehabilitate *the sexually abusive parent* and to improve parental and family functioning, and (5) individual and group treatment to decrease post-traumatic and other *symptoms in the victim*.

Even in child victims this ideal model is not always followed, as the following examples illustrate for each of the five problem axes. [1] When confronted by a hypothetical case in which a nine-year-old retracts under pressure a detailed account of long-term oral sex with her father, 75% of pediatricians would recommend that the child be physically examined and screened for gonorrhea and other venereal diseases. Only 40% of psychologists, psychiatrists, and counselors recommended physical examination, although 100% recommended psychological testing for the child (5). [2] In this same survey, professionals in all categories tended to underestimate the 40% likelihood that if this child were abused, her sibling would have been also (7). [3] As recently as 1978, 58% of pediatricians surveyed stated that they would not report to protective services a confirmed case of incest (8). [4] Parents, especially fathers, often flee, avoid, or legally resist evaluation and treatment (9). [5] Child victims who fail to appear for appointments or who continue to function without major behavior problems may not be referred for treatment or even be systematically evaluated (10).

When an adult victim discloses prior incest, the approach to substantiation is even less systematic. Such disclosures typically occur in the middle phase of a treatment begun because of another chief complaint; few survivors disclose until trust is established (11). The therapist may not even conceptualize an investigation phase for the disclosure; a generation ago, some analytically oriented therapists understood such disclosures as "fantasies," a view that focused treatment on internal rather than external realities (12, 13). However, the importance of ascertaining the realities of the abusive incidents is attested by the high proportion of adult victims who question the authenticity of their own often fragmented or derealized memories and set as a treatment goal either the verification of those memories or some sort of confrontation or acknowledgment of those memories from the abuser or other family members (14). With the adult victim, the therapist typically does not (1) require a physical examination, (2) interview siblings, (3) consider possible legal obligations, or (4) evaluate the parents. However, (5) post-traumatic symptoms are targeted here much as they are in a child victim, although the powerful tool of group therapy is less often used (15).

This chapter offers clinical examples illustrating how adult as well as child victims benefit from careful attention to the five designated problem areas. The five-problem model will be applied systematically to assessment and treatment planning for children and adults. Particular attention will be paid to the sometimes perplexing issue of "Did sexual abuse take place?" A two-part section describes a brief screening approach for post-traumatic symptoms in child and adult victims, which differentiates severe from less disabling forms of the disorder.

A PROBLEM-ORIENTED APPROACH TO ASSESSMENT

Several studies show that only 6 to 9% of all incest allegations reflect fabrication by child or parent; the majority of these fabrications are produced by adults (16–20). Despite this relatively low frequency, concern remains that innocent parents will be accused or even convicted. Given the evidence that only 1% of rape events ever result in conviction (2), this last concern is statistically unlikely, albeit tragic when it occurs.

The problem-oriented approach offers a systematic way to organize clinical data in those perplexing incest allegations, often arising in custody disputes, when accusations and denials may be mutual, unrelenting and enraged, and when it is unclear whether the child suffers primarily from sexual abuse or whether the ongoing battles associated with divorce have produced post-traumatic symptoms. Clinicians can be misled in these situations if they place too much weight on the accounts of any single family member or if they neglect evidence from medical examination, witnesses, or other physical evidence such as photographs (20).

Applying the five-problem model to the substantiation question requires a balanced review of: (1) the *physical findings* on medical examination, (2) *investigatory data* such as the statements of witnesses and physical evidence such as photographs, diaries, and pornographic materials, (3) the potential *victim's statements* and competency to witness in a *legal* setting, (4) data about the suspected *abuser* and the *violence history* in the nuclear and extended family, and (5) data about the victim's *post-traumatic symptoms* and whether these can be linked specifically to details of the traumatic experience described.

The Physical Examination

Physical findings indicative of abuse are present in 50 to 75% of children who have been vaginally or anally penetrated (21–23). Physical signs may be subtle: delayed growth or anemia may reflect malnutrition; absent or incomplete inoculations and/or untreated dental problems can indicate medical neglect; bruises or burns can be signs of inappropriate discipline; a toxicology screen may reveal chemical abuse of the child. Undiagnosed or undertreated medical problems may be found in these children; seizure disorders are the most common (24). Although motile sperm is a rare finding in these chronically sexually abused children, examination of the genital region using magnification (colposcopy) may reveal anal scarring or dilatation, vaginal scarring or dilatation, hymenal stretching or scarring, and microscopic tears. Syphilis, gonorrhea, herpes, *Chlamydia*, genital warts, and other venereal infections are virtually diagnostic of sexual abuse, as is pregnancy. Review of past pediatric records is always indicated. This can reveal hospitalizations in infancy that were related to unrecognized neglect or abuse. Some abused children develop hysterical conversion symptoms or chronic somatic complaints such as headache or stomach ache (25, 26); these also may have led to prior treatment.

Investigation: Finding Other Victims, Witnesses, and Physical Evidence

Statements from witnesses are sought in child cases in part because of the need to identify other child victims. Intrafamilial sexual abusers were once thought to represent a separate category of offenders, quite different from pedophiles. However, we now recognize that some incestuous offenders sexually abuse many children, experience sexual arousal when fantasizing about children, use coercive strategies identical to those employed by pedophiles, and tend to accept treatment only under legal mandate (27). Grandfathers who sexually abuse have histories of victimizing numerous grandchildren and often children outside the family as well. They also tend to have victimized their own children, and those who accept treatment describe sexual contacts as adolescents with siblings or other relatives (28). Sometimes siblings are found to have been sexually abused by the identified victim or by family members other than the identified abuser. Siblings often have witnessed elements of the sexual abuse; for example, after a 12-year-old incest victim refused her father for the first time, she heard him go into the next bed and sodomize her brother.

School and neighborhood friends of the identified victim may also have been approached sexually by the abuser. Peers are sometimes told about the abuse by the victim, long before adults are consulted. This kind of witness data can be useful, especially if the credibility of the victim is in question owing to disclosure of incest during a crisis such as a marital separation or in the midst of a disciplinary dispute involving the victim. Valid disclosures are commonly made in precisely those circumstances in which the victim is least likely to be believed. Evidence that the child has told a peer long before decreases the likelihood that the complaint is an improvised manipulative fabrication. I recall one case in which a second grader told her best school friend about the sexual abuse by her father. Her friend was shocked by this and developed a plan to extricate her from the situation. Their plan was to go to school during the day and camp at night in a tent on the school playground. They would do yard work to earn money for food. On the first afternoon, when the two failed to come home on time from school, they were found by frantic parents and punished. The incest problem which had precipitated the "runaway" was not disclosed to the adult world until two years later when the girl contracted gonorrhea. In an even more grim and tragic case, when an adolescent girl disclosed severe physical and sexual abuse to her peers, they arranged for the father's murder.

Assessing the Credibility of the Child's Account

Legal involvement is routine in these cases. Courts or attorneys often ask a psychiatrist or psychologist to assess the credibility of a child's complaint about sexual abuse (29). Some jurisdictions prohibit expert testimony about credibility on grounds that this determination should be reserved for the trier of fact; however, since clinicians must assess whether a child has been abused as part of making a diagnosis and planning treatment, they will usually have an opinion. In some cases, refusal to reinterview the child is the best response to a request for an expert credibility assessment. For example, consider the case of a child who is five years old or under, whose abuse took place more than three months ago, and who has been interviewed by more than three evaluators. Children under five often have difficulty distinguishing what actually happened from what they thought or wished at the time, and from what has been said about the event (30). There is some evidence that distortions increase with elapsed time and number of evaluators (31, 32). Investigation and evaluation are best kept separate from treatment (33). If evaluation is still ongoing three months after an allegation, it is probably displacing needed treatment. Before submitting a young child to a repeated reinterview with yet another 'expert," the evaluation to date can be reviewed to determine whether the four problem areas other than the child's statement have been carefully pursued. Has a thorough physical examination been completed? Have its results been properly interpreted and integrated? Are there journals, photographs, prior medical records, or witnesses that have not yet been reviewed? Have other family members, including the possible abuser, been interviewed and evaluated? Is there a complete family violence history for all family members? Reevaluation of the child's account can include interventions other than a reinterview of the child, such as: (1) interviews of all individuals that the child has told about the sexual abuse or (2) observation of investigative videotapes or of one of the child's therapy hours to assess the child's developmental stage, intellectual capacity, communicative style, emotional state, and continued involvement with the sexual abuse complaint. In some difficult cases, it becomes apparent that the child himself has never made any complaint about abuse; the entire history of concern may be based on the preoccupations of one of the adults in the family.

When a reinterview is deemed necessary, this interview should be designed to respect the child's developmental capacities and the child's right to freedom from coercion. Children can be coerced by interviewers just as they can be by abusers. Abusers ensure silence and cajole retractions by a process Roland Summit (34) has termed the "accommodation syndrome." I use the mnemonic BLIND as a shorthand for five of the elements involved in the process of traumatizing a child: Brainwashing, Loss, Isolation, "Not awake or alert," and Death fears. Abusers brainwash and confuse the child with misinformation or disinformation ("All fathers do this"). They threaten loss of love or loved ones ("It would kill your mother if she knew"). They isolate the child from other sources of information or nurturance ("No one will believe you if you tell"). They initiate or escalate abuse when a child's awareness and concentration are at their lowest (during sleep, during an illness, after a severe punishment). They create an atmosphere of ultimate threat, which may be overt ("I'll kill you if you tell") or unstated but unmistakable to the child.

Coercive evaluations employ subtle variations on the BLIND tactics.

The child is not informed about the legal issues at stake. The child's concrete questions, like "Why is there a television camera here?" are not
answered. The child is isolated during the evaluation process from sources
of nurturance and stability — parents, siblings, extended family, school,
neighborhood — and may be threatened with permanent loss of these attachments. Evaluation sessions are prolonged beyond the child's range of
attention span or allowed to interfere with eating or sleeping. Death fears
can be stimulated by ill-timed, frightening questions (for example, immediately after a denial that sexual abuse occurred, "Are you hearing voices
now?") or by outright coercion ("That's not what you said on the videotape").

Step-by-step protocols can be helpful in preventing coercive interventions, as can structured and semistructured interviews, structured protocols for use of anatomically correct dolls, and lists of nonleading questions
(35–37). However, any system can be misused if the interviewer loses his or
her focus on the child's own reality and endeavors instead to manipulate
the child to meet adult needs.

Assessing the Abuser

The evaluator may find, that while the four-year-old in the case has
been evaluated repeatedly, the alleged adult abuser has refused interviews
with everyone. In England and the United States such refusal is based on
rights against self-incrimination. Nevertheless, collateral sources can often
be used to document a previous pattern of sexual, physical, and emotional
violence. In one case military records revealed a court martial for pedophilia. In another case family members had witnessed the father holding a
rifle to the mother's head and threatening to kill the entire family and then
himself. Hospital records and police reports may document spousal violence or rape, or previous investigations for child sexual abuse in previous
marriages. In some of the complex divorce custody cases, a pattern
emerges in which the abuser uses the legal system to intimidate and harass
the former spouse. School records may document paternal overinvolve-
ment with the child, jealous rage reactions, or a pattern of intimidation of
teachers by the father. These fathers may appear on the surface as the
exemplary, "endogamic," involved fathers described in the older literature
on incest (38, 39). It is only with more detailed history taking that their
involvement is understood as rooted in feelings and fantasies of persecution
and grandiosity rather than in an adult capacity to parent (40).

Screening for Post-Traumatic Symptoms

Various studies report that 20 to 100% of sexually abused children are acutely symptomatic at the time of the allegation (41–43). Some children present with severe psychosis or characterological problems that seem to predate the sexual abuse and may reflect constitutional factors or the result of neglect, emotional abuse, or battering that interfered with development in earlier years of life (44). Some children are completely asymptomatic. The most frequently described syndrome of symptoms includes intrusive memories and feelings about the abuse interspersed by numbing of responsiveness. This syndrome is described in the current diagnostic manual as post-traumatic stress disorder (PTSD) (45, 46).

I use the mnemonic FEARS to list five basic symptoms of PTSD. These are the five symptoms originally described by Kardiner in his study of "shellshocked" World War I veterans (47). They remain the core of present definitions of the syndrome. F stands for Fears and anxiety. Phobias are found and may encompass all men or may focus on a particular feature of the abuse, such as the room where incest occurred. Fears about sexuality are common, with over two-thirds of symptomatic incest victims reporting sexual dysfunction (48, 49). Dysfunction can be pervasive, such as avoidance of all kissing in a patient where oral sex had been prominent or avoidance of all penile contact in victims who maintain the capacity for satisfying sexual experience with females. Sometimes the fears are more circumscribed and can be gotten around by avoiding certain specific sexual practices. Easy startle is characteristic of PTSD. One incest victim blacked her roommate's eye when approached suddenly. Adolescent and adult victims may take fear for granted when it becomes chronic and may lose sight of the connection between incest-related fears and such coping strategies as alcohol or drug abuse or keeping the lights on all night. Certain fears are predictable: female victims will worry about pregnancy; male victims will have concerns about being homosexual. All victims at some level assume that the abuser's threats about disclosure will "come true" if they break their pledge of secrecy; thus, anxiety and fears will increase as disclosures are made in treatment.

E stands for Ego constriction, the phrase Kardiner used to describe the numbing processes used by the victim to avoid overwhelming anxiety. In young children, the constriction appears as loss of recently acquired developmental gains, such as exploration or toilet training in a toddler or adaptive school performance in an older child. Parents or teachers may be able to pinpoint a time, when the child changed or "faded," which coincides with the onset of sexual abuse.

A stands for Anger dyscontrol. A mildly affected victim often has difficulty expressing anger, masking it with compliance and perfectionism, which are punctuated by angry outbursts usually more terrifying to the victim herself than to her targets. Tantrums in young children or "hysterical" outbursts in older children manifest these problems in expression of anger.

R stands for Repetition, usually reflected, in mild cases, in repetitive thoughts, feelings, or images of the events. "Flashbacks" to incest during sexual activity are characteristic. Places, odors, or anniversaries may trigger perceptual reliving of traumatic events. Phobias and numbing often reflect strategies for avoiding flashbacks.

S reminds the evaluator of the importance of Sleep disturbance in PTSD and also stands for Sadness. Repetitive, post-traumatic nightmares are an important feature of PTSD; in very young children, frequent night terrors are an indicator of abuse. Post-traumatic nightmares may incorporate specific elements of the sexual abuse experience (the image of a large penis; the sensation of being crushed; the color of the childhood bedclothes) and are accompanied by physiological arousal or awakening. Modification and eventual disappearance of these dreams is a good indicator of therapeutic success (50). Incest victims and other victims of PTSD usually have some vegetative signs of depression, including crying spells, insomnia, appetite disturbance, or morbid self-reproach. Antidepressant medication is helpful in some patients with PTSD (50).

Screening for Severe Post-Traumatic Symptoms

In a small percentage of victims, symptoms are quite severe and potentially disabling. Severe symptoms have been associated with (1) presence of a parental perpetrator, (2) long duration of abuse, (3) serious threat or violence associated with the abuse (51), and (4) degree of family disruption (28). A modified FEARS mnemonic describes this severe symptom pattern.

In this syndrome, F represents Fugue and other dissociative symptoms. Rather than experiencing anxiety, these victims use fugues, amnesia, depersonalization, and derealization to distance and insulate themselves from the fear-provoking situation. Adolescent victims may become runaways with fuguelike qualities. Many victims use dissociative strategies in emergency situations, but in the severe cases, dissociation has become habitual and uncontrolled. The success of these defenses in combating fears and phobias is illustrated by data from incest victims with multiple personality disorder (52, 53). Despite other severe disabilities, only 10% of these victims have orgasmic dysfunction (54), probably because sexuality often is handled by a specialized alterpersonality insulated by dissociation from incest-related sexual fears.

Ego fragmentation replaces ego constriction in severely affected victims who may fragment completely into multiple personalities (MPD) or more complexly into the "part-object/part-self" representations found in borderline personality disorder (BPD). Ninety-seven to ninety-nine percent of MPD patients report abuse in childhood. Preliminary surveys indicate that 75% of patients with BPD have sexual abuse histories (55). It is intriguing to try to conceptualize the alternating idealizing and devaluing relationships that characterize the borderline patient as related to difficulties integrating the "public," often "perfect" parent with the secretly abusive parent known only to the child (56, 57).

A in the severe syndrome represents Antisocial acting out. Rather than struggling to repress and control anger, these victims often simply act on angry impulses. Such actions may include paraphiliac sexual activities, prostitution, and repeated family violence in adulthood, as spousal or child abuse.

R refers to the Reenactments that occur in these victims in lieu of the predominantly sensory repetitions seen in less severe cases. Repetitive reenactments include experiencing multiple rapes or choosing multiple mates who are physically abusive or multiple mates who incestuously abuse the victim's children (in some cases at exactly the same age of the mother was when she was incestuously victimized). Incest also may be reenacted in a therapeutic relationship in the form of therapist-patient sex (58).

For the severe syndrome, S refers to Suicidality and Somatization. Patients who present with multiple suicidal attempts or self-mutilations should be screened for both prior incest and the other manifestations of the severe FEARS syndrome, especially dissociative symptoms. Suicidality and somatization tend to appear together in incest victims.

In a study of 50 women treated in an adult incest victims group, 10% had multiple personality disorder. All five with MPD had multiple prior suicide attempts, severe multimodal abuse in their childhoods, and prior psychiatric hospitalization. Three had lost custody of their own children because of abuse and neglect. All had prominent somatic symptoms, including two with Briquet's syndrome and one with Munchausen's syndrome (59). Somatic symptoms could often be interpreted as somatic memories of the sexual abuse.

When somatization is part of a severe syndrome, close cooperation between psychotherapist and general physician may be necessary.

Applying the Model to Treatment: Planning for the Adult Incest Victim

In the introduction I described the clinical dilemmas that occur when an adult patient discloses prior incest midway in a treatment begun for another reason. Should the therapist proceed as if nothing had happened? Halt the treatment and reassess? This final section uses the problem-oriented approach to suggest options.

Inquiry is always indicated about physical intactness, bodily sensations, physical pain, and physiological indicators of fear occurring during disclosure to the therapist. Review of physical problems in adulthood may reveal patterns of pelvic pain or headache, which are common in incest victims. Review of pediatric records may uncover patterns of abuse that the victim has minimized or dissociated. One patient had been treated for multiple vaginal infections by her pediatrician. In another case, a brother's death certificate confirmed the patient's memory that he had been beaten to death.

Informal investigation is often undertaken by the adult incest victim, especially if amnesia obscures her own memories. Siblings are often the first collateral informants to be interviewed. In one case in which the victim had been completely amnestic for the incest for many years, a family servant was able to describe the induced abortion that had terminated the patient's forgotten incest pregnancy. Revisiting the former family home or reviewing old photo albums can clarify fragmentary memories. If entire years are lost to amnesia, I recommend that the patient make a notebook for the lost years, including photographs, old report cards, and information gained from family members, neighbors, and friends.

Legal complications are still possible, even if the disclosure comes from an adult victim (60). Younger siblings, nieces and nephews, or the adult's own children may continue to be at risk from her abuser or other victims in the family. Potential abusers include the victim herself, who may have been driven to disclosure by her impulses to physically abuse or neglect her own child. Protective service referrals may be necessary. Other legal involvements may arise. I have treated victims who have been able with treatment to mobilize the family to have the incestuous father civilly committed for psychiatric treatment. In cases where amnesia has deprived the victim of memory of the event, adults still have three years, in most jurisdictions, after recovering the memory to initiate a civil suit against the parent for damages caused; even if a parent is dead, the estate may be liable. The therapist is most helpful if aware of these potential legal entanglements.

Some adult incest victims pursue a role of family therapist, remaining concerned and involved with the abuser and his pathology and with other dysfunctional family members. Therapists narrowly focused on increasing autonomy and assertiveness may try simply to discourage such involvement. A more tolerant approach reveals multiple motives for continued involvement with the family: (1) the (sometimes unconscious) perception of the severity of the parent's pathology and realistic concerns about suicide or psychosis, (2) an attempt to use adult skills to see the family as it really is, (3) a realization that confrontation of the feared father is a direct way to challenge the entire array of fears and phobias related to victimization, and (4) an unconscious realization that many of the symptoms reflect an identification with the aggressor and an internalization of his actions, feelings, and thought patterns. The techniques of individual family therapy (61) are useful in exploring these issues. Sibling group sessions can also be helpful. Parents thought to be hostile and unapproachable can sometimes cooperate if approached in a nonthreatening way for historical information.

Confrontation and apology sessions with the abuser or with the nonprotective mother can be very useful but require extensive preparation of both parties (62). The victim needs extensive work around her fantasy that the apology will occur in such a complete and perfect way that the victim can believe that the parent never abused her at all. Similarly, the abuser needs to understand all the ways he can admit what he did without really admitting that he really did it and that it was seriously wrong and harmful. The victim's fears of the abuser cannot be overestimated. Many victims are extremely adept at concealing their fearfulness in a face-to-face interview. However, the victim's symptoms can be reactivated by a letter, a photograph, or a gift. Confrontation at times must be approached gradually through a process akin to systematic desensitization. Use of one-way mirrors or videotape to allow physical distance during confrontation and the presence of a supportive person can ease the victim's fears (63). If the father is realistically intimidating, even to established authority figures, a clarification of this quality can be a great relief to the victim, who may have misinterpreted her own fears as due to weakness.

In adults, the post-traumatic symptoms are dealt with by systematically linking them to the traumatic abuse. Severely symptomatic victims are vulnerable to treatment-related relapse into self-mutilation, eating disorders, suicidal depressions, and other behaviors that punish them for their defiance of the abusive parent by disclosure. Hospitalization, multimodal treatment, multiple therapists (working collaboratively), and time-intensive treatments (four or more hours per week) are indicated in these severe cases.

CONCLUSION

A five-point problem-oriented approach to assessing and treating incest victims provides a useful framework for initial assessment of incest complaints and for planning treatment. In adults as well as in children the therapist should be alert for (1) physical, physiological, and psychosomatic effects of the abuse, (2) the possibility that there are additional victims, (3) the possibility of legal consequences, (4) serious pathology in the abuser and in the family, as well as (5) post-traumatic symptoms in the victim.

REFERENCES

1. GOODWIN, J. M., McCARTY, T., & DIVASTO, P. (1982). Physical and sexual abuse of the children of adult incest victims. In J. Goodwin (Ed.), *Sexual abuse: Incest victims and their families*. Boston: Wright/PSG.
2. RUSSELL, D. (1984). *Sexual exploitation: Rape, child sexual abuse, and workplace harassment*. Beverly Hills, CA: Sage.
3. GOODWIN, J., ATTIAS, R., McCARTY, T., CHANDLER, S., & ROMANIK, R. (in press). Routine questioning about childhood sexual abuse in psychiatry inpatients. *Victimology*.
4. GOODWIN, J. (1985). Family violence: Principles of intervention and prevention. *Hosp. Comm. Psychiatry, 36*, 1074.
5. ATTIAS, R., & GOODWIN, J. (1985). Knowledge and management strategies in incest cases: A survey of physicians, psychologists, and family counselors. *Child Abuse Neglect, 9*, 527.
6. SGROI, S. M. (1982). *A handbook of clinical intervention in child sexual abuse*. Lexington, MA: Lexington Books.
7. HERMAN, J. (1981). *Father-daughter incest*. Cambridge, MA: Harvard University Press.
8. JAMES, J., WOMACK, W., & STRAUSS, F. (1978). Physician reporting of sexual abuse of children. *JAMA, 240*, 1145.
9. RYAN, T. (1986). Problems, errors, and opportunities in the treatment of father-daughter incest. *J. Interpers. Violence, 1*, 113.
10. ADAMS-TUCKER, C. (1984). The unmet psychiatric needs of sexually abused youths: Referrals from a child protection agency and clinical evaluations. *J. Am. Acad. Child Psychiatry, 23*, 659.
11. WESTERMEYER, J. (1978). Incest in psychiatric practice: A description of patients and incestous relationships. *J. Clin. Psychiatry, 39*, 643.
12. MASSON, J. M. (1984). *The assault on truth*. New York: Farrar, Strauss & Giroux.
13. GOODWIN, J. (1985). Credibility problems in multiple personalities and abused children.

In R. Kluft (Ed.), *Childhood antecedents of multiple personality*. Washington, DC: American Psychiatric Association Press.

14. HERMAN, J. (1986). Recovery and verification of memories of childhood sexual trauma. Unpublished manuscript.

15. TSAI, M., & WAGNER, N. N. (1978). Therapy groups for women sexually molested as children. *Arch. Sexual Behav.*, 7, 417–427.

16. PETERS, J. (1976). Children who are victims of sexual assault and the psychology of offenders. *Am. J. Psychother.*, 30, 398.

17. GOODWIN, J., SAHD, D., & RADA, R. T. (1979). Incest hoax: False accusations, false denials. *Bull. Am. Acad. Psychiatry Law*, 6, 269.

18. CANTWELL, H. (1981). Sexual abuse of children in Denver, 1979: Reviewed with implications for pediatric intervention and possible prevention. *Child Abuse Neglect*, 5, 75.

19. JONES, D. P. H., & McGRAW, J. M. (1987). Reliable and fictitious accounts of sexual abuse to children. *J. Interpersonal Violence*, 2, 27.

20. CORWIN, D. BERLINER, L., GOODMAN, G., GOODWIN, J., & WHITE, S. (1987). Allegations of child sexual abuse in custody disputes: No easy answers. *J. Interpersonal Violence*, 2, 91.

21. WOODLING, B. A., & KOSSORIS, P. D. (1981). Sexual misuse: Rape, molestation, and incest. *Pediatr. Clin. North Am.*, 28, 481.

22. RIMSZA, M. D., & NIGGEMAN, E. H. (1982). Medical evaluation of sexually abused children: A review of 311 cases. *Pediatrics*, 69, 8.

23. DURFEE, M., HEGER, A., & WOODLING, B. (1986). Medical evaluation. In K. MacFarlane, J. Waterman, et al. (Eds.), *Sexual abuse of young children*. New York: Guilford.

24. TILLELI, J. A., TUREK, D., & JAFFE, A. (1980). Sexual abuse of children: Clinical findings and implications for management. *N. Engl. J. Med.*, 302, 319.

25. GOODWIN, J., WILLETT, A., & JACKSON, R. Medical care for male and female incest victims and their parents. In J. Goodwin (Ed.), *Sexual abuse: Incest victims and their families*. Boston: Wright/PSG.

26. LUSK, R., & WATERMAN, J. (1986). Effects of sexual abuse on children. In K. McFarlane, J. Waterman, et al. (Eds.), *Sexual abuse on young children*. New York: Guilford.

27. GROTH, A. N. (1978). Patterns of sexual assault against children and adolescents. In A. Burgess, A. N. Groth, L. Holmstrom, & S. Sgroi (Eds.), *Sexual assault of children and adolescents*. Lexington, MA: Lexington.

28. GOODWIN, J., CORMIER, L., & OWEN, J. (1983). Grandfather-granddaughter incest: A trigenerational view. *Child Abuse Neglect*, 7, 163.

29. AMERICAN BAR ASSOCIATION NATIONAL LEGAL RESOURCE CENTER FOR CHILD ADVOCACY AND PROTECTION (1981). *Child sexual abuse and the law*. Washington, DC: American Bar Association.

30. ETH, S., & PYNOOS, R. S. (1985). *Post-traumatic stress disorder in children*. Washington, DC: American Psychiatric Association Press.

31. GOODMAN, G. S. (1983). The child witness: Conclusions and future directions for research and legal practice. *J. Soc. Issues*, 40, 169.

32. TERR, L. C. (1981). The child psychiatrist and the child witness: Traveling companions by necessity if not by design. *J. Am. Acad. Child Psychiatry*, 25, 462.

33. SATTERFIELD, S. (1985). The legal child abuse in the Jordan, Minnesota, sex ring case. Presented at the Annual Meeting of the American Academy of Psychiatry and the Law, Albuquerque, NM.

34. SUMMIT, R. (1982). The reluctant discovery of incest. In M. Kirkpatrick (Ed.), *Women's sexual experience*. New York: Plenum Press.

35. MACFARLANE, K., & KREBS, S. (1986). Techniques for interviewing and evidence gathering. In K. McFarlane, J. Waterman, et al. (Eds.), *Sexual abuse of young children*. New York: Guilford.

36. ADAMS-TUCKER, C. (1984). Early treatment of incest victims. *Am. J. Psychother.*, 38, 505.

37. GOODMAN, G. S. (1984). The child witness. *J. Social Issues*, 40, 2.

38. WEINBERG, S. (1955). Incest behavior. New York: Citadel.
39. LUSTIG, N., DRESSER, J., & SPELLMAN, S. W. (1966). Incest: A family group survival pattern. Arch. Gen. Psychiatry, 14, 31.
40. GOODWIN, J. (1985). Persecution and grandiosity in incest fathers. In P. Pichot, P. Berner, R. Wolf, & K. Thaw (Eds.), Psychiatry: The state of the art, Vol. 6. New York: Plenum Press.
41. MRAZEK, P. B., & MRAZEK, D. A. (1981). The effects of child sexual abuse: Methological considerations. In P. B. Mrazek & C. H. Kempe (Eds.), Sexually abused children and their families. New York: Pergamon Press.
42. ADAMS-TUCKER, C. (1981). Proximate effects of sexual abuse childhood: A report on 28 children. Am. J. Psychiatry, 139, 1252.
43. MAISCH, H. (1972). Incest. New York: Stein & Day.
44. EMSLIE, G. T., & ROSENFELD, A. A. (1983). Incest reported by children and adolescents hospitalized for severe psychiatric problems. Am. J. Psychiatry, 140(3), 708.
45. GOODWIN, J. (1985). Post-traumatic symptoms in incest victims. In S. Eth & R. S. Pynoos (Eds.), Post-traumatic stress disorder in children. Washington, DC: American Psychiatric Association Press.
46. American Psychiatric Association (1987). Diagnostic and statistical manual of mental disorders (3rd edition-revised). Washington, DC: American Psychiatric Association Press.
47. KARDINER, A. (1959). The traumatic neuroses of war. In S. Arieti (Ed.), American handbook of psychiatry, Vol. 1. New York: Basic Books.
48. MEISELMAN, K. (1981). Incest: A psychological study. San Francisco: Jossey-Bass.
49. GELINAS, D. (1983). The persisting negative effects of incest. Psychiatry, 46, 312.
50. VAN DER KOLK, B. (1987). Psychological trauma. Washington, DC: American Psychiatric Association Press.
51. HERMAN, J., RUSSELL, D., & TROCKI, K. (1986). Long-term effects of incestuous abuse in childhood. Am. J. Psychiatry, 143, 1293.
52. WILBUR, C. (1984). Multiple personality and child abuse: An overview. Pediatr. Clin. North Am., 7, 3.
53. SALTMAN, V., & SOLOMON, R. S. (1982). Incest and multiple personality. Psychol. Rep., 50, 1127.
54. COONS, P., & MILSTEIN, V. (1986). Psycho sexual disturbances in multiple personality: Characteristics, etiology, and treatment. J. Clin. Psychiatry, 47, 106.
55. HERMAN, J., & VAN DER KOLK, B. (1987). Traumatic antecedents of borderline personality disorder. In B. van der Kolk (Ed.), Psychological trauma. Washington, DC: American Psychiatric Association Press.
56. MILLER, A. (1984). Thou shalt not be aware: Society's betrayal of the child. New York: Farrar, Straus & Giroux.
57. SHENGOLD, L. L. (1979). Child Abuse and deprivation: Soul murder. J. Am. Psychoanal. Assoc., 27, 533.
58. DEYOUNG, M. (1983). Case reports: The sexual exploitation of victims by helping professionals. Victimology, 6, 92.
59. GOODWIN, J. (in press). Recognizing multiple personality disorder in adult incest victims. Victimology.
60. MACFARLANE, K., & KORBIN, J. (1983). Confronting the incest secret long after the fact: A family study of multiple victimization with strategies for intervention. Child Abuse Neglect, 7, 225.
61. FRIEDMAN, E. H. (1971). The birthday party: An experiment in obtaining change in one's own extended family. Fam. Process, 10, 345.
62. TREPPER, T. S. (1986). The apology session. In T. S. Trepper & M. J. Barrett (Eds.), Treating incest: A multimodal perspective. New York: Haworth Press.
63. DALE, P., WATERS, J., DAVIES, M., ROBERTS, W., & MORRISON, T. (1986). The towers of silence: Creative and destructive issues for therapeutic teams dealing with sexual abuse. J. Fam. Ther., 8, 1.

4

AGGRESSION IN THE CLASSROOM

NEIL FRUDE, PH.D.

Head of Department of Psychology,
University College, Cardiff, Wales, U.K.

The number of recent books and articles on disruption and aggression in schools is evidence of a growing concern with such problems. Media presentations have frequently portrayed schools as 'blackboard jungles' in which wild behavior and terrorism flourish. Tabloid newspapers have fired a "moral panic," extrapolating from isolated incidents to present the impression that serious bullying, organized attacks, and "extortion rackets" form the general social backdrop against which the educational process struggles. When the matter is assessed in the light of empirical evidence, however, a less remarkable picture emerges (11). There *are* serious incidents of aggression in schools, and severe injuries *are* inflicted by pupils on teachers and other pupils, but such incidents are fortunately rare. Similarly, mass rioting by pupils, with vicious fighting and serious vandalism, occurs only very infrequently.

There are a number of reasons why classroom aggression merits legitimate concern, however, and why it is important to understand the nature of such behavior and to develop strategies for managing and containing it. Many pupils suffer emotionally from the aggression directed toward them by school bullies. Classroom aggression can seriously disrupt the educational process, thereby affecting the educational achievement of many pupils. And in its most extreme form classroom aggression can lead to physical injury.

There is also a sense in which the continued aggressive behavior of a pupil indicates a failed opportunity to socialize that individual. Schools are complex social institutions in which, by and large, pupils are educated successfully and socialized positively, learning to be both cooperative and competitive. Pupils generally learn to behave in a way that reflects their own needs and wishes while having due regard for the needs of others and for the restrictions imposed by legitimate authority. Teachers' expectations, reflecting the standards of the wider society, are powerfully conveyed by example, the application of rules, and the operation of certain sanctions. Thus the school, like the family, is a powerful agent of socialization. The pupil who consistently opposes the influence of the school is also likely to reject the legal constraints of the wider society. There is evidence that children who are seen by their teachers as highly aggressive are likely to be involved in criminal activity in later life (9). Indeed, from the results of an important 20-year study, West (37) concluded that "being perceived as an above average nuisance by teachers and peers was . . . the best predictor of juvenile delinquency."

Disruption and aggressive behavior are also major sources of stress in the lives of many teachers. Surveys by Kyriacou and Sutcliffe (18), Dunham (6, 7), and others show consistently that many teachers find their classroom duties extremely stressful and that disruptive and aggressive behavior by their pupils is the most significant source of such stress. In a large-scale study of teachers in England, Dierenfield (5) found that one in three regarded classroom disruption as a "severe" problem. In a bid to protect their members, teachers' unions have repeatedly called attention to the problem of disruption.

Thus, although we must avoid accepting the more colorful portrayals of school life as chaotic and violent, there seems to be a legitimate cause for concern. Classroom aggression needs to be understood realistically. On the one hand, we should accept that some degree of aggression is a natural part of school life. The classroom is used by pupils as a social laboratory in which they explore and test aspects of self-presentation. Feedback from peers and teachers provides the "social mirror" which affects how they choose to behave. Social responses to their behavior may help to build their confidence and affect their management of feelings of rebelliousness and aggressiveness. Vital issues in the "hidden school agenda" of social experimentation include power, tolerance, justice, and retribution. When bold experiments are attempted, and when things go wrong, aggression is likely to be the result. It is often an error in a process of trial and error that is vital to the learning process. Such aggression, then, is fully to be expected.

On the other hand, bullying and aggressiveness toward teachers can be a chronic and serious problem. But in seeking to identify individuals who need special professional help we need to understand the nature of "normal" classroom aggression and of teachers' responses to it. When an individual pupil's case is reported, usually without the full context and perhaps highly influenced by the attitudes of an individual teacher, it may be too easy to assume that the child is "neurotic" or "antisocial." A degree of aggression is normal in the day-to-day life within many classrooms. The best explanation for the behavior of individuals who assume a central role in such disruption may focus on peer pressures, classroom atmosphere, and teacher-pupil interactions rather than on individual psychopathology. There is thus a need, in dealing with the individual client, to be aware of the wider social and ecological factors that so often determine the nature of aggressive incidents within the classroom.

"NORMAL" CLASSROOM AGGRESSION

Fun

Much disruption, even that with a clear aggressive element, is a manifestation of a classroom sport known as "messing about" or "having a laugh" (3, 39). Goading the teacher and engaging in mock aggression are ways of disrupting the normal lesson, and through such antics pupils provide themselves with fun and entertainment. Generations of school children have indulged in disruptive games, in strategies aimed at breaking the flow of the lesson and distracting the teacher from the formal agenda. Some such behavior is spontaneous. Any interruption or irregularity is leapt upon as an opportunity to start a scene. Other disruptions are planned by groups of pupils before the lesson. The target teacher and the mode of disruption are selected and key pupils are elected to start the action. Sequences of behavior are gleefully rehearsed and designed to provide a welcome distraction from lesson periods that otherwise would be boring.

"Sussing Out"

New teachers are frequently special targets for disruptive action. If the teacher is newly trained, s/he may lack confidence and lack the skills to contain inappropriate behavior. Such a teacher, then, is an easy target, and maximum entertainment payoff may come from disrupting the class s/he teaches. But new teachers are also likely to be systematically harassed in order to test their threshold of tolerance and their means of dealing with offenders. Without a track record, and with pupils having neither direct experience of the individual nor accounts handed on by pupils in other classes, the teacher is an unknown quantity. Certain pupils may be appointed by their peers to see how far they can push the teacher. Uneasy with the ambiguity of the situation, the class needs to know how far it can go. The testing of new teachers in this way is well documented and has been labeled "sussing out" (1, 2).

Justice

Children will rarely acknowledge that their disruptive behavior is irrational. They generally see it as reasonable in the circumstances. Detailed analysis of individual incidents of classroom aggression supports the view that there is often a grammar or internal logic to events that may at first appear random or chaotic. Such incident analysis stresses the individuals' perception of the social events.

A common sequence in disruptive classroom incidents is one in which an offense by the teacher leads to retribution by a pupil or pupils (23). Common offenses of teachers include forgetting children's names and being arrogant or distant. A particularly heinous offense involves administering unjust or inconsistent punishment—the disruption results when a pupil feels that he or she has been picked on. Similarly, a teacher who shows favoritism—who has a pet—is guilty of an offense. Marsh et al. (23) maintain that pupils' retribution is not haphazard but is governed by a rule structure in which the key element is reciprocity.

This analysis is useful in explaining how low-level conflict may quickly escalate to a high level of aggression. The initial attitudes and outlooks of teacher and pupil are different. An event takes place that is judged differently, and the contrast in interpretation causes conflict. The teacher seeks to assert control, but this response reinforces the pupil's view that the teacher is taking an unjustified stance. If, in response to the pupil's protests, the teacher backs down, this may be seen as a sign of weakness and is likely to merely postpone trouble. If the teacher repeats the accusation, generalizes it, or imposes sanctions, then the pupil identifies the response as yet a further offense. The two antagonists may soon be in a state of serious conflict, and the situation is made more intense by the fact that both actors are aware that they are playing before an audience eager to see which will win.

Classes

Just as individual teachers are viewed by classes of pupils according to their tolerance, their fairness, and their ability to keep control, so different classes are judged by teachers differently. Each class may be experienced as having a different "personality" or "atmosphere" Classes, like individual pupils, may acquire reputations, and there will be a tendency for all pupils within a class to be tarred with the same brush. The groups may be addressed, congratulated, or blamed collectively. Finlayson and Loughran (10) found that in high-delinquency schools poor relationships tended to develop between teachers and classes as well as between teachers and individual pupils.

Peer Groups

Pupils may identify to some extent with their class as a whole, but they also have a keen appreciation of the sociometric structure within it. Each class evolves as a minisociety with its key figures, its heroes, its scapegoats, its stars, and its isolates. An appreciation of this structure is fundamental to an understanding of much aggressive and disruptive behavior, for the presence of such subgroups can lead to strong intergroup rivalries and ingroup solidarities.

Peer groups exert strong pressures. An individual pupil's peer group membership will depend on characteristics such as ability, interests, and attitude to authority. Once a pupil identifies with a group there will be strong pressures on him or her to adopt the consensus attitudes of the group. One of the strongest differences between classroom subgroups seems to be whether their general orientation is pro- or antischool (25, 31, 38). Some groups have a positive attitude toward school, authority, teachers, and work, while others have decidedly negative attitudes. Intergroup rivalries and intragroup processes lead to polarization around these clusters of attitudes. Thus Willis (38) distinguished between "the lads" and "the 'ear 'oles," and Pollard (31) found that groups of conforming pupils were referred to by rebel groups as "puffs," "goody-goodies," and "teacher's pets."

It is not difficult to see how the existence of such groupings may promote aggressive behavior. An antisocial act by a member of one gang or rebel group may be recognized and reinforced by the group as heroic or brave, with the teacher's discomfort seen as "just desserts" or as poetic justice. Aggressive behavior may result from imitation and goading. Certain peer groups, therefore, will act as social facilitators of aggressive behavior by their members. The individuals who are most likely to respond to such social backing for aggression include the group leader or hero, who represents and speaks for the group, and the more impressionable child. The peripheral member of a rebel group, as yet unsure of his acceptance by his peers, may exhibit defiance toward the teacher in a bid to gain approval by the group.

The existence of strong groupings within the classroom means that some pupils are left out and become isolated. They may make desperate bids for recognition and acceptance, or their frustration and loneliness may lead to withdrawal or disturbed behavior. Galloway et al. (14) found that a third of a sample of suspended pupils were isolates.

The Teacher-Pupil Relationship

There seem to be important differences between teachers in the extent to which they attract disruption. Hargreaves et al. (17) have provided an ideal typology with categories of deviance-provocative and deviance-insulative teachers. Marsh et al. (23) found that pupils had their own typology. There were good teachers and soft teachers and some, those who merited retribution, who were "a load of rubbish."

Sometimes an unfortunate relationship develops between a teacher and a particular pupil. Galloway et al. (14), for example, found that among a population of suspended pupils a large proportion reported an intense dislike for one particular teacher. They report: "It sometimes seemed as if a long-standing personality clash was at the root of the problem."

Once a teacher has clashed in an incident with a pupil, the relationship between them may be permanently damaged. Each may be wary of the other, and each will be likely to have a lowered threshold for judging the other's subsequent behavior as "offensive." The pupil is likely to seek agreement from his or her peers that the teacher is "mad" or "bad." Similarly, the teacher is likely to seek confirmation within the staff room, or to broadcast that this particular pupil is maladjusted or conduct disordered. The teacher has the advantage of being able to characterize the pupil, by word or deed, as deviant in the public arena of the classroom. Much attention has been given to the process by which teachers label deviant pupils (16).

Of particular concern has been the process by which such labeling may produce a self-fulfilling prophecy. Having once perceived the pupil as deviant, the teacher will be more likely to reapply the label. Such pupils will be regarded with suspicion and their behavior monitored more closely. The threshold for judging an action as deliberate and offensive is likely to be lowered. When a child is aware that s/he is seen as deviant, s/he may behave especially well, in order to have the label removed, or may seek to live up to the label. Hargreaves (16) suggested that the degree to which a child accepts the teacher's judgment of deviancy will depend on how frequently, consistently, and publicly the label is applied. If the judgment appears to be constant and is shared by many teachers, then the child is likely to respond to the stigmatization by living up to the public expectation.

Although labeling theory has been widely used to explain deviant behavior at school, Furlong (12) has provided the useful reminder that the label of deviancy is often applied only after several disruptive incidents. This suggests that the main effect of labeling may be to amplify a disruptive tendency that has already been in evidence.

The School

Many of the analyses explored so far contribute to the understanding of classroom aggression by emphasizing elements of the social situation (peer group influences, teachers' attitudes, etc.) that help to determine the individual's aggression. This emphasis on background determinants, rather than on the personality or psychopathology of individuals, is in keeping with much of the current literature in the field. Most classroom aggression, it is stressed, is not the result of an individual operating in vitro, but is essentially situationally determined. An understanding of the aggressive behavior, it is further emphasized, must involve an appreciation of the social realities of the classroom context and of the meaning of such aggression.

Some writers, particularly sociologists, have also been concerned to include in such analyses elements from the wider context. They have emphasized the relevance of the climate of the school and of the nature of the school system. In its most extreme form such a view leaves little room for explanations and interventions centering on the individual. Thus Polk and Shafer (30) put forward the view that "underachievement, misbehaviour and early school leaving are properly and most usefully to be seen as adverse school-pupil interactions, and not simply as individual acts carried out by students as natural responses to damaged psyches or defective homes."

Although it would not seem appropriate to extend such a view to cover *all* acts of classroom aggression, the influence of school factors in particular is well worth examining. There is evidence that aspects of school organization and ethos are significantly associated with the frequency of disruptive acts. A number of impressive studies indicate that schools vary markedly in the frequency of antisocial acts committed within their walls (14, 32, 35). Such studies indicate that physical aspects (size of buildings, class size, teacher-to-pupil ratio, etc.) are not as important as the less tangible aspects of the school ethos. Thus Rutter et al. (35) showed the importance of such factors as the emphasis of reward rather than punishment, the immediacy of action on indiscipline, and the democratic organization of the teaching staff.

Reynolds and Sullivan (34) found more disruption in "coercive schools" than in what they term "incorporative schools," and a number of studies have indicated that the most important factors contributing to the school ethos are the attitudes and behavior of the principal, particularly with respect to the less academically successful pupils. In some way the rather global variable of school ethos would seem to be represented in the classroom environment such that it influences the behavior of individual pupils. The matter may be rather complex, however, for the atmosphere of a school is likely to reflect, as well as to help determine, the behavior of its pupils. The results of one recent study (37) suggest that differences between schools in contributing delinquents are largely a reflection of differences in the pupil intake.

"The System"

Many school problems, including aggression and truancy, increase in frequency with age. The fact that older boys, in particular, are often involved in the most serious aggressive acts has led some writers to suggest that, particularly for the less academically gifted teenager, the school is an unnatural environment. The biological fact of the earlier onset of puberty and the social fact of the emergence of a teenage culture mean that young adults are now confined within a type of social organization originally designed to contain and educate children.

Older pupils may exercise considerable personal power and independence in their lives outside school and have to suspend many of their adult powers and privileges while in school. Much disruptive behavior can be seen as a bid to be adult (to heckle, to choose to be uncooperative, to smoke, to dress unconventionally, etc.) in a context in which such normal behavior for 15-year-olds is judged to be inappropriate. There is also strong evidence that many secondary-school pupils, especially those of lower ability, find much of their schoolwork boring and pointless (33). They may express their frustration through acts of aggression and vandalism and use disruption to make life more entertaining.

Analyses that highlight the salience of peer factors, teachers' personalities, and school influences on classroom aggression may have the effect of making the characteristics of individuals seem almost irrelevant. However, within any school, and within any group, there are likely to be wide differences in individual levels of antisocial behavior. It seems likely that some pupils will be more aggressive than others whatever classroom or school they are in and with whatever peers or teachers they meet. Such children and adolescents may be isolates or may be ringleaders of an antischool group. In the current emphasis on analyses of the school rebel or the disaffected pupil who acts to disrupt lessons, too little attention may have been paid to those whose target is not the offending teacher or the restrictive school system, but other pupils. Relatively little has been written on the phenomenon of bullying.

THE BULLY

Some children repeatedly attack or terrorize other children. Olweus (26, 28) has studied the "bully" and his target children (whom he labels "whipping boys"). It has become clear from his research that whipping boys are not random targets but have certain characteristics that lead bullies to select them as victims. On the basis of a number of studies (mostly with Swedish boys between 13 and 15 years old), Olweus believes that the most appropriate explanation of bullying centers on the personalities of the boys involved. Thus his findings regarding bullying contrast with work on normal classroom aggression that has tended to deemphasize personality features.

Olweus found that there was a considerable consensus between teachers in their view of which children were bullies and which were frequent targets for aggression. Furthermore, these identifications remained stable over a three-year period (despite changes of school, teachers, and classmates). Bullies were shown to have a strong need to dominate and were characterized by what Olweus labeled a "spirit of violence." They were aggressive both physically and verbally, confident and tough, and lacked empathy for their victims. Their aggressive behavior, then, was reflected in their attitudes and much of their general behavior.

Whipping boys were often unpopular, anxious, and low in self-esteem, and they seemed incapable of aggression or even of self-defense. Whereas most were passive, a few did seem to actively provoke irritation. Whipping boys also tended to be weak physically and thus in many respects they were safe, easy targets.

Retrospective interviews were conducted with the mothers and fathers of bullies, whipping boys, and control children in an attempt to establish likely antecedents of the relevant personality patterns. The results indicated that the mother's treatment of and attitude toward the boy (primarily up to the age of five years) were strongly related to the child's level of aggression in early adolescence. The mothers of many of those identified as bullies had tended to treat their offspring with indifference. If they *were* "involved" with the child, their involvement tended to be markedly negative. The element of indifference was associated with "permissiveness" or freedom from constraint during the early years, and maternal hostility to the child was reflected in the frequent use of physical punishment.

The early maternal response to those who eventually became whipping boys seemed to have been quite different, with the mothers tending to be overanxious and overprotective. Olweus suggests that the way in which whipping boys were treated by their mothers in the early years may have lead them initially to lack confidence and to appear defenseless. The aggression and lack of respect that might then be shown toward them by their peers (and especially by the bullies) would lead to further loss of confidence and self-esteem and thus make them increasingly vulnerable to victimization at school.

Nursery Studies

Thus temperamental and early family environmental factors seem to account for a considerable amount of the variance of aggressiveness among adolescent boys. Olweus (28) concluded that "the basis for this set of problems is in large measure to be found in developmental periods preceding the start of school." In view of this, studies of the aggressiveness of very young children are of special interest.

On the basis of observational studies, Manning and Sluckin (21) have shown that by the age of three years there is a considerable variation in the amount and type of aggression practiced. Although most children exhibit aggression at times, the aggression of well-adjusted children tends to be manipulative and instrumental (e.g., a means of getting a toy from another child) whereas the aggression exhibited by less well-adjusted children tends to be hostile and destructive.

Examining nursery-school children who were reported by their teachers as "difficult," Manning and Hermann (20) found that "aggressive" children were hostile, dominating, attention-seeking, and boastful. Another group—the "demanding" children—were difficult, unpopular, and dependent. The typology used by these authors, and the clusters of characteristics they found to be associated with aggressive and demanding children, have certain parallels with the bully and whipping-boy roles examined by Olweus. Manning, like Olweus, suggests that factors in the homes of the children may be responsible for the differences in level and type of aggression, with rejecting and disturbed homes tending to produce aggressive children, and overcontrolling and overprotective homes tending to produce demanding children.

Stability

Manning and Sluckin (21) report a "remarkable stability" in aggressive tendencies over two years of nursery schooling. Because the individual differences remained stable from the time when nursery schooling commenced to the period after two years of such schooling, these authors conclude that these tendencies are not learned at school. Olweus, in a series of studies with much older boys, found a similarly high degree of stability for the bully and whipping-boy identification over a three-year period despite changes in school, teachers, and classmates. In a review of the published longitudinal studies of aggression, Olweus (27) reported a consensus indicating a substantial degree of stability "not much lower than that found in the intelligence domain."

Certain studies in the field of general school aggression add support to the stability hypothesis. Children regarded as highly aggressive by their teachers are likely to have criminal records in their adult life (9). From the results of his 20-year study West (37) found that being involved in disruption and aggression in school as an 8- or 10-year-old was the *best* predictor, among the many variables included at that stage of the study, of whether the child would later become delinquent.

Although there is a good deal of evidence supporting the view that much of the general aggression and disruption found in classrooms is heavily influenced by teachers, peer-group pressures, and wider organizational characteristics, such factors appear to be less important in determining the behavior of bullies and whipping boys. Olweus included in his analysis several structural and system variables relating to both school (school size, class size, curricula, etc.) and the physical conditions of the home (social class, parental income, housing conditions, etc.) but found that these were *not* significantly related to the boys' levels of aggression.

The consensus of evidence, therefore, supports the stability hypothesis, and it is tempting to infer that a high degree of stability in levels of aggressiveness is to be found across the entire age range between early childhood and adulthood. Although such evidence is consistent with the view that there might be a genetic basis for individual differences in aggressiveness, studies that have attempted to test this directly have not yielded positive results. Twin studies and adoption studies on normal and criminal populations have failed to find evidence of the genetic transmission of aggressiveness or violent criminality (24, 29).

On the other hand, there is considerable evidence supporting the view that the family atmosphere and attitudes toward the child (particularly those of the mother) during the early years may be of key importance in determining the child's level and style of aggressiveness. Many authors, writing on the basis of studies of children in different age groups and different social environments, and using a wide spectrum of methodological approaches, conclude from their evidence that there is a significant association between parental coldness and rejection of the child and high aggressiveness as shown at school. Children from this type of family background tend to have an aggressive personality. They are likely to react angrily to many different kinds of situation and not to exercise restraint in their hostile behavior. Indeed such children seem, from quite an early age, to have a positive view of violence.

SYNTHESIS AND IMPLICATIONS FOR TREATMENT

Classroom aggression is not a simple or indeed a single phenomenon. Although normal classroom aggression would appear to be quite different in many ways from bullying, it is clearly unsatisfactory to think of these things as entirely separate. Within any classroom there are likely to be bullies and whipping boys (in terms of the criteria employed by Olweus, for example, roughly 5% of boys are bullies and 5% whipping boys). There are also likely to be peer groups of which bullies and whipping boys are members. There will be a general class atmosphere which will evolve continuously, and the hour-to-hour activities of the class will largely be a response to the actions and offenses of teachers. The class operates within a particular school with its own ethos. Schools differ markedly in the degree to which they monitor bullying and in the means they use to deal with it.

For the professional who is asked to advise on classroom aggression, or to treat the aggressor (or victim), there are a number of guidelines that can be drawn from the analyses presented in this chapter. It is important not to *assume* that school aggression indicates that one or more children have a behavior disorder. The school is a complex social institution in which some degree of aggression is to be expected. Depending on how things are handled, even normal aggression can easily escalate to crisis proportions. Teachers are not dispassionate witnesses to class aggression but are often heavily emotionally involved. Aggressive children threaten the professional role and status of the teacher and may be a source of considerable stress. Not least, teachers are often the direct targets of pupils' aggression.

When a teacher asks for help, whether from the principal or from an outside agent, s/he is likely to be seeking, among other things, confirmation that the complaint is justified. It can be threatening for the teacher to have to admit that things are out of control, and a referral may be couched in terms of "either they're abnormal . . . or I am." The process by which teachers label children as deviant is fairly well understood, and colorful accounts of the misdeeds of a particular child may reflect such labeling and stereotyping. Sometimes the personal relationship between pupil and teacher will have broken down to such an extent that a psychiatrist or educational psychologist is brought in by the teacher to back his or her judgment that the child is "wrong" and that they themselves are "right." It is all too easy for an innocent professional to become embroiled in the power politics of a particular classroom.

The professional helper is likely to be regarded by the child as a confederate of the teacher, and therefore as a threat. It would seem to be of key importance that the child's account of incidents be heard sympathetically, for children will generally cite grievances against the teacher and often be able to provide a convincing rationale for behavior that at first report might have seemed irrational (4). In view of the evidence reviewed above, the importance of assessing the influences of home background and peers groups hardly needs emphasis. In some cases the evidence will reveal a dysfunction not of an individual child, but of the general pattern of relationships within the class or between pupils and one or more teachers. In some cases it will be possible to bring about a positive effect on the system's dynamics within the class through an intervention with the teacher or with the class as a whole. Advice might be given on changing aspects of the curriculum, the seating arrangements, or the rules that operate within the school. Gillham (15) has provided several useful examples of how changes in school organization can be implemented as a means of preventing disruptive incidents.

Consideration of situational and interpersonal factors is essential for any assessment of a child reported as aggressive in the classroom. Such consideration is likely to be vital for understanding the child's behavior and might also indicate ways in which the frequency of further aggressive outbursts might be prevented. When such an analysis reveals a specific incompatibility between the child and a teacher, or when things have developed to such a state that recovery of normality within the specific context seems unlikely, a recommendation might be given that the child change class or change school. A fresh start may be all that is needed to radically improve behavior, particularly if the child is encouraged to regard the change as an opportunity rather than as a punishment or as confirmation of a diagnosis of deviancy.

Without an ecological awareness in the analysis of a case of classroom aggression it might be too easy to assume that the child's aggressive behavior stems from a personality defect rather than reflecting specific situational factors. If a child does not fit in one class, then it might be too readily assumed that s/he will not fit happily in any normal classroom. Although a further chance of a fresh start should always be considered as an option, however, some children will fail repeatedly to improve in their behavior.

In recent years increased provision has been made in many countries for special units for dealing with children whose behavior has proved, in the longer term, unacceptable to schools (19, 36). Because of their smaller classes and the increased availability of specially trained personnel, such units — often dubbed "sin bins" — are able to provide a therapeutic input in addition to the closer monitoring and containment of children. Whether attempts at prevention and treatment take place in the school or in a special unit, however, the most effective interventions are likely to be those which focus on the child's *social* behavior and outlook.

Olweus (28) stresses the role that schools can play not only in controlling victimization by bullies (the limiting goal) but also in fostering improved nonaggressive and nonexploitative relationships between bullies and their peers (the integrating goal). Noting that a number of conventional treatment methods for dealing with bullies have been "relatively or entirely unsuccessful," he argues that the methods most likely to succeed in changing the behavior of such children will be those which focus on the social environment. Thus although favoring an individual *analysis* of bullying, Olweus nevertheless suggests that the best *treatment* is likely to center directly on the bully's *relationships*. Peers may prove the most effective therapeutic agents, providing ideal models and shaping the behavior of their disruptive classmates by the manner in which they treat the aggressive outbursts.

In taking a wider view of classroom aggression than that which is limited to the disordered individual, it is inevitable that the plight of victims of such aggression will be considered. The main casualties of aggression in the school context are teachers and whipping boys (and girls). Teachers frequently suffer stress as a result of prolonged disruption by particular pupils or by classes as a whole. Dunham (8) has shown how such stress can lead to lack of confidence, depression, and various psychosomatic ailments, and he reported that stress had led some teachers to take sick leave or to opt for early retirement. It is clear that much more could be done during the training of teachers to equip them for coping with the difficulties that may arise in the management of classes. Marland's book *The Craft of the Classroom: A Survival Guide* (22) describes a number of useful class management strategies. A number of writers have emphasized the importance for the morale of a besieged teacher of support from colleagues and particularly from the principal.

Analyses of the bullying phenomenon have also drawn attention to the fact that the *victims* of school aggression are themselves different from most children, and that the formation of the bully/whipping boy relationship depends on a complementarity between *two* types of personality. Victims may be anxious, underassertive, and low in self-esteem *before* the bullying occurs and are likely to become more disturbed as a result of the aggression directed toward them. They may settle into a victim role in which they will remain throughout their lives. Their years at school, therefore, provide a special window of opportunity for change. Teachers are in an especially powerful position to encourage such children to become more assertive and to boost their self-confidence. Although victims may create fewer problems for the teacher than disruptive children, their need for help may be at least as great. Their vulnerability to victimization may result from their early treatment at home, but even if their experiences at school are not responsible for the *formation* of this aspect of their personality, their school career may allow them to grow in personal strength.

REFERENCES

1. BALL, S. J. (1980). Initial encounters in the classroom. In P. Woods (Ed.), *Pupil strategies*. London: Croom Helm.
2. BEYNON, J. (1982). Ways in and staying in. In M. Hammersley (Ed.), *The ethnography of schooling*. Driffield: Nafferton.

3. BEYNON, J., & DELAMONT, S. (1984). The sound and the fury: Pupil perceptions of school violence. In N. Frude & H. Gault (Eds.), *Disruptive behavior in schools*. Chichester: Wiley.

4. BOLGER, A. (1986). Counseling in the treatment of disruptive pupils. In D. Tattum (Ed.), *Management of disruptive pupil behaviour in schools*. Chichester: Wiley.

5. DIERENFIELD, R. (1982). All you need to know about disruption. *Times Educational Supplement*, London, Jan. 29, 1982.

6. DUNHAM, J. (1976). *Stress in schools*. Hemel Hempstead: National Association of Schoolmasters and Union of Women Teachers.

7. DUNHAM, J. (1977). The effects of disruptive behaviour on teachers. *Educ. Rev.*, *29*, 181–187.

8. DUNHAM, J. (1984). *Stress in teaching*. London: Croom Helm.

9. FARRINGTON, D. (1978). The family backgrounds of aggressive youths. In L. A. Hersov & M. Berger (Eds.), *Aggression and antisocial behaviour in childhood and adolescence*. Oxford: Pergamon.

10. FINLAYSON, D. S., & LOUGHRAN, J. L. (1976). Pupils' perceptions in high and low delinquency schools. *Educ. Res.*, *18*, 138–145.

11. FRUDE, N. (1984). Children's disruption at school: Cause for concern? In N. Frude & H. Gault (Eds.), *Disruptive behaviour in schools*. Chichester: Wiley.

12. FURLONG, V. J. (1985). *The deviant pupil: Sociological perspectives*. Milton Keynes: Open University Press.

13. GALLOWAY, D. M. (1980). Exclusions and suspension from school. *Trends Educ.*, *2*, 33–38.

14. GALLOWAY, D. M., BALL, T., BLOMFIELD, D., & SEYD, R. (1982). *Schools and disruptive behaviour*. London: Longman.

15. GILLHAM, B. (1984). School organization and the control of disruptive incidents. In N. Frude & H. Gault (Eds.), *Disruptive behaviour in schools*. Chichester: Wiley.

16. HARGREAVES, D. H. (1976). Reactions to labelling. In M. Hammersley & P. Woods (Eds.), *The process of schooling*. Oxford/London: O.U.P./Routledge and Kegan Paul.

17. HARGREAVES, D. H., HESTER, S. K., & MELLOR, F. J. (1975). *Deviance in classrooms*. London: Routledge and Kegan Paul.

18. KYRIACOU, C., & SUTCLIFFE, J. (1978). Teacher stress: Prevalence, sources and symptoms. *Br. J. Educ. Psychol.*, *48*, 159–167.

19. LAWRENCE, J., STEED, D., & YOUNG, P. (1986). The management of disruptive behaviour in Western Europe. In D. Tattum (Ed.), *Management of disruptive pupil behaviour in schools*. Chichester: Wiley.

20. MANNING, M., & HERMANN, J. (1981). The relationships of problem children in nursery schools. In S. Duck & R. Gilmour (Eds.), *Personal relationships 3: Personal relationships in disorder*. Brighton: Harvester.

21. MANNING, M., & SLUCKIN A. (1984). The function of aggression in the pre-school and primary school years. In N. Frude & H. Gault (Eds.), *Disruptive behaviour in schools*. Chichester: Wiley.

22. MARLAND, M. (1975). *The craft of the classroom: A survival guide*. London: Heinemann Educational.

23. MARSH, P., ROSSER, E., & HARRE, R. (1978). *The rules of disorder*. London: Routledge and Kegan Paul.

24. MEDNICK, S. A., POLLOCK, V., VOLAVKA, J., & GABRIELLI, W. F., JR. (1982). Biology and violence. In M. E. Wolfgang & N. A. Weiner (Eds.), *Criminal violence*. Beverly Hills, CA: Sage.

25. MEYENN, R. J. (1980). School girls' peer groups. In P. Woods (Ed.), *Pupil strategies: Explorations in the sociology of the school*. London: Croom Helm.

26. OLWEUS, D. (1978). *Aggression in the schools: Bullies and whipping boys*. Washington, DC: Hemisphere.

27. OLWEUS, D. (1979). The stability of aggressive reactions in males: A review. *Psychol. Bull.*, *86*, 852–875.
28. OLWEUS, D. (1984). Aggressors and their victims: Bullying at school. In N. Frude & H. Gault (Eds.), *Disruptive behaviour in schools*. Chichester: Wiley.
29. PLOMIN, R., FOCH, T. T., & ROWE, D. C. (1981). Bobo clown aggression in childhood: Environment not genes. *J. Res. Personality*, *15*, 331–342.
30. POLK, K., & SHAFER, W. E. (1972). *Schools and delinquency*. Englewood Cliffs, NJ: Prentice-Hall.
31. POLLARD, A. (1980). Teacher interests and changing situations of survival threat in primary school classrooms. In P. Woods (Ed.), *Pupil strategies: Explorations in the sociology of the school*. London: Croom Helm.
32. POWER, M. J., ALDERSON, M. R., PHILLIPSON, C. M., SCHOENBERG, E., & MORRIS, J. M. (1967). Delinquent schools? *New Society*, Oct. 19, 1967.
33. RAVEN, J. (1978). School rejection and its amelioration. *Educ. Res.*, *20*, 3–9.
34. REYNOLDS, D., & SULLIVAN, M. (1979). Bringing schools back in. In L. Barton & R. Meighan (Eds.), *Schools, pupils and deviance*. Driffield: Nafferton.
35. RUTTER, M., MAUGHAN, B., MORTIMORE, P., & OUSTON, J. (1979). *Fifteen thousand hours: Secondary schools and their effects on children*. London: Open Books.
36. TATTUM, D. (1982). *Disruptive pupils in schools and units*. Chichester: Wiley.
37. WEST, D. J. (1982). *Delinquency, its roots, careers and prospects*. London: Heinemann.
38. WILLIS, P. (1977). *Learning to labour*. Farnborough: Saxon House.
39. WOODS, P. (1979). *The divided school*. London: Routledge and Kegan Paul.

5

CHILDHOOD FIRESETTING

G. ADAIR HEATH, M.D.
VAUGHN A. HARDESTY, PH.D.
PETER E. GOLDFINE, M.D.
ANDREW HINKENS, M.D.
NANCY AMELIA LIND, M.D.

and

ANDREW STROMBERG, M.D.

Department of Psychiatry,
Maine Medical Center, Portland, Maine

REVIEW OF THE LITERATURE

Fire is a necessity for life, inspiring awe, myth, and dependence. Each family and culture has had to find ways to teach its young the proper and safe use of fire. Childhood firesetting represents a breakdown in this process of socialization and education. Childhood firesetting is an important and not uncommon clinical problem that inspires considerable anxiety in the parent and treating clinician alike, but is often neglected in discussions of child psychiatric emergencies and treatment. This article offers the psychiatric practitioner a concise review of the literature on childhood firesetting; case examples of three of the most common ways childhood firesetters present; discussion of treatment issues involved and our view of this important, and often neglected, clinical area.

The modern literature on childhood firesetting can be divided into three eras. The analytic era began with Freud (10), who proposed a link between enuresis, sexual problems, and firesetting. This was hypothesized as a result of his work with his famous patient Dora and his analysis of the

The authors gratefully acknowledge the encouragement and support of Alan M. Elkins, M.D., and the clerical assistance of Marie A. Aceto and Mary M. Rutherford.

Prometheus myth. Later analysts perpetuated this linkage as a result of their own analyses of adults, supplemented by occasional child observations. Later observations were made on the relationship of firesetting to aggressive impulses (6, 11, 23, 39).

The second era, which utilized descriptive studies of firesetting in children, began in 1940. Yarnell (45), Lewis and Yarnell (28), and others found that firesetters tended to be male and to come from disorganized and possibly impoverished families (12, 22, 23, 32, 41). Two groups of firesetters were identified: a younger group, who set fires at home and were immature and asocial, and an older group of children, who set fires in pairs away from home (28). These studies emphasized aggression, rather than sexual issues, and the investigators saw firesetting cutting across diagnostic boundaries (42). These studies were limited methodologically, failing to have control or comparison groups, lacking in defined indexing criteria, mixing firesetters from inpatient, outpatient, and nonpsychiatric settings in a single study group, utilizing nonstandardized and/or nonquantifiable measuring instruments and nonuniform diagnostic classification schemes.

The third era, that of empirical studies, overcame many of these methodological problems. Many of the empirical studies have been conducted with inpatient populations of childhood firesetters (20, 26, 27, 40). Although varied methodologies make comparisons difficult, no consistent picture emerges with reference to the demographic, individual, and family characteristics of these firesetters. Firesetting was found to have a rate of 27.5% in the Kuhnley, Hendren, and Quinlan (27) study, 48% in the Jayaprakash, Jung, and Panitch (20), study and 49.2% in the Kolko, Kazdin, and Meyer (26) study. Age was not found to differentiate firesetters, but this may have been due to the customary age range of child inpatient units (5 to 13 years) exerting a biasing effect. Kuhnley et al. (27) found significantly more males in the firesetting group. The diagnostic picture was also inconsistent. Kuhnley et al. (27) reported significantly more conduct disorder and attention deficit disorder in the firesetting group. In the Kolko et al. (26) study, firesetters were found to be more aggressive and externalizing, regardless of whether they were conduct-disordered or not. However, the higher frequency of the DSM-III diagnosis of conduct disorder was not significant in this study. Thus, there was a discrepancy in this study between the measuring instruments, which showed a conduct-disordered picture, and the diagnostic category into which the child was placed.

A somewhat more consistent picture emerges when one looks at studies of outpatient populations of firesetters. Heath, Hardesty, Goldfine, and Walker (15) have found firesetters to be more externalizing and less internalizing and to come from larger and poorer families. Firesetting had a rate of 15.5%, with only 31% of the firesetters referred for firesetting as the primary problem. Conduct disorder was significantly overrepresented in the firesetting group, and there was a significant interaction between firesetting and conduct disorder, with conduct-disordered firesetters being more pathological and less competent than the conduct-disordered controls (16). Jacobson (18, 19), in the largest controlled study of firesetters, found a 2.45% rate of firesetting and only 13.3% of the firesetters were referred for the symptom of firesetting. Firesetters differed from nonfiresetters in the following ways: younger age, increased frequency of males, having significantly higher rates of conduct disorder, specific reading retardation, incidence of parental discord, and increased aggressive and antisocial behavior. Further analysis revealed a group of younger firesetters who were more often male and set fires more frequently at home. The older group of firesetters had a higher rate of associated behavior problems and generally set fires away from home. Jacobson also grouped the firesetters according to whether they were referred for the symptom of firesetting or for other problems. The group referred specifically for firesetting were all boys who tended to have a short history of setting more costly and more dangerous fires but were less aggressive in general.

A similar picture emerges when one considers delinquent and court populations of firesetters. Strachan (41) studied two groups of court-referred children. One group of 79 children had been referred for firesetting and the other group was not referred for firesetting. Strachan found a rate of 4.6% for firesetting, and a significant sex and age difference between the groups. The firesetters were more often male (99%) and had a mean age of 12.5 years. This is an older age than found in psychiatric populations, but is, undoubtedly, skewed because of the legal cutoff of eight years and older before a child can be referred to the courts. Firesetting occurred in groups and the fires were set to commercial property and rarely at home. There was a high association with other delinquent problems, and few referrals to mental health services, in spite of the seriousness of their offenses. The firesetters tended to come from very poor and large families, with significantly more unemployed or absent fathers, absent mothers, and disruptive homes. Ritvo, Shanok, and Lewis (36) studied incarcerated male firesetters with an appropriate comparison group and found a firesetting rate of 27.8%. Firesetters and nonfiresetters were similar with regard to psychiatric, neurological, and IQ characteristics, but firesetters had a significantly higher rate for mother's absence from the home and previous placements out of the home. The investigators were struck by the number of firesetters who had severely burned themselves. They also felt that firesetters were basically similar to other violent youth in having severe neuropsychological impairments, together with a history of physical abuse and emotional abandonment, which had led to multiple forms of violent behavior, one of which was firesetting.

While we are beginning to get a clearer picture of firesetters from different population groups, questions remain regarding the natural history of firesetting, including its development from the stage of curious fireplay to actual destructive firesetting; why some children go on to persistent firesetting; and why some children are referred to mental health or juvenile justice systems while others are handled by their parents in their natural environment. We have little information with regard to the natural history of firesetting in nonclinical populations. Kafry (21) has found that 45% of an unselected sample of normal children play with matches, with about half of these (often in the five- to seven-year age group) going on to actually setting fires that cause damage. Invariably, children who set fires started by playing with matches. Further information on the natural development of firesetting will have to await the results of longitudinal studies.

With regard to referral patterns, we again have little information. Winget and Whitman (44) have shown that the public and professional attitude toward firesetters results in, at best, only one-third receiving any kind of mental health referral. This referral bias results in firesetting being most likely underreported in clinical populations. Social class and family structure (parental absence) may also determine why some children are referred to juvenile justice or welfare systems versus mental health systems. Jacobson (18) has pointed out that Berkson's statistical bias may operate to cause the association between conduct disorder and firesetting to be artificially elevated, as the referral probability of a conduct-disordered firesetter is the combined probability of the referral for firesetting and conduct disorder.

The natural history of firesetting with regard to response to treatment and follow-up is also far from clear. Only two follow-up studies could be found in the literature. Stewart and Culver (40) found that one-quarter of the firesetters continued setting fires during a follow-up interval averaging three years. Those who continued setting fires were more antisocial and set more fires at the time of admission. The risk of continuing to set fires was not related to placement after admission, family structure, or parental psychopathology. Heath, Hardesty, and Goldfine (14) followed 32 firesetters and 32 matched control subjects over a 15-month period. Results included the finding that 66.7% of firesetters seen in follow-up had stopped setting fires. The firesetters who continued to set fires were significantly less competent and more externalizing than the firesetters who discontinued this behavior.

A number of studies describing treatment approaches have appeared in the literature in the last 15 to 20 years. Many of these have been behavioral approaches to firesetting (3, 4, 17, 24, 29, 35, 37, 43), as well as crisis-oriented family therapy (5, 30, 31). Unfortunately, these are all single case study reports, which do not allow generalization with respect to the characteristics of patients that would predict response to treatment. Bumpass, Fagelman, and Brix (2) describe a "graphing" technique, which correlates external stress, firesetting, and other acting-out behaviors with feelings. This technique was found useful in the treatment of a group of 29 firesetters, 21 of whom were brought in with firesetting as a referral problem. Informal follow-up showed that 93% of the firesetters stopped firesetting in an average follow-up interval of two and a half years. Unfortunately, there were no standard measures or descriptions of patients, nor an appropriate comparison group.

Fineman and the Fire Prevention Committee of the California State Psychological Association and selected firefighters (7, 9) have created a series of interesting manuals and teaching materials, applying much of what is known to helping fire service personnel deal more effectively with juvenile firesetting. These materials aid fire service personnel in interviewing children and parents; recognizing problems that can lead to firesetting; distinguishing, through structured interviews, "curiosity" firesetters from those displaying more serious signs of psychological problems; educating "curiosity" firesetters; and referring those with psychological problems to appropriate mental health professionals. This work is exciting, necessary, and worthwhile. It is hoped that careful evaluation of the program's effectiveness will be conducted to further our understanding of firesetting.

Finally, it is difficult to discuss firesetting without mentioning its supposed connection to enuresis and cruelty to animals. Jacobson (18, 19), Heath et al. (15), Heath, Hardesty, and Goldfine (13) and, Ritvo et al. (36) have all pointed out the lack of an association between enuresis and cruelty to animals to firesetting. When compared to appropriate controls, the rates for enuresis, cruelty to animals, or both are similar in firesetting populations and controls. The predictive value of the triad with respect to violence has not been tested by any anterospective study or by any well-designed retrospective study.

TREATMENT AND CASE HISTORIES

We view childhood firesetting as a symptom that occurs in children with a number of different psychiatric diagnoses, constitutional vulnerabilities and strengths, and family and environmental situations. The treatment approach to each case of childhood firesetting must be individualized and designed with these variables in mind. However, a number of general principles are common to most cases of childhood firesetting. For purposes of communication, we divide these issues into the acute or emergent issues and long-term treatment issues.

Emergent or acute issues primarily involve concerns about safety for the child, his family, and his living environment. Childhood firesetting is a potentially dangerous symptom and, like other dangerous behaviors, needs to have a thorough and immediate evaluation with regard to the potential for harm to self and others. The examination should focus on issues that are similar to those for a suicidal, potentially homicidal, or out-of-control child. These include: base rate of firesetting behavior; presence or absence of psychosis, depression, or other clinical conditions that might impair judgment and impulse control; the motivation for the firesetting; whether the firesetting has succeeded in communicating to the child's family the need for help, understanding, and control of impulses; the ability of the family to control matches; and other factors that might further excite or exacerbate the child's impulsivity. We have found it helpful to view firesetting and to help the family see firesetting as the child's maladaptive attempt to communicate feelings of helplessness, the need for understanding, and a desire for control of impulses.

The family who is unable and/or unwilling to hear this message and take appropriate action, such as obtaining control of ignitable materials, obviously presents a greater risk for the continuation of firesetting behavior than the family who can adopt a more helpful and authoritative stance to the child and the symptom. An environment that is itself out of control in terms of either the family or a community with provocative peers also presents a high risk. A child who is psychotic, consumed with suicidal or homicidal rage, or experiencing lack of controls due to organic conditions presents a high degree of risk. When the clinician judges that the risk is great enough, hospitalization or removal from home to a safe environment may need to be considered. Finding such a safe environment for a child with a known firesetting problem often presents a test of the clinician's imagination and ingenuity. Many families, however, with motivation and support from outside persons, are able to garner enough strength to provide the support and controls necessary to weather the firesetting crisis. During these times, we have found specific behavioral assignments to the child and the family to be helpful. We have used behavioral treatment techniques such as a work penalty for having matches or positive reinforcement techniques for the child who returns ignitable material to the parent. The child who has set only one fire, has no history of collecting flammable materials, has attempted to extinguish the fire or seek help, and has no psychological problems himself may qualify as a so-called "curiosity firesetter" (7–9). In this case, an educational approach with an attempt not to stigmatize the child is appropriate.

The second phase of treatment involves the long-term treatment issues. In general, these issues are similar to the treatment issues encountered when treating the underlying psychiatric disorders, such as adjustment reaction of childhood and/or conduct disorder, and will be further explored in the case history section.

A final general treatment intervention issue must be stressed at this time. We have already referred to the extreme degree of anxiety that is engendered by firesetting behavior in the clinician, family, and community. The reason for the anxiety is quite understandable. The potential for destruction, including loss of life, always exists in firesetting. Any therapeutic intervention must recognize the attendant high levels of anxiety in family and community members. Frequently, this can be addressed as part of the treatment program for the child and family. When the firesetting behavior has occurred in the community, it may be necessary to hold community meetings, or possibly extended family meetings, to address questions of attendant anxiety. Straightforward discussions of the precipitants of the behavior and the possibilities for recurrence are often helpful. In addition, addressing the issues of safety in the treatment of firesetting youngsters also goes a long way toward alleviating concomitant anxiety in the family and community.

The following section deals with clinical issues bearing on the treatment of juvenile firesetters. The case histories presented are illustrative of three distinct subgroups of juvenile firesetters. These cases are synthesized from numerous firesetting cases seen in our clinic over the years.

"Curiosity" Firesetter

Josh is a six-year-old boy referred to the clinic by his mother. Psychiatric evaluation had been recommended by the fire department after their investigation of a small fire in the family's tool shed revealed that the fire had been set by Josh. The patient had no prior history of firesetting behavior, behavior problems, or psychiatric difficulty, and his two older siblings exhibited no firesetting or behavioral disturbance. Josh's parents had been married 12 years and worked outside the home on a split-shift schedule. Significantly, the family had recently installed a woodstove in their home, and Josh had been enthusiastically involved with helping his parents in the operation of the stove. Psychiatric evaluation revealed that the DSM-III criteria for adjustment disorder with disturbance of conduct or conduct disorder were not fulfilled. Mental status examination showed no remarkable features, and the family appeared stable.

Since the parents had discussed appropriate caution with Josh and emphasized the seriousness of his behavior, no psychiatric treatment was recommended. Follow-up at two months revealed no further problems, and Josh was, in fact, responsibly fulfilling an appropriate daily task related to the operation of the stove. This task had been assigned to Josh by his therapist. Josh is representative of the subgroup "curiosity firesetter" (7–9). As previously discussed, children in this group tend to be younger, have no history of collecting flammable materials, attempt to extinguish the fire or seek help, and exhibit a lack of psychological problems. The families are generally healthier and intact. A significant question with this group of youngsters is actually when to treat? In this case an educationally based program was used. Parents discussed the seriousness and potential consequences of the behavior and discussed appropriate cautions to be taken by the child. This appeared to be sufficient, and as noted, a two month follow-up revealed no further instances of firesetting. If such a straightforward and educational approach is utilized but the behaviors persist, then a more therapeutic intervention utilizing either a psychotherapeutic or a behavioral modification paradigm is needed.

Adjustment Disorder Presenting with Firesetting

Shawn is an eight-year-old boy who was referred to the clinic by his mother because of increased behavioral difficulties. Two months prior to Shawn's evaluation, his parents separated, and Shawn, his mother, and three siblings moved to our area. Shawn's mother reported that Shawn's behavior had deteriorated since the move, with Shawn engaging in inappropriate behavior at home and in school. There had been several incidents of fighting in school, and Shawn had run away from home on two occasions. Finally, Shawn had set his mattress on fire. According to

Shawn's mother, there had been no previous difficulties with Shawn and this was the first fire that he had set.

Our second case illustrates firesetting secondary to an adjustment disorder with disturbance of conduct. There was no preexisting history of psychiatric symptomatology, and there was an identifiable psychosocial stressor, the separation of Shawn's parents within three months of the onset of symptomatology. Symptomatology included a number of behavioral impairments, including aggressive behavior, runaway behavior, and firesetting.

With the exception of ensuring control over the firesetting behavior, the treatment does not differ in major ways from the treatment offered any adjustment disorder in children. By and large, short-term interventions are indicated and intervention efforts are directed at removing the specific stressor if this is possible or helping the child and his family achieve a better adaptation to the stressor, which in this case was parental separation. Interventions are generally shorter and there is more opportunity for individual psychotherapeutic approaches as well as family therapy.

With both of our last two subgroups of firesetters, the adjustment disorder with firesetting and the curiosity firesetter, preventive intervention is often indicated. Because of the seriousness and potential destructiveness of the symptom of firesetting and the anxiety that is generated in parents and other responsible adults, it is not uncommon that such youngsters may be labeled chronic firesetters. This is a variant of the "bad seed" syndrome. Labeling such a youngster by parents or other adults in the environment could lead to a situation where the expectation of continued firesetting actually unconsciously stimulates the child to repeat the action. This, in turn, will set up a vicious cycle. Again, the role of the clinician may be most helpful in differentiating cases of short-term or single instances of curiosity firesetting from more chronic conduct-disordered behavior. Such a simple approach involving a rational explanation and use of prognosis should be sufficient in most cases to prevent the potential for unconscious stimulation of repetitive firesetting behavior.

Conduct-Disordered Firesetter

John is an 11-year-old boy who was referred to the clinic because of his out-of-control behavior. His mother reported that his behavior problems of several years' duration included lying, stealing objects from stores, fighting at home and school, and noncompliance at school.

John had set six fires in the previous five months, including setting leaves on fire on a neighbor's porch, setting a mattress on fire, and setting a fire under a porch, which caused serious damage to a house.

John was the second of two children whose alcoholic and physically abusive parents were divorced when he was five. Developmental milestones were apparently normal, but John has exhibited learning difficulties in school, and his mother notes only one close friend in school.

John is an example of firesetting associated with the presence of a conduct disorder of a socialized aggressive type. In this case, the symptom of firesetting is associated with a cluster of other behavioral problems, including lying, stealing, fighting, and aggressive behavior.

Epidemiologically, conduct disorders are more prevalent in boys. There is a frequent association between educational underachievement with learning disabilities and conduct disorder (38), and effective treatment programs must address this problem with remedial education techniques. Disruptive and dysfunctional families are frequently seen in association with conduct-disordered children. John's parents are noted to have been "alcoholic and physically abusive," and divorce occurred when John was five. Familial psychopathology frequently includes neglect and rejection, a lack of bonding, and the frequent presence of single-parent families or mother with depression or substance abuse, trauma, including physical and sexual abuse, absence of adequate parental role models for identification, unstable marriages, and inconsistent parenting. After the firesetting behavior is under control, the general principles that apply to the treatment of conduct disorders also apply to firesetters from this subgroup. Major treatment efforts must be directed toward stabilizing the disorganized family. This frequently means providing social and economic supports. Patterson et al. (33, 34) outlined a specific program for parental therapy. This included training parents to:

1. Consistently set rules.
2. Monitor children's behavior.
3. Provide nonaggressive contingent punishments and awards.
4. Cope with crises.
5. Negotiate compromises.

Techniques for doing this include modeling effective parental behavior in school or the clinic, home visits, and parent groups.

Therapy for conduct-disordered children must stress the development of attachment with parents, or with parental surrogates who can function as adult role models in the school or the clinic. While the treatment of these cases is difficult, therapy that emphasizes behavioral contingencies in the home and school appears most likely to succeed. Individual psychotherapeutic interventions seem less effective because of the high degree of externalizing behavior in these children.

Finally, a word should be said about the diagnostic category of pyromania. This is defined in DSM-III-R (la) as "deliberate and purposeful firesetting on more than one occasion; tension or affective arousal before the act; fascination with, interest in, curiosity about, or attraction to fire and its situational context or associated characteristics; intense pleasure, gratification, or relief when setting fires, or when witnessing or participating in their aftermath; and the fire-setting is not done for monetary gain, as an expression of sociopolitical ideology, to conceal criminal activity, to express anger or vengeance, to improve one's living circumstances, or in response to a delusion or hallucination" (p. 326).* This is a rare condition, particularly in children. In fact, in our studies of clinic populations of firesetters, only one such child was given the diagnosis of pyromania. There is no reported specific therapy for this condition, but behavioral and individual therapeutic interventions employed in the treatment of other impulse-ridden disorders may prove efficacious.

SUMMARY

Childhood firesetting is a relatively common, but serious child psychiatric problem, often neglected in the child psychiatric literature on emergencies and treatment. This chapter has reviewed the literature on the subject, pointing out how the current ideas about childhood firesetting have evolved. Firesetting is seen as emerging from a confluence of many factors, including: learning contingencies that shape and mold normal childhood interest in fire; family and historical factors that can lead to a conduct-disordered problem; and triggering factors that lead to specific instances of firesetting (25). Three case histories are presented that typify common clinical patterns and offer illustrations for discussion of the clinical method of diagnosis and treatment of childhood firesetting. The importance of distinguishing firesetting in the presence of severe psychopathology from firesetting in a curious child or in an adjustment reaction is pointed out with regard to the treatment-planning process and prognosis. The importance of ascertaining the potential for continued firesetting as well as the family and community's ability or lack of ability to control access to ignit-

---

*Reprinted with permission.

able materials is stressed in protecting the patient, family, and community. When appropriate controls cannot be implemented and the risk of continued firesetting is high, hospitalization may be necessary. The use of specific behavioral approaches is discussed as a method of obtaining control of the firesetting process, responding to the child's use of firesetting as a communication for help and controls. Finally, the similarity of the long-term treatment process in childhood firesetting to that of the underlying disorder, such as conduct disorder or adjustment disorder, is discussed.

REFERENCES

1. American Psychiatric Association (1980). *Diagnostic and Statistical Manual of Mental Disorders* (3rd edition). Washington, DC: Author.
1a. American Psychiatric Association (1987). Diagnostic and Statistical Manual of Mental Disorders (3rd edition-revised). Washington, DC: Author.
2. BUMPASS, E., FAGELMAN, E., & BRIX, R. (1983). Intervention with children who set fires. *Am. J. Psychother.*, *37*, 328.
3. CARSTENS, C. (1982). Application of a work penalty threat in the treatment of a case of juvenile firesetting. *J. Behav. Ther. Exp. Psychiatry*, *13*, 159.
4. DENHOLTZ, M. S. (1972). At home: Aversion treatment for compulsive firesetting behavior: Case report. In R. B. Rubin, H. Fensterhein, J. D. Henderson and L. T. Ullmann (Eds.), *Advances in behavior therapy*. New York: Academic Press.
5. EISLER, R. M. (1972). Crisis intervention in the family of a firesetter. *Psychother: Theory Res. Pract.*, *9*, 76.
6. FENICHEL, O. (1945). *The psychoanalytic theory of neurosis*. New York: Norton.
7. FINEMAN, K. R. (1984). Juvenile firesetters handbook: Dealing with children ages 7–14. U.S. Fire Administration, Federal Emergency Management Agency. Washington, DC: U.S. Government Printing Office.
8. FINEMAN, K. R. (1980). Firesetting in childhood and adolescence. *Psychiatr. Clin. North Am.*, *3*, 483–500.
9. FINEMAN, K. R. (1980). Interviewing and counseling juvenile firesetters: The child under seven years of age. U.S. Fire Administration, Federal Emergency Management Agency. Washington, DC: U.S. Government Printing Office.
10. FREUD, S. (1905). *Fragment of an analysis of a case of hysteria*. Standard Edition, Vol. 7. London: Hogarth Press, 1953.
11. GRINSTEIN, A. (1952). Stages in the development of the control of fire. *Int. J. Psychoanal.*, *33*, 416.
12. GRUBER, A., HECK, E., & MINTZER, E. (1981). Children who set fires: Some background and behavioral characteristics. *Am. J. Orthopsychiatry*, *51*, 484.
13. HEATH, G. A., HARDESTY, V. A., & GOLDFINE, P. E. (1984). Firesetting, enuresis and animal cruelty. *J. Child Adolescent Psychother.*, *1*, 97.
14. HEATH, G. A., HARDESTY, V. A., & GOLDFINE, P. E. (1985). Childhood firesetting: A follow-up study. *Syllabus and Proceedings of the 138th Annual Meeting of the American Psychiatric Association* (p. 178). Washington DC: American Psychiatric Association.
15. HEATH, G. A., HARDESTY, V. A., GOLDFINE, P. E., & WALKER, A. M. (1983). Childhood firesetting: An empirical study. *J. Am. Acad. Child Psychiatry*, *22*, 370.

16. HEATH, G. A., HARDESTY, V. A., GOLDFINE, P. E., & WALKER, A. M. (1985). Diagnosis and childhood firesetting. *J. Clin. Psychol., 41*, 571.
17. HOLLAND, C. J. (1969). Elimination by the parents of firesetting behavior in a 7-year-old boy. *Behav. Res. Ther., 7*, 135.
18. JACOBSON, R. R. (1985). Child firesetters: A clinical investigation. *J. Child Psychol. Psychiatry, 26*, 759.
19. JACOBSON, R. R. (1985). The subclassification of child firesetters. *J. Child Psychol. Psychiatry, 26*, 769.
20. JAYAPRAKASH, S., JUNG, J., & PANITCH, D. (1984). Multi-factorial assessment of children who set fires. *Child Welfare, 63*, 74.
21. KAFRY, D. (1980). Playing with matches: Children and fire. In D. Canter (Ed.), *Fires and human behavior*. Chichester, England: Wiley.
22. KAUFMAN, I., HEIMS, L. W., & REISER, D. E. (1961). A reevaluation of the psychodynamics of firesetting. *Am. J. Orthopsychiatry, 31*, 123.
23. KLEIN, M. (1932). *Psychoanalysis of children*. London: Hogarth Press.
24. KOLKO, D. (1983). Multi-component parental treatment of firesetting in a six year old boy. *J. Behav. Ther. Exp. Psychiatry, 1*, 349.
25. KOLKO, D. J., & KAZDIN, A. (1986). A conceptualization of firesetting in children and adolescents. *J. Abnorm. Child Psychol., 14*, 49.
26. KOLKO, D. J., KAZDIN, A. E., & MEYER, E. C. (1985). Aggression and psychopathology in childhood firesetters: Parent and child reports. *J. Consult. Clin. Psychol., 53*, 377.
27. KUHNLEY, E. J., HENDREN, R. L., & QUINLAN, D. M. (1982). Firesetting by children. *J. Am. Acad. Child Psychiatry, 21*, 560.
28. LEWIS, N. D. C., & YARNELL, H. (1951). Pathological firesetting (pyromania). *Nerv. Ment. Dis. Monthly*, No. 82, 8.
29. MCGRATH, P., MARSHALL, P. G., & PRIOR, K. (1979). A comprehensive treatment program for a firesetting child. *J. Behav. Ther. Exp. Psychiatry, 10*, 69.
30. MINUCHIN, S. (1974). *Families and family therapy*. Cambridge: Harvard University Press.
31. MORRISON, G. (1969). Therapeutic intervention in a child psychiatric emergency service. *J. Am. Acad. Child Psychiatry, 8*, 542.
32. NURCOMBE, B. (1964). Children who set fires. *Med. J. Aust., 1*, 579.
33. PATTERSON, G. R. (1974). Interventions for boys with conduct problems: Multiple settings, treatment and criteria. *J. Consult Clin. Psychol., 4*, 471.
34. PATTERSON, G. R., REID, J. B., JONES, R. R., & CONGER, R. E. (1975). *A social learning approach to family intervention*, vol. 1: *Families with aggressive children*. Eugene, OR: Castalia.
35. PENNEY, R. K., MARCELLA, P., & CHARLTON, D. (1974). Classical and operant conditioning program for a firesetting child. *J. Ontario Assoc. Children's Aid Soc.*, 1–4.
36. RITVO, E., SHANOK, S. S., & LEWIS, D. O. (1982). Firesetting and non firesetting delinquents: A comparison of neuropsychiatric, psychoeducational, experiential, and behavioral characteristics. *Child Psychiatry Hum. Dev., 13*, 259.
37. ROYER, S. L., FLYNN, W. F., & OSADACA, B. S. (1971). Case history: Aversion therapy for firesetting by a deteriorated schizophrenic. *Behav. Ther., 2*, 229.
38. RUTTER, M. L., TIZARD, J., & WHITMORE, K. (Eds.) (1970). *Education, health and behavior*. London: Longman. (Reprinted, 1981, Huntington, NY: Krieger.)
39. SIMMEL E. (1949). Incendiacism. In K. R. Eissler (Ed.), *Search-lights on delinquency*. New York: International Universities Press.
40. STEWART, M. A., & CULVER, K. W. (1982). Children who set fires: The clinical picture and a follow-up. *Br. J. Psychiatry, 140*, 357.
41. STRACHAN, J. C. (1981). Conspicuous firesetting in children. *Br. J. Psychiatry, 138*, 26.
42. VANDERSALL, J. A., & WIENER, J. M., (1970). Children who set fires. *Arch. Gen. Psychiatry, 22*, 63.

43. WELSH, R. S. (1971). The use of stimulus satiation in the elimination of juvenile firesetting behavior. In A. M. Graziano (Ed.), *Behavior therapy with children*. Chicago: Aldine-Atherton.
44. WINGET, C. N., & WHITMAN, R. M. (1973). Coping with problems: Attitudes toward children who set fires. *Am. J. Psychiatry, 130*, 442.
45. YARNELL, H. (1940). Firesetting in children. *Am. J. Orthopsychiatry, 10*, 262.

6

VOLATILE SUBSTANCE ABUSE

ITTIACANDY SOURINDHRIN, M.B.B.S.,
M.R.C. PSYCH.

Dykebar Hospital,
Paisley, Scotland, U.K.

The voluntary inhalation of substances for the purpose of mood alteration is not a new phenomenon. Hebrews regarded the breathing of vapors
from burning spices as an integral part of worship. Greeks at Delphi
induced states of ecstasy by inhaling gases from clefts of rocks. South
American Indians have for centuries employed hallucinogeniclike snuffs
(containing tryptamine derivatives) in mystical religious ceremonies (55).

The recreational use of nitrous oxide (N_2O, laughing gas) discovered in
1776 by Sir Joseph Priestley was popularized by, among others, Coleridge,
Southey, and Wedgewood (55).

Exhibitions of effects of ether took place in the eighteenth century. In
the early nineteenth century, ethyl ether parties enjoyed some popularity
and notoriety (34). In the latter half of the century ether was used in
considerable quantities as an inexpensive alcohol substitute in certain
counties of Ireland and Great Britain (40).

Amyl nitrite, indicated for the relief of angina, was used as an agent for
getting "high" and as an aphrodisiac (55).

Several societies seem to have discovered independently that inhalation
is an extremely efficient and rapid method of self-intoxication. Inhalation
is a favored method of self-administration for some users of heroin, cocaine, and a wide variety of volatile substances.

The American solvent epidemic first observed in the late 1950s spread to
the Midwest in the early 1960s and finally reached the East Coast with its
full impact in the mid 1960s (2). The first cases described in America
involved the inhalation of gasoline fumes in the 1950s. In the majority of
reported cases, intoxicating effects of gasoline inhalation were discovered

89

accidentally while working with cars (6) or siphoning gas from one lawn-mower to another (18). Addiction to gasoline sniffing was observed by Nitsche and Robinson (54) and Faucett and Jensen (22). Gasoline sniffing was also reported among children in a Pueblo indian village by Kaufman (37).

The first cases of glue sniffing were reported in California, but the practice seems to have spread to the Midwest in the early 1960s. By 1965, it was reported to be occurring in every state of the United States (12). By the end of 1960s it had involved children and adolescents in numerous countries, including Africa, Australia, Canada, Finland, Japan, Mexico, South America, and Western Europe (84).

Solvent misuse is a comparatively recent phenomenon in Great Britain, with one of the first reports being by Merry and Zacchariadis in 1962 (53). They described the case of a 20-year-old man who had been sniffing plastic cements for a period of 18 months. He gradually increased this habit until he was sniffing one-third of a tube every night; ultimately, he increased this amount to two tubes every night. He subsequently developed withdrawal symptoms whenever he decided to stop sniffing.

The police in the west of Scotland first commented on the existence of the problem in 1970. The first study of solvent abuse in Scotland was conducted in Lanarkshire by Watson, who noticed that this was largely a group activity, predominantly involving males between ages 9 and 17 years with antisocial tendencies (80).

DEFINITION AND TERMINOLOGY

"Glue sniffing" appeared in the *Index Medicus* in 1969. It may be a misnomer as it is not "glue" that is inhaled, but its vapors. The clinical effects are due to the inhalation of volatile hydrocarbons contained in the solvents. A wide variety of products including glue can be used. Finally, the vapor can not only be "sniffed," but also inhaled through the mouth (huffing). Other popular terms are "solvent abuse," and "solvent misuse." "Volatile substance abuse" (VSA) may be a more appropriate term.

PREVALENCE

The prevalence of solvent abuse varies greatly from population to population and from time to time. Barnes provides a useful summary of solvent abuse surveys conducted in America in the 1970s (3). The prevalence of use can range from less than 1% to over 60% in certain populations. The highest recorded prevalence (62%) seems to be for gasoline sniffing (37).

The prevalence of volatile substance abuse in Britain is uncertain and is not restricted to any one area. Francis et al. (25), in a survey of solvent abuse cases referred to the Poison Unit, Guy's Hospital, London, found that requests originated from every Health Authority Region in England. Ramsay (65) found a point prevalence of 9.8% for boys aged 13 to 15 attending a Glasgow secondary school. A quarter of them reported sniffing solvents regularly, another quarter sporadically, and the rest only once. It is possible that underreporting in school surveys may give erroneous prevalence figures. In the county of Avon, Gay et al. (28) identified 304 abusers during a six-month period from a population of 250,000 individuals at risk; 77% of the subjects were aged between 14 and 17 years.

Skuse and Burrel (71) reviewed solvent abusers referred over a three-year period to the Department of Child Psychiatry at the Maudsley Hospital. A total of 45 solvent abusers were identified (28 boys and 17 girls) of whom eight were first recognized in 1979, 15 in 1980, and 22 in 1981. This figure represented 3.5% of all referrals to the Child Psychiatric Services over that period.

CHARACTERISTICS OF ABUSERS

Age

Volatile solvent abuse occurs mainly in the young with a peak in those aged 13 to 15 (64, 73, 74). Press and Done (64) noted that significant numbers of children under 10 years of age were involved in the activity. Most survey data tend to show that the use of solvents decreases with age and/or grade in school (3). Hershey and Miller (32), in a sample of 160 patients with drug-related problems attending an emergency department in Cleveland, Ohio, found that six of them presented with solvent abuse. The average age of these six patients was 26 years, with a range of 17 to 33 years. A shift to adults can thus occur at times.

Sex

Numerous studies have shown that there are more male sniffers than female sniffers (3, 29, 52, 61). Masterton and Sclare (52), in a survey of patients referred to a Glasgow Psychiatric Clinic with a presenting complaint of persistent solvent abuse over a period of 15 months, noted that all

29 were males. Glaser and Massengale (29) noted that the number of arrests of children for glue sniffing increased in the city of Denver from 30 in 1960 to 134 in 1961. They identified a total of 130 children in this two-year period. They ranged in age from 7 to 17, with a mean age of 13 years, and all but six were boys. In several cases, more than one child in a family was charged with glue sniffing, and in fact, 13 of the younger children had older siblings who at some time were picked up for the same offense. In a study of police statistics on solvent abuse by Watson (81) a total of 180 cases were identified. The age range was 6 to 17 years for males and 13 to 16 years for females. The average age for males (13.8 years) was less than that for females (14.2 years). The ratio for males to females was 1.8 : 1 in 1970, 4.3 : 1 in 1971, 5 : 0 in 1972, 1 : 1 in 1973, 35 : 1 in 1974, and 22.8 : 1 in 1975. Sourindhrin and Baird (73), in a study of 134 cases of "glue sniffers" seen at a special clinic in Glasgow, found that 109 were males and 25 were females. The male-to-female ratio was thus 4.4 : 1. Furthermore, of 166 who attended the clinic in 1980, 132 were males and 34 were females, giving a male-to-female ratio of 3.8 : 1.

In numerous studies a sex difference in the prevalence of solvent misuse has not been found (3, 42, 55). An increasing number of female users have also been reported in some studies (55). Goldstein (30) reported that almost twice as many females as males use inhalants among the Pueblo tribes of New Mexico. Johnson et al. (35), in a study of 2752 High School students in Portland, Oregon, who used inhalants, found a greater use in boys. Girls showed a sharp decrease in use with advancing age. Galli (26), in a study of 517 students who sniffed glue at Champaign County, Illinois, found no sex difference. Klinge et al. (42), in a study involving 143 inpatient male and female adolescent drug abusers who sniffed volatile agents, in Detroit, noticed no significant sex differences. Also, they did not find any correlation with other types of drug use. Strimble and Sims (76), in a study of 24,609 college and junior college students in Georgia, sniffing glue, found a male preponderance. Stybel et al. (77), in a study of 551 students at the Poverty Youth Program, Dallas, Texas, found more males than females among sniffers. Jouglard et al. (36), in a survey of 49 "sniffers" carried out in Marseille, France, noticed that three-fourths were males and the mean age was 15 years.

Race

It has frequently been observed that Spanish-American groups tend to be overrepresented in populations of sniffers. In a study of 130 cases arrested for glue sniffing in 1960–1961, Glaser and Massengale (29) noted that

85% of the children were of Spanish-American origin. Specially high rates have been reported by Kaufman (37) among native Indian groups. He found that 62% of a sample of 72 elementary school Pueblo Indian children had inhaled gasoline. Strimbu and Sims (76), in a study of 24,609 college and junior college students in Georgia, found a high preponderance in solvent users in American-Indian groups. Nurcombe et al. (56), in a study of psychosocial background of petrol inhalation, reported high rates of use in an Australian aboriginal population. Langrod (46), in a study of 422 male heroin users in New York State (45% black, 30% Puerto Rican, 25% white), found that 22% used airplane glue and that the use was less common in blacks. In Sterling's study (75), which covers six months in 1962, there was not a single black among the 47 "glue sniffers" in spite of the fact that the 1965 Census figures for the Chicago Elementary School system indicated 52.5% as being nonwhite.

In a study carried out in Marseille by Jouglard et al. (36), 80% of students were from the immigrant population from Europe, Southeast Asia, and Central Africa.

Socioeconomic Factors

A high incidence of sniffing was observed in most impoverished groups by Angle and Eade (2a) in a study of 564 students of Cree and Inuit origin in Manovane and Great Whale River, Quebec. Strimble and Sims (76) found in a University College students' study that a low amount of spending money was positively related to the use of glue. Ellison (20) observed that sniffers came from low socioeconomic backgrounds. Sokol and Robinson (72) observed that sniffers came from low socioeconomic backgrounds and large families. Gossett et al. (31), in a study of 56,745 junior- and senior-high-school students in Dallas, found no relationship between volatile substance abuse and socioeconomic factors. Press and Done (64), in their Salt Lake City study, noted that the most chronic users were from middle-class and upper-class homes; the father of one was vice president of a major corporation and the father of another was a prominent physician. Barker and Adams (4) found that among 28 "sniffers" at a school for boys in Colorado, there was an average of 7^1/$_2$ children per family as compared to 4^1/$_2$ among "controls" from the same school.

Press and Done (64) found a high incidence of family disorganization among the family of sniffers in their study. They were able to obtain sufficient information through repeated interviews of the subjects and their families and from various social agencies to make a reliable evaluation of the 10 most serious offenders. Five of these boys came from broken homes from which the father was missing because of either divorce, death, prolonged institutionalization, or desertion. The most consistent and striking finding was that in every instance the father was, for all practical purposes, "missing" from the boy's life insofar as any effective relationship is concerned. If the father was not physically missing from the home, he at best had little or no positive relationship with the boy and played no role, except perhaps a punitive one, in the rearing of the boy. Sokol and Robinson (72) pointed to the frequency with which the father was missing from the boy's life and considered other factors to be: worries regarding school, inadequacy, small stature, reaction to such frustrations as being unable to meet goals set by parents, the failure of parents to meet emotional needs, the lack of parental love and understanding, and a feeling of insecurity because of frequent quarrels between parents. Massengale et al. (51) found that one or both parents were missing from the homes of three-fourths of glue sniffers, and in nearly one-half of their cases, one or both parents were alcoholics. Sterling (75) found a 26% incidence of physically broken homes among glue sniffers in Chicago. Borozovsky and Winkler (8) found an incidence of 56% broken homes among glue sniffers in Chicago. Nylander (57) reported an even higher incidence of broken homes (70%) among lacquer thinner sniffers in Stockholm. Kaufman (37) did not find any difference in the incidence of alcoholism and broken homes between his sniffers and nonsniffers. Sourindhrin and Baird (73), in a comparative study of 134 glue sniffers and 100 nonsniffers matched for age and sex, found that 83% of nonsniffers had both parents living together, as compared to 61% of sniffers; 39% of sniffers came from single-parent families, compared to 17% of nonsniffers. This was found to be statistically significant. In the same study it was found that 51% of fathers of sniffers were unemployed, as compared to 23% of fathers of nonsniffers. Again, this was statistically significant.

The observed results concerning socioeconomic factors have thus been inconsistent.

PRODUCTS USED IN SOLVENT ABUSE AND THEIR PRINCIPAL COMPONENTS

A wide variety of organic solvents have been inhaled for the intentional induction of intoxication. The volatile solvents contained in the products are responsible for the clinical effects. The products that may be used include adhesives (Evostick, time bond), model cement, polysterene cement, puncture repair outfit, dry-cleaning substances, deodorants, antiperspirants, pain relief spray, hair spray, fly spray, paint spray, gas spray, gas, lighter refills, fire extinguisher agents, nail polish, antifreeze, paint thinners, cleaning fluids and amyl nitrites, correcting fluids, fuel gases (Butane), windshield washers, and dyes (3, 25, 73).

Table 1 lists the products that can be used for sniffing and their principal components. The type of solvent abused varies from place to place and is susceptible to peer group influence, fads, and availability of products.

PRACTICE AND METHOD OF INHALATION

Volatile substance abuse seems to be predominantly a group activity. Kaufman (37) observed that 42 of 45 gasoline sniffers sniffed with others. They tended to congregate around unattended gasoline sources such as abandoned tractors, power saws, and parked cars. Each would take turns sniffing for several minutes and then fall back and experience the effects. The activities associated with solvent inhalation and abuse require seclusion and privacy.

Preferred places for sniffing sessions include public toilets, derelict properties, railway carriages, public parks, and woodland. Watson (85), in a review of 400 cases of solvent abuse from the west of Scotland, observed that 340 (85%) individuals had been involved in groups, 40 (10%) had been sniffing usually in a group but occasionally on their own, and 20 (5%) were involved only in solitary sniffing.

Sourindhrin and Baird (73), in a study of 134 children seen at a special solvent abuse clinic in Glasgow, observed that 124 (92.5%) indulged themselves in this practice as a group activity. In seven cases (5.2%) it was both a group and/or solitary activity, and in only three cases (2.2%) it was solely a solitary activity. The children reported that relief from boredom, peer group pressure, curiosity, and gain of status were the main reasons for their involvement in the practice.

The practice seems to afford a form of social activity that caters to the needs for acceptance, status, and regard of children who feel lonely, rejected, or friendless. Cohen (10) noted that in many instances of solvent abuse it is easy to identify the "cri du coeur" (cry for help) similar to that evinced in suicide attempts by children.

The method of inhalation varies according to the inhalant used. Hydrocarbon sniffers surveyed by Stybel et al. (77) preferred the "bagging" technique to other modes such as sniffing soaked rags, cotton, tissues, or from a cup filled with the substance. The authors warn of the danger associated with this method due to the tendency of sniffers to inhale carbon dioxide fumes along with the hydrocarbon gases.

Table 1
Products Used in Solvent Abuse

Products	Solvents Detected
Adhesives	Toluene acetone, trichlorethylene, naphthalene, benzene
Aerosols (paint, hair spray, etc.)	Fluorinated hydrocarbons, dichlorofluoromethane, trichlorofluoromethane, isobutane
Lacquer thinners	Toluene, aliphatic acetates, methyl, ethyl, or propyl alcohol
Lighter refills	Naphthalene, perchlorethylene, carbon tetrachloride, trichlorethane
Gasoline	Petroleium hydrocarbons, benzene, toluene, zylene, n-hexane, n-heptane
Nail polish remover	Acetone, ethyl acetate, amyl acetate
Antifreeze	Methanol, isopropanolol
Paint thinner	Methanol, ethanol, Isopropanolol, ethyl acetate, n-propyl acetate, acetone, methylethyl ketone, methylbutyl ketone, benzene, toluene, naphthalene, n-heptane, methylene chloride
Windshield washers	Methanol
Dry-cleaning substances	1 or more: trichloroethylene, trichloroethane, tetrachloroethylene, carbon tetrachloride
Dyes	Acetone, methylene, chloride
Fire extinguisher agents	Bromochlorodifluoromethane (BCT)
Butane gas container Calor gas Gas lighter fuel }	Butane

Sources: (1) Sharp, C. W., & Brehm, M. L. (1977) *Review of inhalants: Euphoria to dysfunction*, Pub. No. ADM 77. Washington DC: Department of Health, Education and Welfare. (2) Oliver, J. S., & Watson, J. M. (1977). Abuse of solvents "for kicks"— A review of 50 cases. *Lancet*, *1*, 84. (3) Anderson, H. R., Dick, B., MacNair, R. S., Palmer, J. C., & Ramsay, J. D., (1982). Death from volatile substance abuse. *Hum. Toxicol.*, *1*, 207.

"Huffing," inhalation through the mouth, is another method utilized, especially when the inhalant used may irritate the nasal membranes if sniffed. Dry-cleaning substances can be inhaled from their containers or their tops or alternatively from rags or handkerchiefs saturated with the fluid. Watson (85) reported that fire-extinguishing contents were decanted into empty beer cans and the vapors inhaled from the can. Aerosols can be sprayed directly into a bag or cloth rags and inhaled. Less cautious users sniff directly from the original containers. Sourindhrin and Baird (73) noted that the majority of 134 sniffers inhaled glue from potato chip bags and a few from plastic bags. The associated CO_2 rebreathing places the user at risk of hypoxia and hypercarbia (85).

TYPOLOGIES OF VOLATILE SOLVENT ABUSE

Two main types of volatile substance users can be distinguished. The first, the largest group, includes those who use solvents on an experimental basis. These children sniff as a new experience but do not continue with the habit. There may be acute behavior problems at the time of the acitivity but they do not affect the child's development and welfare.

The second, much smaller group is the problem-centered group. These children might use a wide variety of solvents for one to five years or more. They might sniff solvents almost every day and in increasing amounts. Some may be considered in need of psychiatric care because of prolonged habitual and/or solitary solvent sniffing with disturbance of emotions and relationships and persistent impaired personal functioning. Some may be psychologically and physically dependent on solvents. They may also get involved in antisocial activities. However, as pointed out earlier, the vast majority of people sniff solvents on an experimental basis, and "maturing out" of the solvent habit is a well-established phenomenon (33).

Skuse and Burrel (71), in a study of 45 solvent abusers referred to the Child Psychiatric Department at Maudsley Hospital, London, considered three groups of abusers: "chronic abusers" (16), "periodic solvent abusers" (14), and "experimental users" (15). The criteria for chronic users were: first, reported use of at least once a day; second, quantity of at least one pot (250 mg) or two large tubes of glue, or equivalent, each day; third, a duration of continuous solvent abuse prior to referral of at least six months. "Periodic users" did not by definition abuse solvents daily, on a regular basis, although they may have been involved with the activity for several months. "Experimental users" by definition used glue, or another solvent, on only one or two occasions.

Personality Characteristics of Users

At the outset a distinction must be made between the experimenter and the person who has become well habituated in the practice. There are few systematic investigations of personality characteristics of sniffers. The characteristics that are most frequently mentioned are anxiety, alienation, depression, and passivity (3). Fejer and Smart (23) found that sniffers had higher scores on the Taylor Manifest Anxiety Scale than did users of any other drug.

They also found that sniffers reported having been treated for psychological problems more often than did nonsniffers (23). Nurcombe et al. (56) obtained the Nutter Behaviour Questionnaire ratings on aboriginal gasoline sniffers. They found higher scores on tension discharge and anxiety inhibition among sniffers than nonsniffers. Sourindhrin and Baird (73), in a study of 134 children involved in glue sniffing, found that relief from boredom, peer group pressure, curiosity and gain of status were, in the majority of cases, the main reasons for their involvement in the practice.

MODE OF ACTION OF SOLVENTS

Volatile solvents are central nervous system depressants. They are lipid soluble and are rapidly absorbed across the large surface area of the lungs. Inhalation is the fastest method of incorporating solvents into the body tissue. At constant air levels, blood concentrations reach 60% of their maximum within 10 to 15 minutes of exposure, and an asymptomatic curve is reached in about half an hour. The concentration in richly vascularized organs such as the brain rises at a similar rate to that in the blood, although the concentrations are at least four times greater. Although some toluene is eliminated unchanged through the lungs, most of it is oxidized to benzoic acid and by conjugation with glycine is converted into water-soluble hippuric acid, which is eliminated through the kidneys. During constant exposure to toluene hippuric acid levels reach 60% of their maximum after 40 to 60 minutes and the elimination curve becomes asymptomatic in two or three hours. Toluene cannot be detected in blood four to six hours after the cessation of exposure, by which time the concentration of hippuric acid in urine has decreased to 30% of its maximum value.

A second peak in blood toluene representing the release of lipid-bound toluene has been described as occurring days after the cessation of exposure

(41). Thus, the interval between exposure to toluene and sampling is important when interpreting results. Toluene assay is the most sensitive indicator of exposure to toluene. The analysis can be carried out by using a Pye Model 104 gas chromatograph equipped with a heated flame ionization detector (61). There is a definite correlation between blood concentrations of toluene and clinical features (48). Thus, concentrations of between 1 and 2.5 μg/g are accompanied by marked intoxication, those between 2.5 and 10 μg/g by greater disturbance of consciousness often requiring hospital admission, and those at higher levels result in coma and death. For toluene, the threshold limit value of airborne concentration to which industrial workers can be repeatedly exposed without adverse effects is 100 ppm (parts per million). Toluene abusers are exposed to concentrations approximately 50 times greater, although the duration of exposure is usually shorter (68).

SUBJECTIVE EFFECTS

Subjective effects vary from person to person, on expectation of the user, on the amount of solvent inhaled, and on the duration of inhalation. The clinical features of solvent intoxication are similar to those of alcohol intoxication, with initial stimulation followed by depression. Reported symptoms occurring within a few minutes of inhalation include a sense of well-being, euphoria, blurring of vision, tinnitus, slurring of the speech, ataxia, feelings of omnipotence, headache, abdominal pain, anorexia, nausea, vomiting, jaundice, chest pain, sneezing, coughing, bronchospasm, impaired judgment, irritability, and excitement. Clouding of consciousness, illusions, and hallucinations can occur in a variable proportion of subjects (41, 73, 85). In a survey of 19 patients admitted to the Royal Hospital for Sick Children, Glasgow, King et al. (41) noted that seven had a history of euphoria or hallucinations. The remainder presented with coma (four), ataxia (three), convulsions (three), and behavior disturbance with diplopia (two). Sourindhrin and Baird (73), in a survey of 134 glue sniffers, noted that hallucinations occurred in 17 patients (12%), of whom 14 described visual hallucinations, one had auditory hallucinations, and two experienced both visual and auditory hallucinations. Watson (85) noted that hallucinations occurred in 168 cases, of a total of 400 solvent abusers (42%).

The combination of intoxication, disorientation, and hallucination can be responsible for accidents, particularly if sniffing sessions occur in places such as bridges, high apartments, rooftops, and in proximity of water. The effects last for 30 to 45 minutes after cessation of exposure. Skuse and Burrel (71) reported that many chronic users had transient symptoms of toxic psychosis, which frequently had a marked affective component often depressive in character. Convulsions, status epilepticus (1), and coma may occur (25). Unlike alcohol intoxication, there is no hangover, or the hangover is not as bad as that of alcohol intoxication.

TOLERANCE AND DEPENDENCE

Psychological dependence and tolerance may develop, but physical dependence is rare (53, 83). Psychological dependence, manifested by a compelling need to inhale and/or anxiety about not being able to, is frequently seen in solvent abusers. Psychological dependence was observed in abusers of paints, thinners, and aerosols by Comstock and Comstock (11). Tolerance can develop. Merry and Zacchariadis (53) describe the case of a 20-year-old man who inhaled at first one-third of a plastic cement tube once a week and gradually increased this habit until he was sniffing one-third of a tube every night; ultimately he increased the amount to two tubes every night. He also developed withdrawal symptoms on cessation of the habit the day after his admission to hospital. He complained of painful cramps of both hands; on examination the hands were rigid and flexed at the metacarpophalangeal joints and extended at the interphalangeal joint (53).

Physical withdrawal symptoms occurring on cessation of the habit have also been described by Watson (83). She reports the case of a 13-year-old boy who has been sniffing an adhesive containing toluene for two years and who developed withdrawal symptoms 36 hours after admission. The reported symptoms were abdominal cramps, aching limbs, fatigue, and nausea, which continued daily over the next five days (83). However, Sourindhrin and Baird (73) did not find any evidence of physical dependence in a sample of 300 glue sniffers.

VOLATILE SOLVENT ABUSE AND ACADEMIC PERFORMANCE

Numerous studies have commented on the relationship between poor academic performance and solvent abuse (3). Press and Done (64), in their study of 16 boys who had been habitual sniffers for periods ranging from three months to more than three years, noted that school adjustment and scholastic performance were poor in nearly all subjects. Barker and Adams (4) noted that 28 glue sniffers were underachievers and averaged two grades less than controls of the same age. Truancy had been common, even prior to the onset of sniffing activities with many, and was frequently associated with other types of delinquent behavior. Galli (26) reported that there was a higher incidence of absenteeism among sniffers. Press and Done (64) observed that sniffers do not appear to be substantially less intelligent than other students. They pointed out that intellectual endowment per se is not likely to be the chief determinant of addictive behavior of this type. Dodds and Santofefano (17) used detailed psychological procedures, such as assembling, ability to maintain attention and concentration in the face of distractions, and exercising visual motor coordination, to investigate various cognitive functions of chronic glue sniffers. They found no evidence of adverse effects.

A study of cognitive functioning of solvent abusers was carried out by Mahmood (49) in Glasgow. Twenty-eight nonactive solvent-abusing youngsters with a mean age of 14½ and 20 nonabusing adolescents were given tests of nonverbal and verbal intelligence, arithmetic, literacy, and learning ability. The results clearly indicated that the two groups did not significantly differ in potential abilities.

Observed performance decrements in solvent abusers are more likely due to poor motivation and poor school attendance. IQ's within the normal range have been reported in uncontrolled (Massengale et al. [51]) and retrospective (Skuse and Burrel [71]) studies of solvent abusers. Fornazzari et al. (24) described cognitive impairment in 16 of 24 solvent abusers two days after admission to hospital. In this uncontrolled study, cognitive impairment was found to correlate significantly with the presence of neurological signs and CT scan abnormalities.

RELATIONSHIP WITH OTHER TYPES OF DRUG USE

In studies that have examined the relationship between solvent use and other types of drug use, a relationship has generally been found. Single et al. (70) found that the use of inhalants correlated significantly ($p < .001$) with the use of all legal and illicit drugs. Whitehead (86) observed an interrelationship between various types of drug users. In a survey of 902 drug users he found that solvent users were higher than nonusers of solvents in virtually every type of drug use with the exception of tobacco. Klinge et al. (42) found no relationship between the use of volatile solvents and the use of hallucinogens, stimulants, depressants, and narcotics in 143 drug-abusing adolescent psychiatric inpatients. Skuse and Burrel (71) reported that of 13 chronic solvent abusers referred to the Child Psychiatric

Unit at Maudsley, seven drank alcohol regularly and four used multiple illicit drugs, including cannabis (three), amphetamine (two), and barbiturates (one).

PROGRESSION IN DRUG USE

There is no firm evidence to date that glue sniffing leads directly to abuse of other solvents (33). The problem of demonstrating a progression in drug use from one drug to another, such as the use of marijuana to the use of heroin, has caused much debate. Similarly, the question of whether solvent abuse leads to other forms of drug use remains clouded. In most cases, solvent misuse is a transient phenomenon. Davies et al. (15), however, highlighted the fact that a few chronic solvent misusers do subsequently take illicit drugs. These authors are undertaking a much-needed follow-up study of a sample of solvent misusers to identify the characteristics of this minority group. Whitehead and Brook (87) found that over one-third of the persons seen at drug treatment units in London, Ontario, reported using solvents. Kramer (45) found that many of the heroin addicts in his sample had started with glue; 68% of the younger addicts in his study had used glue, while only 22% of the older addicts had used glue. Langrod (46) found that 27% of his sample of 422 male heroin users had used glue. Langrod also found that 65% of the group who had been using heroin for less than five years had also used glue. However, this high prevalence of volatile substance abuse among heroin addicts is not indicative of a pattern of progression from solvent abuse to heroin use. Little information is available on the progression of solvent abuse to alcohol abuse.

Watson (82), in a retrospective study involving 102 solvent users and 102 nonsniffing deviant controls matched for age and sex, found that 16 of the test cases and one control case had been involved within two to three years of the initial referral (for solvent abuse) in drug or alcohol abuse.

PHYSICAL SEQUELAE OF SOLVENT MISUSE

There is general agreement that solvent abuse is one of the most dangerous types of drug use. Erythematous spots around the nose and mouth ("glue sniffer's rash") may be observed when a plastic bag is used for inhalation. This is due to chemical irritation of the skin by the volatile hydrocarbons. This might be a useful sign in the detection of glue sniffing. Irritation of mucous membranes and respiratory tract can also occur. The ketones produce sharp irritation usually sufficient to prevent acute overexposure. Exposure to high concentrations can, as expected, lead to central nervous system depression.

Hematological abnormalities as a result of solvent abuse have been reported (3, 55). Aplastic anemia secondary to glue sniffing has been reported (63). Benzene is generally considered to be myelotoxic (55). Acute hemolysis due to naphthalene inhalation has been observed (78). Aplastic anemia particularly may be a risk in those having sickle cell disease.

Transient, reversible, acute hepatic and renal damage as a result of solvent abuse has been reported (58). O'Brien et al. (58) reported the case of a 19-year-old boy who had been sniffing glue for three years and who presented with transient jaundice and reduced urinary output.

Grabski (27) described a cerebellar syndrome with the main symptoms being nystagmus, tremor, and ataxia in a patient who inhaled toluene regularly and gasoline occasionally for two years. At follow-up these symptoms had improved transiently during periods of abstinence (27). Prolonged cerebellar dysfunction as a result of paint sniffing has been observed by Kelly (39). Persistent cerebellar ataxia in toluene abusers has also been reported (Boor and Hurtig [7]). Equilibrium disorders as a result of long-term toluene sniffing have been reported by Sasa et al. (69). King et al. (41) reported that toluene inhalation may cause encephalopathy and may lead to permanent neurological damage. Nineteen children aged 8 to 14 years were admitted to Yorkhill Hospital, Glasgow, during 1974 to 1980 with an acute encephalopathy due to toluene intoxication. Thirteen recovered completely and one had persistent cerebellar signs a year after the acute episode (41). Fornazzari et al. (24) observed cerebellar signs in 11 of 24 toluene abusers admitted to a Canadian drug treatment unit. The mean age of the subjects was 23, and the fact that they were involved in severe and prolonged abuse might be responsible for the high frequency of cerebellar abnormalities. The presence and severity of the cerebellar signs were significantly correlated with the width of cerebellar sulci and superior cerebellar cisterns in the CT scan.

Escobar and Aruffo (21) described loss of Purkinje cells with ballooning of the remaining axons, gliosis of the molecular layer, and demyelination of the white matter in a postmortem study of a case of chronic thinner intoxication.

In summary, transient cerebellar signs are a common feature of acute toluene intoxication, and in some cases persistent cerebellar abnormalities can occur.

Optic neuropathy has been reported on rare occasions. Keane (38) and Fornazzari et al. (24) reported optic neuropathy in association with cerebral and cerebellar anomalies in the CT scan. Progressive optic neuropathy and sensorineural hearing loss due to chronic glue sniffing were reported by Ehyai and Freemon (19).

Peripheral neuropathy has been reported in toluene abusers when they start abusing products containing n-hexane (44). Korobkin et al. (44) noted that improvement took place while the subject continued to inhale an adhesive containing toluene. The clinical picture of the peripheral neuropathy caused by n-hexane and other volatile solvents is fairly constant. Symptoms usually start within weeks or months of exposure, with fairly rapid deterioration continuing for some weeks after its cessation. The resulting neuropathy is usually symmetrical and predominantly motor. Electrophysiological studies have demonstrated slow conduction velocities and delayed latencies. Paranodal swellings with accumulation of neurofilaments and secondary demyelination have been observed in biopsies of peripheral nerves (68).

Toluene may thus cause optic neuropathy and sensorineural deafness. However, unlike n-hexane, toluene's potential for causing peripheral neuropathy is low.

Widening of the cerebral and cerebellar sulci and basal cisterns with enlargement of the ventricular system has been reported in some cases of volatile substance abusers. Radiological abnormalities have been found in some cases of volatile substance abusers by using pneumoencephalography (Knox and Nelson [43]; Sasa et al. [69]) or computerized tomography (Boor and Hurtigh [7]; Escobar and Aruffo [21]). Normal CT scans have also been reported in severe abusers (Kelly [39]; Malm and Lying-Tunell [50]; Channer and Stanley [9]).

Fornazzari et al. (24) scanned 14 toluene abusers during the second week of abstinence and compared the scans with those of 20 neurological patients reported as normal matched for age and sex. Using linear measurements, toluene abusers were found to have significantly wider cerebral and cerebellar sulci and larger ventricular systems. The cerebellar abnormalities correlated significantly with the presence of neurological symptoms such as ataxia and tremor, but no significant correlations were found between the severity of the radiological abnormalities and the frequency and duration of toluene abuse. The neuropathological changes that may account for the CT scan abnormalities are unknown, and the possibility that radiological appearances could improve with abstinence, as in the case of alcoholics (Ron [67]), needs to be explored. Furthermore, as with chronic alcoholics, isolated CT scans must be interpreted with caution.

PSYCHIATRIC MORBIDITY

Behavioral changes and perceptual abnormalities occur commonly during acute solvent intoxication. They need to be distinguished from the sequelae of solvent abuse and preexisting or existing psychiatric disorders. In a specially set-up clinic in Glasgow, Sourindhrin and Baird (73) found that only nine children of 134 (6%) were considered to be in need of psychiatric care because of prolonged, habitual, and/or solitary glue sniffing with disturbances of emotions and relationships and persistently impaired personal functioning. Of these nine children, three were already attending a psychiatric unit in the area and the remaining six were followed up at a local psychiatric clinic.

Skuse and Burrel (71), in a retrospective study of 45 solvent abusers, found a much higher frequency of psychiatric disturbances. Approximately two-thirds of the subjects received the diagnosis of conduct and emotional disorders. The authors pointed out that toluene abuse does not appear to be a cause of psychiatric disturbance, but that it occurs in a group of individuals with high psychiatric morbidity.

Lockhart and Lennox (47) compared a group of 23 delinquent boys in a regional secure unit who had abused solvents once a week for three months with a group of nonabusers from the same area, matched for age and IQ. On a questionnaire dealing with psychiatric and psychosomatic symptoms, both groups scored above the cutoff point for the general population, but no significant differences were detected between abusers and nonabusers (47).

In populations of drug and alcohol abusers, those who also abuse solvents appear to be more severely disturbed. Crites and Schuckit (13) studied a large sample of subjects detained for alcohol-related offenses and classified them according to their use of solvents and other drugs; 120 subjects had used volatile solvents and other drugs, 411 were polydrug users but had not used solvents, and the remainder (255) had used only alcohol and cannabis. The three groups were of similar age, sex, race, and family backgrounds and came from the same area. The volatile solvent abusers had more severe drug and alcohol problems than the rest and received the diagnosis of antisocial personality more often than other groups. The antisocial activities of the solvent abusers preceded the onset of the practice and were considered to be the cause of the more severe drug and alcohol problems. The prevalence of affective symptoms was the same in all groups, and no cases of schizophrenia were diagnosed. In a similar study D'Amanda et al. (14) found that heroin addicts who abused solvents were more severely addicted to heroin than those who did not abuse solvents. Suicidal ideation was more common in volatile substance abusers, but there was no evidence of increased frequency of depressive or other psychiatric symptoms in this group.

In summary, the reported rates of psychiatric morbidity vary according to the population under study. Glue sniffing appears to be essentially a socialized disturbance of conduct, and in only a few individuals is there a mixed disturbance of conduct and emotions for which psychiatric intervention is warranted (74).

ACCIDENTS AND ANTISOCIAL BEHAVIOR

Self-destructive and antisocial acts may be carried out while under effect of solvents (64). Accidents can occur while the subjects are under effect of solvents. Impaired judgement, incoordination, clouding of consciousness, and feelings of omnipotence can lead to serious accidents. Automobile accidents and homicides while under the effect of solvents have been reported by Press and Done (64). However, the relationship of any of these practices to subsequent criminality, narcotic addiction, and alcoholism is as yet unclear.

MORTALITY ASSOCIATED WITH SOLVENT MISUSE

In Britain from 1971 to 1981 some 140 deaths were identified from abuse of volatile substances (2). Death rates were highest in conurbations and in Scotland, northern Ireland, and northern England. The chief substances were butane (28%), solvents in adhesives (23%), other solvents (26%), aerosols (15%), and fire-extinguishing agents (5%). Most deaths occurred alone at home. In 41% of cases death was only indirectly associated with solvent abuse (trauma 8%, plastic bag over the head 19%, and inhalation of stomach contents 14%). In nearly half the cases death was attributed to the direct toxic effects of the substances; this proportion was highest with aerosols and lowest with solvents in adhesives (2). An epidemic of 110 sudden deaths without plastic bag suffocation in American youths was reported by Bass (5). Severe cardiac arrhythmias, intensified by hypercapnia, stress, or activity, are thought to be the most likely explanation for sudden death after inhalation of aerosols (5). The lack of morbidity and mortality in a group of 300 glue sniffers seen at a Glasgow clinic is reassuring (73). Solvent abuse may kill the first time, as in a game of Russian roulette.

THE ROLE OF THE LABORATORY
IN THE INVESTIGATION OF SOLVENT ABUSE

A wide range of compounds that may be abused by inhalation, such as the butanes, the halons, 1,1,1,-trichloroethane, trichloroethylene, and toluene, can be detected and identified in blood specimens by means of headspace gas chromatography (66). The measurement of urinary concentrations of benzoic and hippuric acids (metabolites of toluene) and of toluric acids (metabolites of the xylenes) by high-performance liquid chromatography may provide useful information. In general, a hippurate/creatinine ratio of greater than 1 is indicative of recent toluene exposure (Ramsay and Flanagan [66]). The toluric acids are not normally present in urine, but hippuric acid (derived primarily from a metabolism of the food preservative sodium benzoate) is a normal urinary constituent.

PROPHYLAXIS

Prevention Through Education

The subject of solvent abuse could be part of a broad health education program. It is important to organize discussions with parents, teachers, social workers, youth workers, medical staff, and other agencies coming in contact with children and adolescents. Schoolteachers observing irritability, inattentiveness, poor performance, and truancy should suspect the possibility of solvent abuse. The resemblance of solvent intoxication to alcoholic intoxication often draws the attention of the police to the child. Parents should be made aware of the signs of glue sniffing: breath smell, glue sniffer's rash, spillage marks on clothes, erratic mood swings, and general air of furtiveness. Educational leaflets and videotapes on solvent abuse can have a useful role in prevention of the habit.

Prevention of Solvent Misuse

Restriction on sales, reformulation of solvent products, and addition of aversive substances have all been found to be impracticable; a voluntary informed code of conduct practiced by retailers has been shown to be of some benefit (73). The controls of the Misuse of Drugs Act or similar legislature controls would probably be inappropriate (16).

The Solvent Abuse Scotland Act (1983) allows a child being found by more than one person to be under the influence of solvents to be referred to the children's panel as being perhaps in need of compulsory medical care. The Intoxicating Substances (Supply) Bill (1985) prohibits the supply to persons under the age of 18 of certain substances that may cause intoxication if inhaled.

Health education, thus, plays a vital role in the prevention of solvent misuse.

MANAGEMENT OF VOLATILE SUBSTANCE ABUSE

Acute solvent intoxication is usually a brief and self-limiting illness. The child is best kept under observation in a place of safety. The child may need to be resuscitated if necessary.

In chronic users, a complete history, physical, and neurological examination and relevant laboratory investigations should be carried out. Particular attention should be paid to the lonely, dependent chronic users with emotional problems who may be using the more dangerous substances (e.g., aerosols) (74).

It is important to reassure children and their parents that for most children, solvent abuse is a transient phase through which they pass apparently unscathed. It is also important to tell children that experimenting with glue or any other solvent-based product is potentially hazardous and that harm can occur at random. However, scare-mongering tactics (e.g., telling children they will suffer from brain, kidney, or liver damage) are unhelpful and inadvisable. Children and adolescents should be made aware of their own responsibilities in relation to their behavior, and parents, should, if necessary, be made conscious of their obligations toward their children. This applies particularly to parents who often do not know where their children go or make little attempt to regulate their activities. In specific cases parents should be made aware of the negative role of parental criticism, rejection, hostility, erratic inconsistent response to bad behavior, threats of abandonment, and severe sanctions (73). It should be pointed out that prompt, regular, positive reinforcement of good behavior and a nondramatic response to deviant behavior might decrease the probability of continued solvent usage (73). The problem is best dealt with by general practitioners, community physicians, social and youth workers, and the community involvement branch of the police. Health education, improved recreational facilities, and help to single parents and those with alcohol, physical, marital, and psychiatric problems have proved to be of benefit (73). Individual therapy, family therapy (71), behavior modification programs (73), and suggestion techniques (60), may be useful in selected cases.

Minimal, nondramatic, nonalarmist intervention at an early stage, with the participation of parents, appears to be effective, and this is consistent with treatment of abuse of other drugs, especially alcohol (62, 73, 74).

REFERENCES

1. ALISTER, C., LUSH, M., OLIVER, J. S., & WATSON, J. M. (1981). Status epilepticus caused by solvent abuse. *Br. Med. J.*, *283*, 1156.
2. ANDERSON, H. R., DICK, B., MacNAIR, R. S., PALMER, J. C., & RAMSAY, J. D. (1982). An investigation of 140 deaths associated with volatile substance abuse in the United Kingdom (1971–1981). *Hum. Toxicol.*, *1*, 207.
2a. ANGLE, M. R., & EADE, N. R. (1975, March). Gasoline sniffing and tetraethyl lead poisoning in a northern native community. Epidemiological and Social Research Division, Research Bureau, Nonmedical Use of Drugs Directorate, Health and Welfare, Canada. Report No. ERD-74-19.
3. BARNES, G. E. (1979). Solvent abuse: A review. *Int. J. Addict.*, *14*(1), 1.
4. BARKER, G. H., & ADAMS, W. T. (1963). Glue sniffers. *Sociol. Soc. Res.*, *47*(3), 298.
5. BASS, M. (1970). Sudden sniffing death. *JAMA*, *212*, 2075.
6. BLACK, P. D. (1967). Mental illness due to the voluntary inhalation of petrol vapour. *Med. J. Aust.*, *2*, 70.
7. BOOR, J. W., & HURTIGH, I. (1977). Persistent cerebellar ataxia after exposure to toluene. *Ann. Neurol.*, *2*, 440.
8. BOROZOVSKY, M., & WINKLER, E. G. (1965). Glue sniffing in children and adolescents. *NY State J. Med.*, *65*, 1984.
9. CHANNER, K. S., & STANLEY, S. (1983). Persistent visual hallucinations secondary to chronic solvent encephalopathy: Case report and review of the literature. *J. Neurol. Neurosurg. Psychiatry*, *46*, 83.
10. COHEN, S. (1975). Glue sniffing. *JAMA*, *231*, 653.
11. COMSTOCK, E. G., & COMSTOCK, B. S. (1977). Medical evaluation of inhalant abusers. In C. W. Sharp & M. L. Brehm (Eds.), *Review of inhalants: Euphoria to dysfunction*. Rockville, MD: NIDA.
12. CORLISS, L. M. (1965). A review of evidence of glue sniffing—A persistent problem. *J. School Health*, *35*, 442.
13. CRITES, D. G., & SCHUCKIT, M. A. (1979). Solvent misuse in adolescents at a community alcohol centre. *J. Clin. Psychiatry*, *40*, 39.
14. D'AMANDA, C., PLUMB, M. M., & TAINTOR, Z. (1977). Heroin addicts with a history of glue sniffing—A deviant group within a deviant group. *Int. J. Addict.*, *12*, 255.
15. DAVIES, B., THORLEY, A., & O'CONNOR, D. (1985). Progression of addiction careers in young adult solvent misusers. *Br. Med. J.*, *290*, 109.
16. Department of Health and Social Security (1982). Report of the Advisory Council in Misuse of Drugs. *Treatment and rehabilitation*. London: HMSO.
17. DODDS, J., & SANTOFEFANO, S. (1964). A comparison of cognitive functioning of glue sniffers and non-sniffers. *J. Paediatr.*, *64*, 565.
18. EDWARDS, R. V. (1960). Case report of gasoline sniffing. *Am. J. Psychiatry*, *117*, 555.
19. EHYAI, A., & FREEMON, F. R. (1983). Progressive optic neuropathy and sensorineural hearing loss due to chronic glue sniffing. *J. Neurol. Neurosurg. Psychiatry*, *46*, 349.

20. ELLISON, W. S. (1964). Portrait of a glue sniffer. *Crime Delinquency, 11*(4), 394.
21. ESCOBAR, A., & ARUFFO, C. (1980). Chronic thinner intoxication: Clinicopathological report of a human case. *J. Neurol. Neurosurg. Psychiatry, 43*, 986.
22. FAUCETT, R. L., & JENSEN, R. A. (1952). Addiction to the inhalation of gasoline fumes in a child. *J. Paediatr., 41*, 364.
23. FEJER, D., & SMART, R. (1973). The knowledge about drugs, attitudes towards them and drug use rates of high school students. *J. Drug Educ., 2*(14), 377.
24. FORNAZZARI, L., WILKINSON, D. A., KAPUR, B. M., & CARLENE, P. L. (1983). Cerebellar, cortical and functional impairment in toluene abusers. *Acta Neurol. Scand., 67*, 319.
25. FRANCIS, J., MURRAY, V. S. J., RUPRAH, M., FLANAGAN, R. J., & RAMSAY, J. D. (1982). Suspected solvent abuse in cases referred to the Poisons Unit, Guy's Hospital, July 1980–June 1981. *Hum. Toxicol., 1*, 271.
26. GALLI, N. (1974). Patterns of student drug use. *J. Drug Educ., 4*(2), 237.
27. GRABSKI, D. G. (1961). Toluene sniffing producing cerebellar degeneration. *Am. J. Psychiatry, 118*, 461.
28. GAY, M., MELLER, R., & STANLEY, S. (1982). Drug abuse monitoring: A survey of solvent abuse in the county of Avon. *Hum. Toxicol., 1*, 257.
29. GLASER, H. H., & MASSENGALE, O. N. (1962). Glue sniffing in children. Deliberate inhalation of vapourised plastic cements. *JAMA, 181*, 300.
30. GOLDSTEIN, G. S. (1978). Inhalant abuse among the Pueblo tribes of New Mexico. In C. W. Sharp & L. T. Carroll (Eds.), *Voluntary inhalation of industrial solvents.* Rockville, MD: Maryland: NIDA.
31. GOSSETT, J. T., LEWIS, J. M., & PHILLIPS, V. A. (1971). Extent and prevalence of illicit drug use as reported by 56,745 students. *JAMA, 216*, 1464.
32. HERSHEY, C. O., & MILLER, S. (1982). Solvent abuse: A shift to adults. *Int. J. Addict., 6*, 1085.
33. HERZBERG, J. L., & WOLKIND, S. N. (1983). Solvent sniffing in perspective. *Br. J. Hosp. Med., 29*, 72.
34. JAFFE, J. H. (1975). *Drug addiction and drug abuse — Pharmacological basis of therapeutics* (p. 284). New York: Macmillan.
35. JOHNSON, K. G., DONNELLY, J. H., SCHEBLE, R., WINE, R. L., & WEITMAN, N. (1971). Survey of adolescent drug use. 1 — Sex and grade distribution. *Am. J. Public Health, 61*, 2418.
36. JOUGLARD, J., JEAN, P., DAVID, J. M., ARDITTI, J., & AICARDI, F. (1984). Le sniffing: Jeu d'écolier ou toxicomanie? Résultat d'une enquête concernant 49 écoliers sniffeurs. *Méd. Hygiène, 42*, 2479.
37. KAUFMAN, A. (1973). Gasoline sniffing among children in a Pueblo Indian village. *Paediatrics, 51*, 1060.
38. KEANE, J. R. (1978). Toluene optic atrophy. *Ann. Neurol., 4*, 390.
39. KELLY, T. W. (1975). Prolonged cerebellar dysfunction associated with paint sniffing. *Paediatrics, 56*, 605.
40. KERR, N. (1980). Ether drinking. *New Rev., 3*, 536.
41. KING, M. D., DAY, R. E., OLIVER, J. S., LUSH, M., & WATSON, J. M. (1981). Solvent encephalopathy. *Br. Med. J., 283*, 663.
42. KLINGE, V., NAZIRI, H., & LENNOX, K. (1976). Comparison of psychiatric in patient male and female adolescent drug abusers. *Int. J. Addict., 11*(2), 309.
43. KNOX, J. W., & NELSON, J. R. (1966). Permanent encephalopathy from toluene inhalation. *N. Engl. J. Med., 275*, 1494.
44. KOROBKIN, R. ASBURY, A. K., SAUMNER, A. J., & NIELSON, S. L. (1975). Glue sniffing neuropathy. *Arch. Neurol., 32*, 158.
45. KRAMER, J. P. (1972). The adolescent addict: The progression of youth through the drug culture. *Clin. Pediatr., 11*(7), 382.

46. LANGROD, J. (1970). Secondary drug use among heroin users. *Int. J. Addict.*, 5(4), 611.
47. LOCKHART, W. H., & LENNOX, M. (1983). The extent of solvent abuse in a regional secure unit sample. *J. Adolescence*, 6, 43.
48. LUSH, M., OLIVER, J. S., & WATSON, J. M. (1980). The analysis of blood in cases of suspected solvent abuse with a review of results during the period October 1977 to July 1979. In J. S. Oliver (Ed.), *Forensic toxicology*. London: Crook Helm.
49. MAHMOOD, Z. (1983). Cognitive functioning of solvent abusers. *Scott. Med. J.*, 28, 276.
50. MALM, G., & LYING-TUNELL, U. (1980). Cerebellar dysfunction related to toluene sniffing. *Acta Neurol. Scand.*, 62, 188.
51. MASSENGALE, O. N., GLASER, H. H., LELIEVRE, R. E., DODDS, J. R., & KLOCK, M. H. (1963). Physical and psychological factors in glue sniffing. *N. Engl. J. Med.*, 269, 1340.
52. MASTERTON G., & SCLARE, A. B. (1978). Solvent abuse. *Health Bull. (Edinburgh)*, 2, 305.
53. MERRY, J., & ZACCHARIADIS, N. (1962). Addiction to glue sniffing. *Br. Med. J.*, 2, 1448.
54. NITSCHE, C. J., & ROBINSON, J. F. (1959). A case of gasoline addiction. *Am. J. Orthopsychiatry*, 29, 417.
55. NOVAK, A., & STASH, S. (1980). The deliberate inhalation of volatile solvents. *J. Psychedelic Drugs*, 12(2), 105.
56. NURCOMBE, B., BRANCHI, G. N., MONEY, J., & CAWTE, J. E. (1970). A hunger for stimuli. The psychosocial background of petrol inhalation. *Br. J. Med. Psychol.*, 43, 3670.
57. NYLANDER, I. (1962). "Thinner" addiction in children and adolescents. *Acta Paedopsychiatr.*, 29(9), 273.
58. O'BRIEN, E. T., YEOMAN, W. B., & HORBY, J. A. E. (1971). Hepato renal damage from toluene in a "glue sniffer." *Br. Med. J.*, 2, 29.
59. O'CONNOR, D. J. (1979). Annotation. A profile of solvent abuse in school children. *J. Child Psychol. Psychiatry*, 20, 365.
60. O'CONNOR, D. (1982). The use of suggestion techniques with adolescents in the treatment of glue sniffing and solvent abuse. *Hum. Toxicol.*, 1, 313.
61. OLIVER, J. S., & WATSON, J. M. (1977). Abuse of solvents for kicks. A review of 50 cases. *Lancet*, 1, 84.
62. ORFORD, J., & EDWARDS, G. (1977). *Alcoholism*. London: Oxford University Press.
63. POWARS, D. (1965). Aplastic anemia secondary to glue sniffing. *N. Engl. J. Med.*, 273(13), 700.
64. PRESS, E., & DONE, A. K. (1967). Solvent sniffing — Physiological effects and community control measures for intoxication from the intentional inhalation of organic solvents. *Paediatrics*, 39, 451.
65. RAMSAY, A. W. (1982). Solvent abuse: An educational perspective. *Hum. Toxicol.*, 1, 265.
66. RAMSAY, J. D., & FLANAGAN, R. J. (1982). The role of the laboratory in the investigation of solvent abuse. *Hum. Toxicol.*, 1, 299.
67. RON, M. A. (1983). The alcoholic brain: CT scan and psychological findings. *Psychol. Med. — Monograph Supplement 3*.
68. RON, M. A. (1986). Volatile substances abuse. A review of possible long term neurological, intellectual and psychiatric sequelae. *Br. J. Psychiatry*, 148, 235.
69. SASA, M., JGARASHI, S., MIYAZAKI, T., MIYAZAKI, T., NAKANO, S., & MATSUOKA, I. (1978). Equilibrium disorders with diffuse brain atrophy in long term toluene sniffing. *Arch. Otorhinolaryngol.*, 221, 163.
70. SINGLE, E., KANDEL, D., & FAUST, R. (1974). Patterns of multiple drug use in high school. *J. Health Soc. Behav.*, 15(4), 344.
71. SKUSE, D., & BURREL, S. (1982). A review of solvent abusers and their management by a child psychiatric out-patient service. *Hum. Toxicol.*, 1, 321.
72. SOKOL, J., & ROBINSON, J. L. (1963). Glue sniffing. *West Med.*, 4, 192, 193, 196, 214.
73. SOURINDHRIN, I., & BAIRD, J. A. (1984). Management of solvent abuse: A Glasgow community approach. *Br. J. Addict.*, 79, 227.

74. SOURINDHRIN, I. (1985). Solvent misuse. *Br. Med. J.*, *290*, 94.
75. STERLING, J. W. (1964). A comparative examination of two modes of intoxication—An exploratory study of glue sniffing. *J. Crim. Law: Crim. Police Sci.*, *55*, 94.
76. STRIMBU, J. L., & SIMS, O. S. (1974). A university system drug profile. *Int. J. Addict.*, *9*(4), 569.
77. STYBEL, L. J., ALLEN, P., & LEWIS, F. (1976). Deliberate hydrocarbon inhalation among low socio-economic adolescents not necessarily apprehended by the police. *Int. J. Addict.*, *11*(2), 354.
78. VALSES, T., DOXIADIS, S., & FESSAS, P. (1963). Acute intoxication due to naphthalene inhalation. *J. Paediatr.*, *63*, 904.
79. WALDRON, H. A. (1981). Effects of organic solvents. *Br. J. Hosp. Med.*, *26*, 645.
80. WATSON, J. M. (1975). A study of solvent sniffing in Lanarkshire. *Health Bull.*, *23*, 153.
81. WATSON, J. M. (1979). A study of the police statistics on solvent abuse. *Strath. Police Guardian*, *3*(3), 29.
82. WATSON, J. M. (1979). Solvent abuse: A retrospective study. *Community Med.*, *1*, 153.
83. WATSON, J. M. (1979). Glue sniffing: Two case reports. *Practitioner*, *222*, 845–847.
84. WATSON, J. M. (1980). Solvent abuse by children and young adults: A review. *Br. J. Addict.*, *75*, 27.
85. WATSON, J. M. (1982). Solvent abuse: Presentation and clinical diagnosis. *Hum. Toxicol.*, *1*, 249.
86. WHITEHEAD, P. C. (1970). The incidence of drug use among Halifax adolescents. *Br. J. Addict.*, *65*, 159.
87. WHITEHEAD, P. C., & BROOK, R. (1973). Social and drug using backgrounds of drug users seeking help: Some implications for treatment. *Int. J. Addict.*, *81*(1), 75.

7

PSYCHOSOCIAL ASPECTS OF ALCOHOL ABUSE

RICHARD J. FRANCES, M.D.

Professor of Clinical Psychiatry,
New Jersey Medical School, UMDNJ,
Newark, New Jersey

and

WALTER STRAUSER, M.D.

Chief Resident in Physical Medicine and Rehabilitation,
Stanford University Medical Center,
Palo Alto, California

The misuse of alcohol across various societies results in tremendous social and economic costs which affect everyone, drinkers and abstainers alike. This chapter outlines the alcohol field's developments in nomenclature, epidemiology, cross-cultural studies, special populations, social policy, and prevention.

Alcohol is used moderately and safely by the majority of people in our society. Yet for certain individuals drinking can be a potentially destructive form of socializing. It is this latter group of vulnerable individuals who suffer the serious consequences of alcohol abuse and impact adversely on the lives of many other members of society. Many of the alcohol-related problems to which this group is prey underlie the ambivalence our society has toward drinking, but since it is unlikely that we will in the near future replace alcohol with another form of entertainment, it is important for us to know as much as we can about this drug and its effects. This chapter reviews the psychosocial aspects of alcoholism, including its definition,

113

epidemiology, social costs, diagnosis, effects on children and other special populations, and prevention.

DEFINITION

Studies of the incidence and prevalence of alcoholism may be affected by the criteria used for the diagnosis of alcoholism, the subpopulation studied, and the tolerance of a particular culture for alcohol-related behaviors. Studying seven different criteria for the diagnosis of alcoholism, Boyd et al. (13) demonstrated excellent agreement between the two most frequently used classifications in the United States and Europe, DSM-III (recently revised) and ICD-9. The latter will also be revised in the next few years. The revision of DSM-III shifts from attempts at use of purely biologically based diagnostic criteria to greater emphasis on sociocultural factors. In DSM-III, alcohol dependence was based solely on the presence of either tolerance or withdrawal symptomatology; however, in DSM-III-R, the concept of dependence has been expanded to embrace nine criteria (Table 1), including several dealing with whether the person frequently performs social or occupational functions while intoxicated and whether the person has missed important social, occupational, or recreational activity because of drinking (72). Referring to the WHO classification, Edwards et al. (24) describe dependence as a "socio-psychobiological syndrome manifested by a behavioral pattern in which the use of a given psychoactive drug (or class of drugs) is given a sharply higher priority over other behaviors which once had significantly greater value . . . " (p. 3). Despite varied definitions, alcoholism is clearly a public-health menace, which in the United States is the third largest health problem, estimated to directly affect 14,000,000 people (83).

EPIDEMIOLOGY

Current epidemiological surveys use data from standardized interviews to estimate the prevalence of psychiatric disorders in the general population. Robins et al. (67) reported on lifetime prevalence rates for psychiatric disorders using data from the Epidemiologic Catchment Area (ECA) Project collected in three United States cities. Substance abuse disorders ranked first among 15 DSM-III diagnoses, with an average of 13.6% of the general population sample having a lifetime prevalence of alcohol abuse or dependence. Myers et al. (57), looking at prevalence rates in a population

Table 1

Diagnostic Criteria for Psychoactive Substance Dependence Disorders*

A. At least three of the following:
   (1) substance often taken in larger amounts or over a longer period than the person intended
   (2) persistent desire or one or more unsuccessful efforts to cut down or control substance use
   (3) a great deal of time spent in activities necessary to get the substance (e.g., theft), taking substance (e.g., chain smoking), or recovering from its effects
   (4) frequent intoxication or withdrawal symptoms when expected to fulfill major role obligations at work, school, or home (e.g., does not go to work because hung over, goes to school or work "high," intoxicated while taking care of his or her children), or when substance use is physically hazardous (e.g., drives when intoxicated)
   (5) important social, occupational, or recreational activities given up or reduced because of substance use
   (6) continued substance use despite knowledge of having a persistent or recurrent social, psychological, or physical problem that is caused or exacerbated by the use of the substance (e.g., keeps using heroin despite family arguments about it, cocaine-induced depression, or having an ulcer made worse by drinking)
   (7) marked tolerance: need for markedly increased amounts of the substance (i.e., at least a 50% increase) in order to achieve intoxication or desired effect, or markedly diminished effect with continued use of the same amount
   Note: The following items may not apply to cannabis, hallucinogens, or phencyclidine (PCP):
   (8) characteristic withdrawal symptoms (see specific withdrawal syndromes under Psychoactive Substance-induced Organic Mental Disorders)
   (9) substance often taken to relieve or avoid withdrawal symptoms

B. Some symptoms of the disturbance have persisted for at least one month, or have occurred repeatedly over a longer period of time.

---

*Reprinted with permission from the *Diagnostic and Statistical Manual of Mental Disorders, Third Edition, Revised*. Copyright 1987 American Psychiatric Association.

for the six-month period prior to study, report a 5% rate of alcohol abuse or dependence.

Blazer et al. (11), using data from the ECA Project, found a lower urban compared to rural prevalence of alcohol abuse or dependence. Lower educational status also predicted higher prevalence rates. When alcohol problems were identified in urban dwellers, those persons were usually older, less educated men who had never married or were separated, widowed, or divorced. The greater rural prevalence is unexpected if based on the prevailing belief that urban conditions of crowding, crime, and poverty are more or less directly correlated with alcohol abuse. Rural dwellers in America are apparently not immune from alcohol problems and for many reasons, "including poverty, unemployment, movement of the younger generation to cities, free-flowing access to information (e.g., cable television), and a more ready access to urban settings through improved transportation" (p. 651) are at substantial risk for abusing alcohol. Alternatively, Helzer et al. (42) suggest that this finding, a low urban/rural ratio of alcoholism for a given area, is found infrequently and may be characteristic only of areas where social sanctions against drinking are strong. Hypothetically, social sanctions may have a greater impact on more densely populated communities than on more widely distributed populations.

Helzer and associates (42) are making a major contribution to advancing our understanding of alcoholism and its effects across different cultures. Using the Diagnostic Interview Schedule (DIS), a highly structured diagnostic interview based on DSM-III criteria and capable of administration by lay interviewers, they have done cross-national comparisons between cities in five countries, the United States, Canada, Puerto Rico, Taiwan, and Korea. With the uniform diagnostic classification, they found lifetime prevalence rates of alcoholism to differ greatly between the cultures, Taiwan being lowest and Korea highest at 23%. Some Asian populations, like Koreans, may have higher rates of alcoholism related to their having a slower, less sickening flushing response (62). In other demographic variables, the five different nations were similar, with far more frequent alcoholism among men, mean age of onset in the third decade (later for women), and comparable symptom complexes.

Warheit and Buhl Auth (81) have reviewed 12 American studies that utilized national samples done between the years 1946 and 1982. Taking the different diagnostic classification schemes into account, the authors found similar percentages of alcohol use across the studies, with approximately 30% of the general population described as abstainers, 10% described as heavy drinkers, and 5% to 10% as problem drinkers (i.e., at least one significant indicator of alcohol-related dysfunction). In the problem drinker group, men were represented four to five times more often than women. The authors found that most alcohol-related problems occurred between the ages of 18 and 30, with the lowest percentage of problems in persons older than 50 years of age. With regard to marital status, the authors found the greatest number of problems for single, separated, or divorced persons. They had too little data to draw specific conclusions with regard to racial, ethnic, and socioeconomic influences, though they did find that abstinence was more frequently seen in lower socioeconomic groups. Edwards et al. (26) state that a single category for abstainers may be misleading, because there can be substantial differences with respect to psychosocial and behavioral factors between past drinkers who are currently abstinent and lifelong abstainers.

ECONOMIC COSTS

Societal costs related to alcohol abuse are diverse. A major study commissioned by NIAAA focused on six major categories of expense (85). Lost production ranked costliest. This included the losses incurred by male alcoholics in the American workforce who suffer a diminished capacity for work, higher rates of absenteeism and industrial accidents, plus less future production secondary to earlier mortality. Health care costs were next, representing the costs of diagnosis, treatment, and prevention of alcohol-related illnesses. The other categories assessed costs attributable to motor vehicle accidents, social responses (e.g., highway safety programs), crime (only homicide, rape, and aggravated assault were studied), and fire losses. A British study assessed somewhat different categories, including the costs of police activities, prison, and judiciary services (53). A 1983 estimate of social costs related to alcoholism in the United States placed the annual total at $116.7 billion (60).

MORBIDITY AND MORTALITY

In a study of a United States sample, Martin et al. (51) found the diagnosis of primary alcoholism to be associated with a threefold greater overall mortality rate regardless of race or gender when compared with a matched control group drawn from the general population. His group reported a nine times greater increase in the mortality rate of alcoholics when unnatural deaths (such as suicide or homicide) were considered alone (52). Berglund (9) found in a Swedish sample that the occurrence of suicides was greatest in alcoholics within two years following hospitalization and decreased in successive years. Peptic ulcer disease was the factor most frequently identified in the histories of those who later killed themselves.

An estimated 50,000 to 200,000 deaths annually in the United States are associated with alcohol abuse (85). Cirrhosis alone accounts for 31,500 deaths, the majority linked to alcohol. In the years 1978–1984, alcohol was cited as a factor in at least 37 % to 43 % of motor vehicle accident fatalities, including pedestrian victims (many of whom are intoxicated when hit), but during Christmas and New Year holiday periods this figure rose to 42 % to 53 % (84).

Excess morbidity associated with alcohol abuse is reflected by a number of health statistics. Alcoholics utilize a disproportionate number of hospital inpatient days compared with nonalcoholics (39). Members of lower socioeconomic groups seem at increased risk for developing alcohol-related illnesses despite a relatively lesser degree of alcohol consumption than higher socioeconomic groups. Alcohol abuse seems to amplify the adverse health effects of tobacco smoking and is associated with hemorrhagic stroke (22), plus oral, pharyngeal, laryngeal, esophageal, and hepatic carcinoma (33). Psychiatric morbidity includes Korsakoff's psychosis and alcoholic dementia, two disabling organic mental disorders linked with chronic alcohol abuse. Alcoholics are at high risk for suicide (31) and homicide (70), especially those alcoholics with a coexistent depression. There is in general an increased association between alcohol use and violent crime, including assault, rape, child molestation, and attempted murder (19, 58).

The effects of alcohol can be significant even before birth. Concern for the use of alcohol during pregnancy dates back to at least the 18th century, although it was not until 1973 that the term fetal alcohol syndrome (FAS) was coined (71). Rosett and Weiner (71) note that more than 400 FAS cases have been reported to date in the literature, and the incidence in women who are heavy drinkers during pregnancy ranges from 2.5 % to 40 % in various studies. FAS does not respect ethnic or socioeconomic boundaries but is linked with chronic alcoholic mothers who drink heavily throughout pregnancy, an estimated 5 % to 10 % of all pregnant women. Rates of FAS vary from 1/1,000 live births in the general population to as high as 1/100 in some American Indian and Eskimo societies (66).

While not pathognomonic, the features associated with the diagnosis of FAS consist of a combination of prenatal and/or postnatal growth retardation, central nervous system involvement (e.g., mental retardation), and a characteristic facial dysmorphology most commonly affecting the eyes, nose, lips, and midface. The facial malformation has been noted to directly correlate with severity of mental impairment and prognosis (Figure 1).

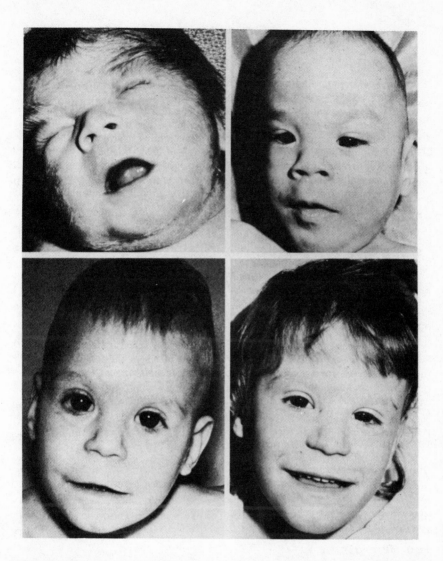

Figure 1. Top: Boy with fetal alcohol syndrome at birth (left) and at age 6 months (right). Bottom: Girl with fetal alcohol syndrome at age 16 months (left) and 4 years (right). Note short palpebral fissures, low nasal bridge with short or upturned nose, epicanthic folds, midface hypoplasia, and long convex upper lip with narrow vermillion border. A narrow bifrontal diameter, ocular ptosis, strabismus, wide mouth, prominent ears, and decreased periocular zone of hair inhibition are common features. (Reprinted with permission from J. W. Hanson, K. L. Jones, and D. Smith (1976), Fetal Alcohol Syndrome—Experience with 41 Patients. *JAMA, 235,* 1459. Copyright 1976, American Medical Association.)

DIAGNOSIS

Alcoholism has been said to have "supplanted syphilis as the great imitator of other diseases" (78, p. 1017). The problem of differing criteria mentioned earlier plus the insidious nature in which primary alcoholism often presents to the clinician complicate the diagnostic process. Greater attention to multiaxial diagnoses in DSM-III research has led to more systematic correlation of other psychopathology with alcohol abuse, and while the question of causation is still indeterminable, alcoholism has been associated with and probably exacerbates a number of other psychiatric conditions, including depression, anxiety disorders, minimal brain dysfunction and attention deficit disorder (30), antisocial personality (18), borderline personality (50), somatoform disorders (12), and other drug abuse (79).

The primary/secondary dichotomy, based usually on chronology or severity, appears to differentiate groups of alcoholics with distinct clinical syndromes and outcomes. Schuckit (73) finds that men with primary alcoholism develop alcohol problems later in life, have lower intensity of drinking, fewer antisocial problems, and less associated drug use. In his review (74) of alcoholism and affective disorder, Schuckit states that primary alcoholics have a significant risk of suffering from a secondary affective illness during periods of heavy drinking, and he believes that 90% of men and women with concurrent symptoms of alcoholism and depression have a diagnosis of primary alcoholism, not primary depression. Conversely, in patients with primary affective disorder, only an estimated 20% are problem drinkers and even fewer (5% to 10%) would meet criteria for a diagnosis of secondary alcoholism. Schuckit argues that alcoholism and affective illness are genetically separate disorders frequently associated owing to the high prevalence of each in the general population. Secondary alcoholism has a prognosis more typical of the associated primary disorder (73) and may carry an even greater risk of suicide than does primary alcoholism (31).

Another useful diagnostic dichotomy appears to be family-history-positive/family-history-negative alcoholism. In a large, multicenter study of male alcoholics, Penick (63) found that two-thirds of family-history-positive and half of family-history-negative alcoholics met criteria for another psychiatric syndrome in addition to alcoholism. Our group (32) has found that familial alcoholics have an earlier onset of problem drinking, more severe social consequences, less consistent stable family involvement, poor academic and social performance in school, more antisocial behavior and a poor outcome in treatment. Donovan (23) views familial alcoholism as a separate diagnostic entity which may be subdivided into bilineal, patrilineal, and matrilineal subgroups. The evidence supports a significant genetic component to the propagation of alcoholism in families, and as Schuckit et al. (75) estimate, the relative risk for alcoholism is increased 10 times in monozygotic twins, four times in first-degree relatives, and two times in second-degree relatives of alcoholics. There appears to be variable penetrance in the phenotypic expression of the unknown gene or genes central to the transmission of alcoholism. Psychosocial influences modulate the expression of the genotype.

CHILDREN AND ALCOHOLISM

Children as a group suffer a great deal from the diverse effects of alcoholism. Early in life they may be exposed to both genetic and environmental factors if raised by an alcoholic parent. Later, they are subject to the hazards associated with alcohol use as they themselves begin to drink. Referred to as "the hidden tragedy" (25), children of alcoholics are vulnerable to various forms of physical abuse, including incest and head trauma. They are also at greater risk for developing psychological difficulties.

Vaillant (80) cites a study done at a children's outpatient clinic that reported that fully half the children had an alcohol-abusing parent. A host of disruptions are frequently identified in alcoholic families, including unpredictability, impulsivity, inconsistent role models, and others that can directly impact on the child's development. Regardless of diagnosis, when a child enters treatment, it is crucial to consider the possibility of an alcohol-abusing parent (56). The significance of this as a potential social problem has not gone unrecognized.

In 1983, in the United States, a group of concerned individuals, many of them children of alcoholics themselves, founded the National Association for the Children of Alcoholics. In addition, Al-Anon reports 500 registered support groups for adult children of alcoholics, and support groups in several centers are beginning to offer both outpatient and brief residential programs for the children of alcoholics.

As the child grows older, he himself begins to drink. One survey (17) of 12- and 13-year-old children from an urban school system found 36% were already using alcohol and 18% were frequent drinkers (two or more drinks per week on average). Unfortunately, there were no significant differences in knowledge of alcohol and its effects between the students who drank frequently and those who did not, suggesting that alcohol education programs in this young age group may not alter drinking patterns. Famularo et al. (27) describe 20 children who met DSM-III criteria for alcohol abuse or dependence by age 13. This group showed a high prevalence of concurrent affective disorders, especially bipolar disorder, plus familial loading for affective disease. Babayan and Gonopolsky (5) suggest that alcohol consumption is increasing among children in the Soviet Union, with 75% of boys and 40% of girls having sampled alcohol by grade 8 and fully 90% to 95% of all children having done so by grade 10.

Plant et al. (65) studied older adolescent students from Scotland and found that 98% had drunk alcohol at some point in their lives, most having their first drink between the ages of 10 and 11, usually offered to them at home by their parents. The rate of questionnaire return was nearly perfect in this study, and it revealed a high level of alcohol consumption in a substantial minority that correlated directly with alcohol-related problems. Girls who were using alcohol to excess were also identified, lending support to emerging evidence for a rising prevalence of alcohol-related problems in females.

Late adolescence and young adulthood are a time of high risk for some of the hazards associated with alcohol-related deaths. The National Center for Health Statistics reported United States data for the year 1980, finding eight deaths in children between the ages of 10 and 14 years, while finding 276 deaths related to alcohol in children between the ages of 15 and 19 (55). Most of the deaths in the older adolescent group were traumatic in nature, specifically, in decreasing frequency of occurrence, motor vehicle accidents, drownings, shootings, stabbings, carbon monoxide inhalation, hanging, poisoning with other drugs or chemicals, falls, and fire. Two things of interest about the data are that over half the deaths represent teenagers who lived in smaller communities (less than 10,000 people) and that while these data represent a national sample, they may grossly underestimate the true frequency of deaths associated with alcohol use because they are based on death certificate data. In studying United States teen and young-adult suicide rates, which have increased two and one-half times in the last two decades, Greenberg et al. (38) noted that the highest death rates were located, surprisingly, in six of the less populous Western states of America.

Motor vehicle accidents are a major cause of morbidity and mortality in this age cohort. The 16- to 24-year age group has the highest frequency of alcohol-related auto accidents (21). Interestingly, this younger age group has been noted to have lower average blood alcohol concentrations when contrasted with older cohorts involved in motor vehicle accidents, suggesting that younger people may be less tolerant to the effects of alcohol on driving skills or perhaps are more likely to take risks when mildly intoxicated than would comparably intoxicated older individuals. Room and Collins (69) have asserted that the basis of disinhibition is more cultural than physiological with respect to alcohol; thus the significance of peer influences in this age group cannot be overemphasized.

Interpersonal violence is another hazard to which this age group is prey. A prospective Danish study (41) of violent assault revealed that the peak incidence for both male and female victims was in the 15- to 19-year age range. Men were represented as victims five times more frequently than women. Alcohol was found to be present in 43% of all victims. Hedeboe et al. (41) note that, unlike other Scandinavian countries, Denmark has few restrictions on the sale of alcoholic beverages; however, their findings show that this less restrictive climate does not seem to increase the frequency of violent behavior. In fact, the rate of violent assaults in Denmark is lower than in either Sweden or Finland. An American study (36) dealing with victims of criminal homicide found alcohol in 46% of the victims. Fully 30% had a blood alcohol concentration greater than 0.10%, the laboratory definition of legal intoxication in most states in America.

OTHER SPECIAL POPULATIONS

Special populations are so designated because of experiences, traits, and often risks shared in common. Cross-cultural psychiatry, sociology, and anthropological studies have delineated the problems of interpretation across cultures in blacks, Hispanics, Jews, and Native Americans. Certain other groups, such as veterans, the elderly, women, and homosexuals, share common sociopolitical roots. It is quite likely that during early life experiences with family and culture a person learns many of the behaviors he will later manifest when intoxicated. As more research is done in this area, we hope to have an increasingly better understanding of cultural influences and to more accurately characterize the drinking patterns of different cultures.

Flasher and Maisto (28) conclude that the generally accepted belief that Jews as a group are immune from alcoholism is misleading and probably false. They cite methodological problems with much of the work, supporting a "stereotype of sobriety among the Jews" (p. 596) and argue that this stereotype may influence Jews to be more reluctant to seek help for drinking problems and make clinicians less alert to recognize problematic drinking in this population. Blacks may develop alcohol-related medical problems such as cirrhosis at a younger age, and they seem at risk for more legal difficulties due to frequent binge-drinking patterns (7). In addition, alcohol use probably plays a role in the high rate of black homicide. Hispanic and Native Americans also have high rates of alcoholism relative to the general population (61). Finally, increasing rates of overall alcohol consumption in the United States may be accompanied by lessening of differential rates of consumption between racial groups (47).

Veterans are at greater risk for alcohol abuse and alcohol-related problems. One survey (14) of veterans in a medical clinic found that over half the sample had met DSM-III criteria for alcohol abuse or dependence at one time in their lives and that one-third of the sample met criteria at the time of the survey. A significant correlation was noted between exposure to combat and level of alcohol consumption, and significantly more patients in the group of alcohol abusers qualified for an associated diagnosis of post-traumatic stress disorder. Hearst et al. (40) found Vietnam veterans to have a 13% increase in mortality from suicide, an 8% increase in mortality from motor vehicle accidents, and a 4% increase in overall mortality at time of follow-up compared with a similar control population.

For a long time, there has been a generally held belief that alcoholism and homosexuality are frequently associated (45). Early writings heavily influenced by psychoanalytic thinking conceptualized homosexuality as a cause of alcoholism through the process of regression to an earlier developmental stage. More recent reviews (59) have not supported this hypothesis and also note that prevalence estimates that have placed problem-drinking rates in the gay population three times higher than rates for the general population have been based only on surveys conducted in gay bars. The association of the gay community with the illness of AIDS is more clearly a factor in making homosexuals an at-risk population.

The interaction between alcohol abuse and AIDS affects all members of the gay community (Table 2). Misconceptions about the disease, including the unfounded fear of casual transmission, have in our experience been associated with major depression, anxiety disorders, and hypochondriasis in gay patients. Even with proper education about the acquisition and transmission of AIDS, alcoholic intoxication, disinhibition, or blackouts probably increase the likelihood of "unsafe" sexual practices (sexual behavior that purportedly places one at greater risk for transmission of the virus). Our group has now observed in four patients the conscious attempt by an individual to contract AIDS through numerous casual sexual contacts facilitated by alcohol use (29). The interaction between alcohol abuse and AIDS can intensify the stigma already directed against the gay com-

Table 2
Interactions Between Alcohol and AIDS

A. Alcoholics with AIDS or in groups at high risk for contracting AIDS (e.g., homosexuals, parenteral drug users)
   1. Increased risk of depression, suicide, and organic mental disorders, especially dementia
   2. Immunosuppression of chronic alcoholism may facilitate acquisition of HIV
   3. Alcohol-related behavioral disinhibition may facilitate acquisition or transmission of HIV
   4. Alcohol can facilitate self-destructive behavior

B. Alcoholics not in groups at high risk for contracting AIDS:
   False positive tests for HIV antibodies have been reported in patients with alcoholic hepatitis (54)

munity. Should the caregiver respond with heightened fears or prejudice, this can lead to suboptimal treatment for the gay alcoholic and refusal for halfway-house placement or residential treatment when indicated.

Two groups that until recently had not been systematically studied with respect to alcohol use are the homeless and the mentally retarded. Recent evidence shows that the homeless population is no longer composed primarily of skid row alcoholics, or single, older, chronic alcoholic men (48). Today the mean age of this population appears to be getting younger, and also greater numbers of women are represented. As many as 90% of this population may have a primary psychiatric diagnosis (3, 6). In the three surveys cited, which sampled different urban populations in the United States, between 20% and 60% of those interviewed reported a history consistent with alcohol dependence. A major problem is that almost by definition these patients are disconnected from a social network and underutilize available social services. Contrary to the generally held view that retarded persons are at greater risk for alcohol abuse is a Swedish study (37) of mildly and severely retarded individuals. Both groups of retarded citizens drank significantly less alcohol than controls, and there were no significant differences from controls in the extent of previous or current alcohol abuse.

A person's choice of occupation may place him at increased risk for alcohol abuse or be conducive to continuing a pattern of abuse already present in the individual. Some of the professions that have been shown in the literature to be associated with high rates of alcohol-related problems are the armed forces, the medical profession, the oil industry (1), and the distilling industry (64). In a review of the literature, Plant (64) found eight factors that he felt explained why certain jobs are associated with high rates of alcohol problems. These deal with how available alcohol is at work, the closeness of supervision, a person's income (very high or very low) and whether or not the person is likely to be separated from his usual social relationships for an extended period of time, as often occurs with salesmen or people in the military. Another predisposing factor concerns unusual stresses placed on an individual by his occupation, such as the large responsibility placed on physicians.

Among physicians, the use and even misuse of alcohol are frequently accepted as a way of coping with job-related stresses. Brewster (15) reviewed the literature dealing with the prevalence of alcoholism among physicians and concluded that available data support a prevalence rate comparable to that of the general population. It has been estimated that between 13,600 and 22,600 physicians in the United States are currently alcoholic or will become alcoholic (10). Johnson and Connelly (46) treated a sample of physicians impaired by substance abuse and found a wide range of psychopathology, the most severe of which occurred in physicians manifesting problems with addiction before the age of 40. They prospectively followed their alcoholic physicians and found that two years after discharge 65% had a successful outcome as measured by abstinence and return to work.

Women, until more recently, have not been well studied in the area of alcohol-related problems. Rising alcohol use in women may be related to the trend in Western societies for greater numbers of women to enter the workforce. As with cigarette smoking, the rates of alcoholism in women over the past 10 years are rising, and this is probably not just an artifact due to more frequent reporting as women become more visible in the workforce (43). As women enter the workforce, they are subject to greater stress in balancing multiple roles (e.g., homemaker versus mother versus businesswoman). On the other hand, housewives often have less opportunity for feeling a sense of achievement and competence than do women in the workforce. In addition, housewives have more opportunities for solitary drinking and fewer of the external controls on drinking that a job provides. Rising rates of alcoholism in women may also be linked more generally with loosening social mores in Western societies (71).

Although prevalence rates for alcoholism among women are still consistently lower than among men, alcoholic women seem to be at greater risk for developing associated medical complications than alcoholic men. Hesselbrock et al. (44) find women to most often have primary alcoholism, frequently accompanied by major affective syndromes and phobias. Their female alcoholics tend to have a later onset of alcoholic drinking patterns but subsequently experience more rapid progression to alcohol dependence than do males. Two long-term follow-up studies (8, 77) showed alcoholic women to have a mortality rate four to five times greater than that of the general population. Berglund (8) reported hepatic cirrhosis to be a far more common cause of death in female alcoholics than male alcoholics, while Smith et al. (77) noted in their sample that the lifespan of alcoholic women was shortened by over 15 years. Hopefully, the underreporting of alcohol-related problems among women is on the wane.

Another group that has been underreported with respect to alcohol problems is the elderly. Atkinson (4) reports that the prevalence of alcohol-related problems decreases at a differential rate for men and women as they age. In women, the prevalence of heavy alcohol use begins to decline during the fifties and sixties, whereas in men, the decline doesn't begin until the mid-seventies. Atkinson notes that general community prevalence estimates for problem drinking in the seventh decade have noted for men a 5% to 12% prevalence but for women only a 1% to 2% prevalence. A subset of individuals, however, may become problem drinkers after lifelong absti-nence (20). Multiple losses to which the elderly are prone, such as retire-ment, death of spouse, financial limitations, and social isolation, seem to play a role in this late-onset alcoholism. Weissman et al. (82) studied a more strictly defined group of problem drinkers in the elderly using DSM-III criteria. In their survey of a predominantly white, urban community sample of people aged 65 and over, they found the six-month prevalence rate for alcohol abuse or dependence to be only 0.7% overall, or 1.7% in males and only 0.1% in females. The reported prevalence for problem drinking in the hospitalized or institutionalized elderly population is high-er and is said to range from 10% to 15% (16).

There are several likely explanations as to why the prevalence of alcohol-related problems declines with age (4). Age-related physiological changes impair a person's ability to metabolize alcohol and make a person more sensitive to alcohol's aversive effects, such as cognitive impairment and dysphoria. In addition, alcoholism is associated with much higher rates of mortality, and to some extent decreased prevalence rates in the elderly may reflect the death of a segment of the younger alcoholic population prior to reaching old age. Finally, underreporting of the diagnosis of alcoholism may be a particular problem in the elderly owing to negative cultural attitudes and to the insidious way in which alcohol-related problems may present clinically in the elderly. While frequent intoxication and withdrawal phenomena are common in younger alcoholics, the elderly alcoholic may show only signs of self-neglect, subtle confusion, labile mood, strange behavior, or more frequent physical problems. These nonspecific symptoms and signs may easily be attributed to reasons other than alcohol abuse in the elderly unless the clinician takes a thorough history of substance use.

PREVENTION

A major development in the area of alcoholism prevention is the shift from tertiary prevention, where the alcoholic is the predominant focus of intervention, to the public-health model of alcoholism, which acknowledges that the effects of alcohol use are widespread throughout society and warrant a more comprehensive approach to prevention with efforts directed at host, agent, and environment (Table 3) (35, 49).

Several factors have contributed to increasing acceptance of the public-health model. Alcohol consumption and alcohol-related problems are increasing worldwide, especially in developing nations. In the United States, greater financial and political backing has come from the publicized support of major entertainers and political figures, in particular, the last three American first ladies. The high social and economic costs of alcoholism as described earlier are now well documented.

Until recently, political support in the United States for alcohol controls has not been as powerful a political lobby as that representing the interests of the alcoholic beverage manufacturing industry. Internationally, alcoholic beverages comprise a major portion of the exports of countries like England and France and alcohol sales and tariff agreements have for years been a valuable commodity in trade negotiations between countries (86). There is surging debate about raising alcohol taxes connected with the realization that alcohol taxation provides an opportunity to accrue revenue to fund treatment efforts for that 10% of the population which consumes 50% of alcoholic beverages purchased (and likewise would assume a major portion of the tax burden). Room (68) states: "There is now no doubt that alcohol controls [regulatory measures affecting the marketplace] can reduce not only consumption but also alcohol-related problems, and that, contrary to common belief, they often most strongly affect the behavior of the heaviest drinkers" (p. 85).

A number of advances in the area of biological research offer promise for prevention through earlier recognition of the at-risk host. Currently, there

Table 3
Prevention of Alcohol Abuse

A. Host factors: Presymptomatic identification and targeted intervention with:
  1. Biologically vulnerable individuals, e.g., children of alcoholics
  2. Groups at risk, for example
    a. Pregnant women
    b. Certain occupations, e.g., military personnel
    c. Various ethnic groups, e.g., American Indians

B. Agent (beverage)
  1. Thiamine fortification of beverages
  2. Health warning labeling
  3. Regulation of beverage distributors, e.g., hours of operation
  4. Minimum drinking age (minimum purchase age)
  5. Alcohol taxation

C. Environmental factors
  1. Mass media
    a. Controls on beverage advertising
    b. Education
  2. Community
    a. Education programs
    b. Greater drunken-driver detection, e.g., road checks
    c. Stricter penalties for drunken drivers
    d. Self-help groups
  3. Workplace, e.g., Employee Assistance Programs

---

is a major quest for a test that would identify early in life those individuals who might later develop alcoholism. Potential genetic markers under study include the finding of low platelet MAO in alcoholics and their first-degree relatives (2). It has now been demonstrated that there are a number of molecular forms of the liver enzyme alcohol dehydrogenase, each metabolizing alcohol at a different rate (75). The genetic control and variable distribution of these isoenzymes may help to explain why certain individuals or groups possess greater vulnerability toward alcoholism. Schuckit et al. (75) have shown that healthy sons of alcoholics experience a lesser subjective sense of intoxication when drinking compared with matched controls without an alcoholic parent. This hypothesized lowered sensitivity of the brain to alcohol in individuals predisposed to developing alcoholism is further supported by electrophysiological studies of alcoholics and healthy sons of alcoholics, revealing decreased P300 amplitude in brain-

evoked potential studies and less alpha rhythm on sober-state EEG record-
ings. Mounting research, including work with animal models, almost confirms that there are people who are biologically vulnerable to alcoholism
owing to heredity, and in the near future this promising branch of the
study of alcoholism may permit us to detect these individuals earlier and
more accurately target our prevention efforts.

An example of attempts in the United States to make preventive changes
in the environment deals with alcohol and the driver. More vigorous attempts have been made to detect drunken drivers by setting up roadblocks
randomly at different sites on weekends and holidays to screen all drivers
passing through for intoxication. Treatment and education efforts plus
stiffer penalties are being mandated for offenders caught driving under the
influence of alcohol as part of drunken-driver-diversion programs (76).
The American Medical Association supports lowering the blood alcohol
concentration considered illegal for driving from 0.10% to 0.05% plus
more frequent driver's license suspension for those convicted of driving
under the influence of alcohol (21). The U.S. federal government recently
passed the National Minimum Drinking Age Law in an attempt to have all
50 states enact a uniform minimum drinking age of 21 years or face the loss
of federal highway fund subsidies. All of these environmental changes are
based on evidence that increasing the minimum drinking age leads to
significantly fewer motor vehicle accident fatalities in the 18- to 20-year
age group (34).

As we stated at the outset, ambivalent societal attitudes toward drinking
underlie many alcohol-related problems in society; therefore, any prevention program in isolation will face substantial resistance, and along the
lines of the public-health model, the best approach to alcoholism and
alcohol abuse prevention necessitates comprehensive social policy changes.
A picture on the front page of the *New York Times* showed the winner of
the 1986 Indianapolis 500 motor race standing, arms raised victoriously,
with the logo of a popular brewery emblazoned across his chest, thereby
associating beer and beer drinking with the youthful, vibrant, triumphant
image of the champion. The media display of images like this weakens the
efficacy of alcohol education programs in our schools and drunken-driver-
diversion programs. An integrated approach to prevention requires coordi-
nating educational programs with the media to promote the message that
alcohol use is potentially dangerous but also a form of entertainment that
can be used appropriately, intelligently, and healthfully. In summary, since
alcohol use is widespread and generally accepted, the best approach to the
prevention of alcohol-related problems should involve a concerted social

policy plan using education, advertising, and mass media with taxation, drunken-driver-diversion programs, and other regulatory measures to foster safe, controlled use of a substance that, when used carelessly, incurs enormous personal and social costs.

REFERENCES

1. AIKEN, G. J. M., & McCANCE, C. (1982). Alcohol consumption in offshore oil rig workers. *Br. J. Addict*, 77, 305.
2. ALEXOPOULOS, G. S., LIEBERMAN, W., & FRANCES, R. J. (1983). Platelet MAO activity in alcoholic patients and their first-degree relatives. *Am. J. Psychiatry*, 140, 1501.
3. ARCE, A. A., TADLOCK, M., VERGARE, M. J., & SHAPIRO, S. H. (1983). A psychiatric profile of street people admitted to an emergency shelter. *Hosp. Commun. Psychiatry*, 34, 812.
4. ATKINSON, R. M. (1984). Substance use and abuse in later life. In R. M. Atkinson (Ed.), *Alcohol and drug abuse in old age*. Washington, DC: American Psychiatric Press.
5. BABAYAN, E. A., & GONOPOLSKY, M. H. (1985). *Textbook on alcoholism and drug abuse in the Soviet Union*. New York: International Universities Press.
6. BASSUK, E. L., RUBIN, L., & LAURIAT, A. (1984). Is homelessness a mental health problem? *Am. J. Psychiatry*, 141, 1546.
7. BENJAMIN, R., & BENJAMIN, M. (1981). Sociocultural correlates of black drinking. *J. Stud. Alcohol*, 42 (Suppl. 9), 241.
8. BERGLUND, M. (1984). Mortality in alcoholics related to clinical state at first admission. *Acta Psychiatr. Scand.*, 70, 407.
9. BERGLUND, M. (1984). Suicide in alcoholism. *Arch. Gen. Psychiatry*, 41, 888.
10. BISSELL, L., & JONES, R. W. (1976). The alcoholic physician: A survey. *Am. J. Psychiatry*, 133, 1142.
11. BLAZER, D., GEORGE, L. K., LANDERMAN, R., PENNYBACKER, M., MELVILLE, M., WOODBURY, M., MANTON, K. G., JORDAN, K., & LOCKE, B. (1985). Psychiatric disorders: A rural/urban comparison. *Arch. Gen. Psychiatry*, 42, 651.
12. BOHMAN, M., CLONINGER, C. R., VON KNORRING, A-L., & SIGVARDSSON, S. (1984). An adoption study of somatoform disorders, III: Cross-fostering analysis and genetic relationships to alcoholism and community. *Arch. Gen. Psychiatry*, 41, 872.
13. BOYD, J. H., WEISSMAN, M. M., THOMPSON, W. D., & MYERS, J. K. (1983). Different definitions of alcoholism, I: Impact of seven definitions on prevalence rates in a community survey. *Am. J. Psychiatry*, 140, 1309.
14. BRANCHEY, L., DAVIS, W., & LIEBER, C. S. (1984). Alcoholism in Vietnam and Korea veterans: A long-term follow-up. *Alcoholism*, 8, 572.
15. BREWSTER, J. (1986). Prevalence of alcohol and other drug problems among physicians. *JAMA*, 255, 1913.
16. BRODY, J. A. (1982). Aging and alcohol abuse. *J. Am. Geriatr. Soc.*, 30, 123.
17. BUTLER, J. T. (1982). Early adolescent alcohol consumption and self-concept, social class, and knowledge of alcohol. *J. Stud. Alcohol*, 43, 603.
18. CADORET, R. J., O'GORMAN, T. W., THROUGHTON, E., & HEYWOOD, E. (1985). Alcoholism and antisocial personality. *Arch. Gen. Psychiatry*, 42, 161.
19. CALIFANO, J. A., JR. (1982). *The 1982 report on drug abuse and alcoholism*. New York: Warner Books.
20. CHRISTOPHERSON, V. A., ESHER, N. C., & BAINTON, B. R. (1984). Reasons for drinking among the elderly in rural Arizona. *J. Stud. Alcohol*, 45, 417.

132   MODERN PERSPECTIVES IN PSYCHOSOCIAL PATHOLOGY

21. COUNCIL ON SCIENTIFIC AFFAIRS (1986). Alcohol and the driver. *JAMA, 255*, 522.
22. DONAHUE, R. P., ABBOTT, R. D., REED, D. M., & YANO, K. (1986). Alcohol and hemorrhagic stroke. *JAMA, 255*, 2311.
23. DONOVAN, J. M. (1986). An etiologic model of alcoholism. *Am. J. Psychiatry, 143*, 1.
24. EDWARDS, G., ARIF, A., & HODGSON, R. (1982). Nomenclature and classification of drug and alcohol related problems: A shortened version of a WHO memorandum. *Br. J. Addict, 77*, 3.
25. EL-GUEBALY, N., & OFFORD, D. (1977). The offspring of alcoholics: A critical review. *Am. J. Psychiatry, 134*, 357.
26. EWARDS, A. M., WOLFE, R., MOLL, P., & HARBURG, E. Psychosocial and behavioral factors differentiating past drinkers and lifelong abstainers. *Am. J. Public Health, 76*, 68.
27. FAMULARO, R., STONE, K., & POPPER, C. (1985). Pre-adolescent alcohol abuse and dependence. *Am. J. Psychiatry, 142*, 1187.
28. FLASHER, L., & MAISTO, S. A. (1984). A review of theory and research on drinking patterns among Jews. *J. Nerv. Ment. Dis., 172*, 596.
29. FLAVIN, D. J., & FRANCES, R. J. (1987). Risk-taking behavior, substance abuse disorders, and the acquired immune deficiency syndrome. *Adv. Alcoholism, 6*(3), 23–31.
30. FRANCES, R. J., & ALLEN, M. H. (1985). The interaction of substance-use disorders with nonpsychotic psychiatric disorders. In R. Michels (Chairman, Ed. Board) & J. O. Cavenar, Jr. (Ed.), *Psychiatry*, Vol. 1 (Chap. 42, pp. 1–13). Philadelphia: Lippincott, Basic Books.
31. FRANCES, R. J., FRANKLIN, J., & FALVIN, D. K. (1987). Suicide and alcoholism. *Am. J. Drug Alcohol Abuse, 13*(3), 327–341.
32. FRANCES, R. J., TIM, S., & BUCKY, S. (1980). Studies of familial and non-familial alcoholism. *Arch. Gen. Psychiatry, 37*, 564.
33. FRAUMENI, J. F., JR., (1982). Epidemiology of cancer. In J. B. Wyngaarden & L. H. Smith (Eds.), *Cecil's textbook of medicine* (16th ed.). Philadelphia: Saunders.
34. GALLANT, D. M. (1982). Alcohol and driving: Changing the laws. *Alcoholism, 6*, 280.
35. GERSTEIN, D. (1984). Alcohol policy: Preventive options. In L. Grimspoon (Ed.), *Psychiatry update, vol. III*. Washington, DC: American Psychiatric Press.
36. GOODMAN, R. A., MERCY, J. A., LOYA, F., ROSENBERG, M. L., SMITH, J. C., ALLEN, N. H., VARGAS, L., & KOLTS, R. (1986). Alcohol use and interpersonal violence: Alcohol detected in homicide victims. *Am. J. Public Health, 76*, 144.
37. GOSTASON, R. (1985). Psychiatric illness among the mentally retarded. *Acta Psychiatr. Scand., 71*(Suppl.), 318.
38. GREENBERG, M. R., CAREY, G. W., & POPPER, F. J. (1985). External causes of death among young, white Americans. *N. Engl. J. Med., 313*, 1482.
39. HALLDIN, J. (1985). Alcohol consumption and alcoholism in an urban population in central Sweden. *Acta Psychiatr. Scand., 71*, 128.
40. HEARST, N., NEWMAN, T. B., & HULLEY, S. B. (1986). Delayed effects of the military draft on mortality: A randomized natural experiment. *N. Engl. J. Med., 314*, 620.
41. HEDEBOE, J., CHARLES, A. V., NIELSEN, J., GRYMER, F., MOLLER, B. N., MOLLER-MADSON, B., & JENSEN, S. E. T. (1985). Interpersonal violence: Patterns in a Danish community. *Am. J. Public Health, 75*, 651.
42. HELZER, J. E., CANINO, G. J., HWU, H., BLAND, R. C., NEWMAN, S., & YEH, E. (1986). Alcoholism: A cross-national comparison of population surveys with the DIS. In R. M. Rose and J. Barrett (Eds.), *Alcoholism: A medical disorder*. New York: Raven Press, 1986.
43. HERR, B. M., & PETTINATI, H. M. (1984). Long-term outcome in working and homemaking alcoholic women. *Alcoholism, 8*, 576.
44. HESSELBROCK, M. N., MEYER, R. E., & KEENER, J. J. (1985). Psychopathology in hospitalized alcoholics. *Arch. Gen. Psychiatry, 42*, 1050.
45. ISRAELSTAM, S., & LAMBERG, S. (1983). Homosexuality as a cause of alcoholism: A historical review. *Int. J. Addict, 18*, 1085.

46. JOHNSON, R. P., & CONNELLY, J. C. (1981). Addicted physicians. *JAMA*, 245, 253.
47. KLATSKY, A. L., SIEGELAUB, A. B., LANDY, C., & FRIEDMAN, G. D. (1983). Racial patterns of alcoholic beverage use. *Alcoholism*, 7, 372.
48. KROLL, J., CAREY, K., HAGEDORN, D., FIRE DOG, P., & BENAVIDES, E. (1986). A survey of homeless adults in urban emergency shelters. *Hosp. Commun. Psychiatry*, 37, 283.
49. LIEBER, C. S. (1982). A public health approach for the control of the disease of alcoholism. *Alcoholism*, 6, 171.
50. LORANGER, A. N., & TULIS, E. H. (1985). Family history of alcoholism in borderline personality disorder. *Arch. Gen. Psychiatry*, 42, 153.
51. MARTIN, R. L., CLONINGER, C. R., GUZE, S. B., & CLAYTON, P. J. (1985). Mortality in a follow-up of 500 psychiatric outpatients, I: Total mortality. *Arch. Gen. Psychiatry*, 42, 47.
52. MARTIN, R. L., CLONINGER, C. R., GUZE, S. B., & CLAYTON, P. J. (1985). Mortality in a follow-up of 500 psychiatric outpatients, II: Cause−Specific mortality. *Arch. Gen. Psychiatry*, 42, 58.
53. MAYNARD, A., & KENNAN, P. (1981). The economics of alcohol abuse. *Br. J. Addict*, 76, 339.
54. MENDENHALL, C. L., ROSELLE, G. A., GROSSMAN, C. J., ROUSTER, S. D., & WEESNER, R. E. (1986). False positive tests for HTLV-III antibodies in alcoholic patients with hepatitis. *N. Engl. J. Med.*, 314, 921.
55. MILLER, R. W., & McKAY, F. W. (1985). Alcohol-associated teenage deaths: United States, 1980. *JAMA*, 254, 3308.
56. MILLER, S. I., & TUCHFELD, B. S. (1986). Adult children of alcoholics. *Hosp. Commun. Psychiatry*, 37, 235.
57. MYERS, J. K., WEISSMAN, M. M., TISCHLER, G. L., HOLZER, C. E. III, LEAF, P. J., ORVASCHEL, H., ANTHONY, J. C., BOYD, J. H., BURKE, J. D., JR., KRAMER M., & STOLTZMAN, R. (1984). Six-month prevalence of psychiatric disorders in three communities. *Arch. Gen. Psychiatry*, 41, 958.
58. MYERS, T. (1982). Alcohol and violent crime re-examined: Self-reports from two subgroups of Scottish male prisoners. *Br. J. Addict.*, 77, 399.
59. NARDI, P. M. (1982). Alcoholism and homosexuality: A theoretical perspective. *J. Homosex.*, 7, 9.
60. NIVEN, R. G. (1984). Alcoholism − A problem in perspective. *JAMA*, 252, 1912.
61. PAINE, H. (1977). Attitudes and patterns of alcohol use among Mexican Americans: Implications for service delivery. *J. Stud. Alcohol*, 38, 544.
62. PARK, J. Y., HUANG, Y-H., NAGOSHI, C. T., YUEN, S., JOHNSON, R. C., CHING, C. A., & BOWMAN, K. S. (1984). The flushing response to alcohol use among Koreans and Taiwanese. *J. Stud. Alcohol*, 45, 481.
63. PENICK, E. (1984). Familial alcoholism and other psychiatric disorders. Presented at APA Annual Meeting, Dallas, TX.
64. PLANT, M. A. (1979). Occupations, drinking patterns and alcohol-related problems: Conclusions from a follow-up study. *Br. J. Addict*, 74, 267.
65. PLANT, M. A., PECK, D. F., & STUART, R. (1982). Self-reported drinking habits and alcohol-related consequences amongst a cohort of Scottish teenagers. *Br. J. Addict*, 77, 75.
66. RICHARDS, W. (1986). Presented at APA Workshop Alcoholism: Future in Psychiatry, Washington, DC.
67. ROBINS, L. N., HELZER, J. E., WEISSMAN, M. M., ORVASCHEL, H., GRUENBERG, E., BURKE, J. D., JR., & REGIER, D. A. (1984). Lifetime prevalence of specific psychiatric disorders in three sites. *Arch. Gen. Psychiatry*, 41, 949.
68. ROOM, R. (1984). The World Health Organization and alcohol control. *Br. J. Addict*, 79, 85.
69. ROOM, R., & COLLINS, G. (Eds.) (1983). *Alcohol and disinhibition: Nature and meaning of the link.* NIAAA Research Monograph 12, Washington, DC.

70. ROSENBAUM, M., & BENNETT, B. (1986). Homicide and depression. *Am. J. Psychiatry*, *143*, 367.
71. ROSETT, H. L., & WEINER, L. (1984). Alcohol and the fetus: A clinical perspective. New York: Oxford University Press.
72. ROUNSAVILLE, B. J., SPITZER, R. L., & WILLIAMS, J. B. W. (1986). Proposed changes in DSM-III substance use disorders: Description and rationale. *Am. J. Psychiatry*, *143*, 463.
73. SCHUCKIT, M. A. (1985). The clinical implications of primary diagnostic groups among alcoholics. *Arch. Gen. Psychiatry*, *42*, 1043.
74. SCHUCKIT, M. A. (1986). Genetic and clinical implications of alcoholism and affective disorder. *Am. J. Psychiatry*, *143*, 140.
75. SCHUCKIT, M. A., LI, T-K., CLONINGER, C. R., & DEITRICH, R. A. (1985). Genetics of alcoholism. *Alcoholism*, *9*, 475.
76. SHORE, J. H., & KOFOED, L. (1984). Community intervention in the treatment of alcoholism. *Alcoholism*, *8*, 151.
77. SMITH, E. M., CLONINGER, R., & BRADFORD, S. (1983). Predictors of mortality in alcoholic women: A prospective follow-up study. *Alcoholism*, *7*, 237.
78. SMITH, J. W. (1983). Diagnosing alcoholism. *Hosp. Commun. Psychiatry*, 34, 1017.
79. SOKOLOW, L., WELTE, J., HYNES, G., & LYONS, J. (1981). Multiple substance use by alcoholics. *Br. J. Addict.*, *76*, 147.
80. VAILLANT, G. E. (1984). Introduction: Alcohol abuse and dependence. In L. Grinspoon (Ed.), *Psychiatry update, Vol. III*. Washington, DC: American Psychiatric Press.
81. WARHEIT, G. J., & BUHL AUTH, J. (1985). Epidemiology of alcohol abuse in adulthood. In R. Michels (Chairman, Editorial Board) and J. O. Cavenar, Jr. (Ed.) *Psychiatry*. Philadelphia: Lippincott, Basic Books.
82. WEISSMAN, M. M., MYERS, J. K., TISCHLER, G. L., HOLZER, C. E., LEAF, P. J., ORVASCHEL, H., & BRODY, J. A. (1985). Psychiatric disorders (DSM-III) and cognitive impairment among the elderly in a U.S. urban community. *Acta Psychiatr. Scand.*, *71*, 366.
83. WEST, L. J., MAXWELL, D. S., NOBLE, E. P., & SOLOMON, D. H. (1984). Alcoholism. *Ann. Intern. Med.*, *100*, 405.
84. Alcohol-related traffic fatalities during Christmas and New Year holidays—United States, 1978-1984 (1985). Morbidity and Mortality Weekly Report, *34*(49), Dec. 13.
85. Institute of Medicine (1980). Report of a study: Alcoholism, alcohol abuse and related problems: Opportunities for research. Washington, DC: National Academy Press.
86. Public health aspects of international production, marketing and distribution of alcoholic beverages. Report of an "informal consultation" held by the World Health Organization (WHO Geneva), June 10-12, 1981 (1982). *Br. J. Addict.*, *77*, 349.
87. DSM-III-R in Development (1985). Workgroup to Revise DSM-III, American Psychiatric Association (R. Spitzer, Chairman), p. 44.

8

PATHOLOGICAL GAMBLING

RICHARD A. MCCORMICK, PH.D.

Assistant Chief, Psychology Service,
Cleveland Veterans Administration Medical Center,
Cleveland, Ohio

and

LUIS F. RAMIREZ, M.D.

Associate Professor of Psychiatry,
Case Western Reserve University School of Medicine,
Cleveland, Ohio

OVERVIEW

Increasing Exposure to Gambling

Gambling has always been a common recreational activity in most societies, but in recent years we have seen a proliferation of gambling options in Western society. The number of locations available for legalized casino gambling has significantly increased in the last 10 years. Sports betting, which has been estimated to exceed 70 billion dollars annually, has expanded to include legalized off-track betting stations. Publicly administered lotteries have become a popular means for national and state or territorial-level governmental bodies to generate revenue. Lotteries are now conducted by most states in the United States, where wagering exceeds 10 billion dollars annually.

This increase in legalized gambling opportunities has been accompanied by tremendous increases in the media coverage of gambling. The lastest multimillion-dollar lottery winner is a common front-page story in most major metropolitan newspapers. The gambling-related difficulties of national sports figures fill the sports pages. Debates about the viability and advisability of legalized casinos in declining recreational centers provide additional media forums for exposure to gambling options. Motion pictures, made-for-television movies, and magazine feature articles capitalize on the revitalized public interest in gambling. Much of this publicity concentrates, even if inadvertently, on the glamour and excitement that accompany the gambling experience.

There have also been significant increases in the more "hidden" forms of gambling. The apparently benign, often church-sponsored bingo games gross unexpectedly large revenues and are increasing in number and frequency. Bingo is legal in 43 states in the United States. In one state alone (Ohio) 1985 proceeds exceeded 200 million dollars. The volatile commodities, futures, and stock markets have become a "game" that is increasingly popular with the more affluent gambler. Often those who use these volatile monetary markets do not label their behavior as gambling.

Definition and Scope of Pathological Gambling

Pathological gambling is defined in DSM-III-R as a "chronic and progressive failure to resist impulses to gamble, and gambling behavior that compromises, disrupts, or damages personal, family, or vocational pursuits" (p. 324) (1). Increases in the prevalence of pathological gambling parallel the increase in public exposure to gambling. A formal study by the U.S. government, the report by the Commission on the Review of the National Policy Toward Gambling (2), estimated that there were over 1.1 million pathological gamblers in the United States. It is likely that this number has continued to climb as more people have been exposed to expanding opportunities to gamble. A recent reevaluation of the Commission's 1978 data indicated that its final estimate of the incidence of the problem may have seriously underestimated the problem (3). The impact of pathological gambling goes well beyond the identified patient. Family and friends are pulled into the whirlpool of this deepening problem. Employers are also acutely affected, with the pathological gambler using funds embezzled from his employer to maintain his addiction. The clinician needs to be aware of the likelihood of underdiagnosing or failing to identify the problem, particularly in its early stages. This is partly due to a lack of familiarity on the part of clinicians, and partly to the denial and mislabeling of the problem by patients and their significant others. Pathological gambling is often a concomitant syndrome present with other psychopathology. It is commonly seen with depression (4) and substance abuse (5). These more commonly recognized emotional disorders may be the presenting problem that the clinician instinctively focuses on, failing to assess or recognize the early signs of pathological gambling.

SELECTED SUMMARY OF CURRENT LITERATURE

Much of the literature devoted to personality studies of pathological gamblers is in the form of case reports and clinical descriptions. It was Freud (6) himself who analyzed the personality of the Russian novelist Dostoevsky, a notorious casino gambler. Psychoanalytically oriented writers have subsequently described the unconscious drives and compulsive tendencies of the gambler (7, 8) in an effort to demonstrate that gambling has symbolic significance. Bergler (7) has carefully synthesized his conclusions based on observations of a series of patients seen in therapy, noting that gamblers search for a sensation or mood which seems to be more important than whether they win or lose. He focused heavily on themes of anger and aggression. Themes of narcissism (9) and depression have also frequently characterized the earlier literature. More recently, the importance of depression and significant traumatic events in the life of the gambler has been highlighted (10).

There have also been a limited number of studies examining the personalities of pathological gamblers through the use of standardized personality tests. Utilizing the Minnesota Multiphasic Personality Inventory (MMPI), investigators have found that pathological gamblers generally have elevated scores on scales measuring depression, anxiety, hyperactivity, and poor impulse control (11–13). Investigators using other personality measures have found gamblers to be relatively high on measures of achievement, exhibitionism, aggressiveness, and narcissism (14, 15).

The addictive qualities of chronic gambling have been reported and accepted as characteristic by many writers (e.g., Ref. 16). Moran (17), in his studies of large cohorts of gamblers, has made special note of their psychological dependence on gambling.

An in-depth sociological study authored by Lesieur (18) offers the reader excellent insight into the general personality characteristics of the pathological gambler. This study highlights the impulsivity, manipulation, and high energy level often characteristic of gamblers. Lesieur gives a vivid account of the deteriorating spiral of decreasing psychological alternatives to gambling, where the gambler comes to see gambling not as the cause of his problem, but as the only possible "solution" for regaining what he has lost.

Literature on the treatment of the pathological gambler is sparse.

Bergler (7) claimed a 75% success rate among the gamblers treated in his practice, although no objective documentation is offered. Behavior therapists have claimed moderately good to poor results, in small samples of gamblers, with aversive conditioning (19, 20), imaginal desensitization (21), and in situ desensitization (22). Limited studies have supported the efficacy of specialized, broadly based treatment programs for pathological gamblers (23, 24).

THE ETIOLOGY AND DEVELOPMENT OF THE DISORDER

Pathological gambling is a complex disorder in which a number of variables interact. Figure 1 presents, in schematic form, a model for the dynamic interaction of key variables in the development of the addictive process. This schematic will be utilized in our discussion of the development of the disorder, its assessment, and its treatment.

Hereditary Vulnerability

The model recognizes the role of inherited vulnerability as a potential contributing factor in the development of pathological gambling. Evidence for the strength of this factor is at this time indirect. Studies of the families of pathological gamblers indicate a high incidence of depression in their relatives (15). Approaching familiar patterns of depression in gambling from the other perspective, Clayton (25) reported unexpected high rates of compulsive gamblers in the relatives of patients with affective disorders. These relationships between pathological gambling and depression parallel the frequently documented relationship between substance abuse and depression, in studies of both substance abusers (26, 27) and their relatives (28, 29). While research has suggested links between serotonergic (30) and noradrenergic (31) markers and depression in samples of clinically depressed patients, studies of biological markers in pathological gamblers are just beginning. Studies of sensation seekers, a more general category, which often includes gamblers and drug abusers, have found low levels of monoamine oxidase (MAO) and cerebrospinal fluid norepinephrine, as well as elevations in urinary 4-methoxy-3-hydroxy phenylglycol (MHPG) (32). In a related finding Brown et al. (33) reported lower cerebrospinal fluid 5-hydroxytryptamine (CSF-5-HT) and elevated CSF-MHPG in a sample of nonalcoholic subjects with personality disorders characterized by impulsivity and aggressiveness.

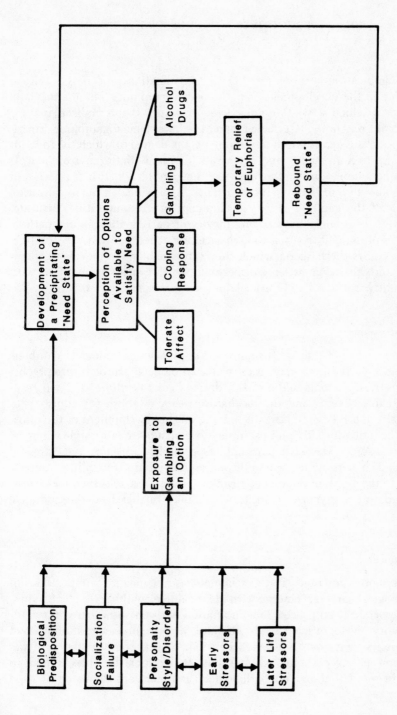

Figure 1. Interaction of variables in the development of the addictive process.

Socialization

It has been our experience that the socialization process is a critical variable in the development of pathological gambling. The manner and degree to which a well-organized set of values is internalized plays a significant role in the later development of pathological gambling. Equally important is ego strength development, the degree to which the individual learns to competently and effectively interact with the environment. It is very common to find in the history of the gambler a well-ingrained set of beliefs about his or her own incompetence. Also critical in the socialization process of the gambler is the development of a "competitive" attitude. Gamblers commonly have a long history of participation in competitive sports. For many it seems as though excelling at competition, very early in life, becomes the basis on which they subsequently evaluate both themselves and others. Their sense of personal worth is heavily enmeshed with competitive successes and the acclaim that these successes provide.

Life Stressors

We have found that for a significant number of pathological gamblers the role of early-life stressors is critical. Pathological gamblers often report highly stressful events in their lives, dating back to childhood. Their reaction to these events and the mechanisms they establish for adjusting to their aftermath have significant bearing on the development of the disorder. The individual may, for example, develop a personality style where he or she assumes excessive personal responsibility for negative, stressful events. This personality style follows the individual through life, contributing to the depth of depressive reactions in response to subsequent stressors and the emergence of guilt, which may further feed the addictive cycle.

Personality Styles

The model portrayed in the schematic is not meant to imply that all pathological gamblers emerge with identical personality styles. The nature of the socialization process in combination with potential hereditary vulnerability and significant environmental factors can lead to a number of personality styles or disorders which help define some of the subtypes common among pathological gamblers. It is critical for the clinician to keep in mind that not all pathological gamblers are the same or even similar on some of these critical dimensions. The personality styles we find to be common and characteristic of a significant number of pathological gamblers include the following.

Avoidant personality style. Gamblers with this personality style present, in times of crisis, with significant symptoms of depression and anxiety. Their case histories often reveal traumatic experiences dating back to their early years. They tend to handle their emotions through repression and denial. They communicate very little about their emotional needs and tend to minimize the intensity of their feelings. Anger is seldom experienced directly. Symptoms of anxiety disorder, including nightmares and intrusive thoughts, may be present, but are seldom volunteered. They experience guilt and remorse, although these feelings generally do little to alter their gambling behavior. Their self-concept is poor and they tend to undervalue their accomplishments and see themselves as underachievers. Patients with this personality style often have periods of their life where they have displayed good coping skills and have acted responsibly. It may, for example, happen that they have extended periods of good vocational adjustment and often still have significant others who are firmly committed to their welfare despite heavy strains on the relationship. While they have periods of significant impulsivity, they tend to have the capacity, at least, for maintaining control. They generally have strong, in fact often overly rigid, value systems. The history may reveal a hard-driving father, who was never satisfied with the patient.

Undersocialized personality style. This personality style typifies the inadequately socialized pathological gambler. These patients tend to have a weak internal value system. They seem to be continually evaluating what other people want, in an attempt to at least take on the appearance of ascribing to these external, often fleeting values. Impulsivity is marked and generally constant across the years and across all the dimensions of their lives. They do not display significant affect, although they may be situationally depressed and discontented. They tend to be verbal, socially adept at a superficial level, and manipulative. Rationalization and projection are used heavily to deflect responsibility for their frequent failures. They project their own mistrust onto others and are constantly on the defense.

Narcissistic personality style. Pathological gamblers in this subtype tend to be verbal and to manage social situations in what often seems to be a commanding manner. Their primary focus is on their own personal needs, and while they can be charming at times, those who come in close contact with them eventually tend to feel used. They are boastful and have an unrealistically high evaluation of themselves. They concentrate on their past successes and learn very little from their failures. These gamblers repeatedly act and speak as though they were "entitled" to whatever they wish or dream of. Thus they feel entitled to the esteem of others regardless of how they behave. They feel entitled to win at any endeavor they undertake regardless of the rules of chance or probabilities. They are constantly striving to be, or appear, superior, in an attempt to compensate for feelings of inferiority and emptiness. This striving results in exhibitionism and unreasonable demands for attention. Common defenses are projection, splitting, devaluing, and hypercriticalness of others, which also serve to avoid intimacy. Sensation seeking is a cardinal feature of this personality type. These patients are easily excited and easily bored.

The angry-aggressive personality style. Pathological gamblers with this personality style are less likely to appear for treatment. These patients have a marked history of angry outbursts, at times including assaultive behavior. Blame for all of their repeated failures is projected outward. They are distrustful of other people and are instinctively interpreting the actions of others in terms of their expectation that people will attempt to take advantage of them. Between angry outbursts they tend to be more passively aggressive. They will freely discuss their past experiences, as though almost to "warn" the interviewer of their potential power and volatility. Significant trauma may be interwoven among their life experiences. They tend to be opinionated and, although less so than the narcissistic gambler, hold themselves in high esteem. Unlike the narcissistic gambler, they can form limited intimate relationships.

The Addictive Cycle

The addictive cycle for the pathological gambler is depicted on the right portion of the schematic. The gambler brings to the cycle the personality and biochemical changes that have been the result of earlier experience. Another necessary condition, of course, is the exposure to gambling as an option. The pathological gambler, most often early in life, has learned that gambling causes some perceived psychological and/or physiological changes, of at least a temporary nature. The pathological gambler then enters a precipitating need state which is brought on by a combination of internal and external cues and events. This need state most often involves some combination of dysphoria, anxiety, and boredom. For example, the "avoidant" gambler may encounter a new failure experience. His tendency would be to ascribe responsibility for the failure to himself. This process would lead to an increase in his negative self-concept, guilt, and depression. Often the depression would be of an agitated variety. The gambler may not be able to articulate these feelings and would merely perceive an unpleasant negative affective state. Another example would be the "narcissistic" gambler who finds little satisfaction with the usual experiences of life. He experiences a subjective state of boredom which is unpleasant. The boredom may reflect, at an unconscious level, underlying feelings of inadequacy. All the gambler perceives is an unpleasant, even overwhelming need for excitement and stimulation.

As the need state increases in intensity, the pathological gambler intuitively assesses the options available to satisfy or ameliorate the unpleasant need state. As the gambler has descended into the spiral of decreasing options, coping, through problem solving or changing his pattern of behavior, may no longer be viable. For example, if the gambler has gambled away large embezzled sums of money, approaching family, friends, or his employer may no longer be a reasonable option. Gamblers vary in the number of options that they see available. This variability has to do both with their prior experience and with the particular events that precipitate the current need state. The pathological gambler increasingly perceives gambling as the best option available. The anticipation and experience of gambling do in fact provide temporary relief for the precipitating need state. This relief is likely both a psychological and physiological phenomenon, since, for example, high-arousal activities have been documented to cause catecholamine changes that have a potentially antidepressant effect. Some patients during the gambling experience will experience an altered state of consciousness that includes euphoria, suggesting the possibility that internal endorphin secretion is occurring as a result of the high arousal and release. Certainly, for many gamblers the experience of gambling allows them to psychologically detach from awareness thoughts of any events other than gambling. This has the effect of being a mechanism for massive repression and denial.

The relief that gambling provides, whether psychological, physiological, or a combination of both, is temporary. Gamblers often report that following this temporary relief there is a rebound of the need state, which is characterized by an increase in the negative affect. This can occur both through psychological mechanisms, since denial and avoidance tend to merely compound the concrete problem at hand, as well as through physiological mechanisms, since the biological system may be thrown further out of balance by the temporary secretion of the endogenous chemicals which provide temporary relief. The gambler then is thrown back to the point of experiencing the need state that was the precipitant of the gambling behavior. The cycle thus continues and the gambling becomes compulsive. Amplification of the addictive cycle can be found in Custer's writings (34).

ASSESSMENT OF THE DISORDER

General Comments

When the patient with pathological gambling presents, multiple biophysical and environmental variables, and their interactions, must be considered. It has been our experience that pathological gamblers who seek treatment in an identified program for pathological gambling provide reliable information during the assessment phase, but when the patient is not coming to the practitioner specifically for treatment of pathological gambling, the clinician must bear in mind that denial and rationalization are hallmark defense mechanisms. The pathological gambler may deny to himself and to others that his gambling is a problem. Many relabel their behavior and deny that it is gambling at all, preferring to term it "investing" or a "profession." As with other addicted individuals, the pathological gambler is likely to project blame onto other individuals. It is important for the clinician conducting the assessment to listen empathically, but to be firm and clear. The story that the pathological gambler presents, even without embellishment, can be so colorful as to be seductive. Although details of the gambling behavior are important, the clinician must be able to concentrate on the core personality variables and the process of the addictive cycle.

Gambling History

It is important that the assessment include a thorough gambling history. When the pathological gambler is not using denial, this portion of the assessment is often the least threatening for the patient. The clinician must be able to identify all the forms of gambling, even if mislabeled as something other than gambling, practiced by the patient. The frequency, intensity (in terms of both time and financial investment), and duration of each form of gambling need to be documented, as does the degree to which the gambling behavior affects other major portions of the patient's life, including family life and vocation. Equally important is a careful assessment of the duration and nature of nongambling behavior, since many pathological gamblers will display a cyclical pattern of pathological gambling. The manner in which the patient accumulates the money necessary to continue gambling also needs to be documented.

Having established the concrete parameters of the gambling behavior, the assessment should next focus on the patient's subjective experience during gambling. Patients report significant mood and perceptual changes as they begin to anticipate the gambling encounter. As they progress through the anticipation phase to the action phase of a particular gambling experience, patients may report a dreamlike, or even euphoric, subjective experience. The patient's perception is generally focused exclusively on the anticipated and ongoing gambling experience during both the anticipation and action phases. Probing and questioning are often necessary to assist the patient to actually put into words the changes in mood state that are experienced. Patients are often best able to describe these feelings through analogies or metaphors and can be productively encouraged to do so.

The Assessment of Biophysical Factors

Since pathological gambling is a stressful life-style, a complete physical examination is critical. A high incidence of cardiovascular and stress-related disorders is to be expected. The identification of psychosomatic conditions, in addition to its obvious medical necessity, also provides supportive data for the assessment of personality style.

A thorough medication and psychoactive substance history is required. Gambling and alcohol use, particularly in the case of the casino gambler, are mutually supported by the gambling environment. The high incidence of alcoholism or other substance abuse among pathological gamblers (5) should sensitize the clinician to the likelihood of actual or incipient substance abuse problems.

It is not uncommon for the pathological gambler to have been treated in the past, with medication, for depression or anxiety. During the denial phase of gambling these may be the symptoms that are presented to the practitioner, who, failing to assess the pathological nature of the gambling, provides symptomatic treatment. The response of the patient to the medication, considered in the context of the patient's continued gambling, can provide important data on the degree and nature of the depression. The high incidence of affective disorders among pathological gamblers justifies the use of the dexamethasone suppression test in order to provide further information on the nature of the depression. The clinician should be aware of the conflicting results found with the dexamethasone suppression test in alcoholics (35, 36) and must consider the patient's possible concomitant substance abuse in assessing the clinical utility of this test with a particular patient.

When the patient presents with either depression or significant hyperactivity, it is important to assess the possibility of endocrine dysfunction. We have identified, over the course of years of providing treatment in a structured program for pathological gamblers, a small number of cases where undiagnosed hypothyroidism was a contributing factor to the patient's pathological gambling cycle. Endocrine treatment of the hypothyroidism had a demonstrably facilitative affect on the treatment process.

A brief neuropsychological testing battery is useful. In the case of the pathological gambler with concomitant substance abuse, such testing may identify cognitive deficiencies and slippage which need to be considered in the treatment and recovery process. An assessment of the patient's intellectual aptitude is also helpful to the clinician, since gamblers, because of their verbal skills, will often seem to be more intellectually superior than they in fact are able to demonstrate on structured, carefully normed tests. Objective measurement of intellectual capacity can be important in long-range planning for the patient's rehabilitation.

The Assessment of Personality Dimensions

Easily administered paper-and-pencil personality inventories offer a unique contribution in the assessment of the pathological gambler. The Minnesota Multiphasic Personality Inventory (MMPI) provides information that is extremely useful in subtyping pathological gamblers. Gamblers fitting the avoidant personality type, outlined earlier, show large elevations on MMPI scales measuring anxiety and depression. While they have elevations on scales measuring impulsivity and acting out that are higher than the normative group for the test, they are relatively low compared to other gamblers. Elevations on scales measuring social introversion are common, even if the avoidant gambler seems, superficially, to be fairly extroverted.

Undersocialized gamblers show little, if any, elevation on scales measuring affect. They have marked elevation on scales measuring impulsivity, hyperactivity, lack of self-control, and extroversion.

The angry-aggressive gambler will have high elevations on scales measuring mistrust, suspiciousness, and impulsivity and may also have elevations on scales measuring affect, although generally at a lower level than the avoidant gambler.

The California Personality Inventory (CPI), which measures personality dimensions of a nonpathological nature, can also be of unique use. The CPI provides measures on dimensions that are directly relevant to the treatment process, such as responsibility, self-control, and socialization.

A semistructured interview can be used to fully assess the socialization history and the development of the patient's value system. Pathological gamblers are generally responsive to questions that probe their beliefs and values, as well as the origin of these beliefs. In the course of the interview it is important to identify the dominant figures in the patient's past history. These are often personages other than their parents. This portion of the assessment also has therapeutic value since the pathological gambler often has little awareness of his inherent value system and of the factors responsible for its development. The introjects of the pathological gambler are often quite strong and are, consequently, readily brought to awareness by probing. While assessing the socialization history of the gambler, it is important to pay attention to the role that competition and competitive values have played. Often the gambler's self-worth is heavily enmeshed with competitive successes. Many gamblers have had few opportunities to develop a sense of their worth that is separate from competition and its outcome.

It is recommended that special focus also be placed on the assessment of narcissistic tendencies. Psychometric scales are available, including a specialized scale from the MMPI (37) and the Narcissistic Personality Inventory (38). An in-depth interview focusing on the patient's tendencies toward overvaluing his worth and eliciting stories of how he "manages" people can also provide insights in this regard.

The Assessment of Significant Life Events

A high incidence of significant life trauma among pathological gamblers and the possible significance of gambling as a means to cope with traumatic memories reinforce the value of carefully assessing the traumatic history of the patient. The written autobiography (39) can be a useful tool in this portion of the assessment. Requiring the autobiography to be written has special advantage with the pathological gambler since many pathological gamblers have overlearned the skill of distorting events during verbal recall. Requiring the gambler to use a written medium seems to have value in breaking through this pattern, at least for the motivated patient. Gamblers often spend extensive periods of time laboring over their autobiographies and gain considerable insight just through the process of writing it. A required format for the autobiography forces the gambler to track his lifeline and to highlight certain significant events at each point during the lifeline. Standardized instruments for the assessment of life trauma are also available (40). It is possible for the clinician to devise his own form which lists a menu of possible traumatic events, have the patient mark those which apply, and then rate each on subjective impact. It is important to obtain the subjective impact of the event since it is our common experience that the events that seem objectively most traumatic are not always the ones that have the greatest subjective impact on the pathological gambler. The interview with the patient should also probe carefully for the cardinal symptoms of post-traumatic stress disorder, including nightmares, intrusive thoughts, and a generalized avoidance of situations or stimuli that elicit recall of the trauma. The clinician's impressions during the interview process, while the traumatic history is being discussed, are an invaluable source of personal data. Often the facial expressions and body language of even the most constrictive gambler provide ready insight into the importance of this variable.

Assessment of the Addictive Cycle

The nature and depth of the addictive cycle, in the present, for the particular pathological gambler need to be understood. We recommend first identifying cues in the patient's perceptual field that seem to trigger gambling behavior. For some patients these are internal phenomena, which can be as vague as an unpleasant, restless boredom or an uneasy, unhappy feeling. For other gamblers there may be concrete outside stimuli, which include sights and sounds, approaches by friends, or angry interchanges with significant others. Once cues have been identified, it is important to assess the strength of potentially competing responses. This may include other addictive behaviors, such as substance abuse, or coping behaviors, such as problem solving, or other more benign avoidant behaviors, such as escapes to seclusion. For some gamblers what seem to be coping responses may also have an addictive quality. It is not unusual to find a workaholic tendency in the pathological gambler. Having assessed the nature and amount of money involved in the patient's gambling behavior, the cues, and the number of currently existing competing responses, it is then possible for the clinician to assess the patient's current stage in the spiral of decreasing options. Both the patient's perception of the options that are available and, based on his life circumstances, the realistic options that exist, even if not recognized clearly at that point by the patient, need to be considered. If earlier portions of the assessment have implicated negative affect (e.g., depression, emptiness, anxiety) or boredom as crucial variables, it is now necessary to assess the degree and duration of relief that gambling provides. It is then generally possible to understand the complete loop of the cycle.

Having carefully assessed the key variables noted above, it is then possible to individualize treatment to the needs of the gambler.

TREATMENT OF THE PATHOLOGICAL GAMBLER

Peer Counseling and Self-Help Groups

Recovering gamblers, who serve as peer counselors, have an important role in the overall treatment of the pathological gambler. For the dysthymic or avoidant gambler, they serve as valuable role models and sources of concrete advice and encouragement. For the undersocialized gambler, they are able to provide the confrontation and harsh feedback necessary, in a manner that is difficult for the pathological gambler to deflect. A good peer counselor is able to effectively read through manipulative patterns and to appropriately share his own life experiences and the lessons learned. However, it is important not to confuse the role of the peer counselor with that of a psychotherapist.

Gamblers Anonymous (GA) has a long history of successful intervention with many pathological gamblers. The stepwork of Gamblers Anonymous, a system for spiritual or psychological growth, appropriately focuses away from gambling behavior and toward the psychological steps necessary for effective recovery. The clinician needs to bear in mind, however, that Gamblers Anonymous meetings will vary greatly depending on the membership of the particular meeting. Gamblers Anonymous meetings may not have the degree of discipline that Alcoholics Anonymous meetings have. Consequently, particularly in the case of gamblers who possess internal self-control, the gambler may find the meetings difficult to tolerate. If the clinician is familiar with the character of a particular Gamblers Anonymous meeting and has done a thorough assessment of the personality dimensions of the particular gambler in treatment, he can carefully prepare the pathological gambler and highlight those aspects of the Gamblers Anonymous experience which are critical to that particular patient's recovery. The clinician can, simultaneously, frankly discuss those aspects of the Gamblers Anonymous experience which will be difficult to accept. In almost all cases, the Gamblers Anonymous experience is, on balance, a positive one for the pathological gambler. Careful preparation can help assure that the unpleasant, or, in some cases, even inappropriate, portions of the experience are not used by the gambler as an excuse to abandon the whole effort. Most gamblers need the support, the external feedback, and even the structure that Gamblers Anonymous provides for their lives during the recovery process.

Group and Individual Psychotherapy

Group psychotherapy has become an accepted mode of treatment for addicted and impulsive patients. Space considerations allow us to highlight only a few characteristics of pathological gamblers in psychotherapy and some of the most common themes with which the therapist must wrestle. Generally early on in the therapeutic relationship, the gambler will raise the issue of whether the therapist can really "understand" him since the therapist has never been a pathological gambler himself. The therapist needs not to become defensive or apologetic. It is often, in fact, advisable for the therapist to take a strong counterposition, as advised by Taber (41), and confront the gambler that the issue is not whether the therapist can understand the pathological gambler, but whether the pathological gambler can come to understand nongamblers. The gambler needs to understand that other people also face coming to grips with urgent impulses but have learned skills in deferring and moderating such impulses.

In the therapeutic process the irrational beliefs of the pathological gambler will emerge. These irrational beliefs can be arbitrarily divided into irrational beliefs regarding the external world and irrational beliefs regarding the self. The irrational beliefs regarding the external world include the belief that, in games of pure chance such as the lottery, the gambler can come out ahead in the long run, despite the large percentage of the pool extracted by the sponsor of the game. Another common irrational belief is that if you gamble long enough, things will have to turn your way and you will regain your losses. The irrational beliefs regarding the self are often similar to those of depressed individuals in general. They include beliefs of unworthiness, such as the belief that the gambler can only be cared about if he is able to bestow large monetary presents on those around him. Also common are irrational beliefs regarding the motives of others. The gambler may easily misinterpret the actions of others and their intent as being against him. The depressed gambler in particular will often tend to overascribe to himself blame for misfortunes and negative events in his life. Interestingly, and perhaps unexpectedly for those who have less experience with gamblers, the depressed gambler will often ascribe credit for his successes to outside forces. This tendency, of course, is much less common in the narcissistic gambler or the undersocialized gambler. The narcissistic gambler often has irrational beliefs about the self which border on grandiosity. He may believe that he has a "system" which makes him superior to the experts who own the game. He may harbor the irrational belief that he is a "professional" gambler, or that he is merely an "investor." Likewise he may believe that the money he embezzles is merely a "loan."

The irrational beliefs of the pathological gambler are often most effectively dealt with in a group therapy situation, where other gamblers can be of assistance in breaking through the irrational belief system. Gamblers are very effective in discerning and confronting the irrational beliefs of other people. The therapist must, of course, construct the framework in which beliefs are carefully extracted in the therapeutic group and examined in terms of reality. This involves dealing with extensive denial, at times supported by the majority of the group, and persevering toward uncovering the irrational basis of the gambler's position. The irrational beliefs of the depressed gambler that center around personal self-doubt can also be dealt with in a group setting. In this case it is also helpful to supplement the group with individual psychotherapy which is aimed at a more in-depth examination of the source of these irrational beliefs.

The therapist who is familiar with substance abusers in a group therapy situation is likely to find the pathological gambler more animated and aggressive than the average alcoholic. This is especially true in the case of the narcissistic or undersocialized gambler. During the therapy process, themes of "entitlement" are likely to emerge. The gambler tends to feel he is entitled to special treatment, entitled to win, and entitled to external respect regardless of his behavior. When the therapy is being conducted in a treatment milieu setting, the daily frictions of living together provide excellent "grist" for the therapeutic mill, particularly around themes of responsibility and entitlement. An issue as mundane as not excusing the gambler's lateness, if pursued appropriately, can uncover feelings of entitlement that can then be dealt with therapeutically. The narcissistic gambler can be expected to react to confrontation with disdain and aggression.

Structured facilitative techniques can be of use provided they are employed thoughtfully and are not overdone. Having the patient present his autobiography verbally in the group setting is a good example. Other techniques that focus the group on a theme are also useful. For example, techniques that place each gambler in a position of being the focus of feedback from the other members regarding his day-to-day behavior and demeanor can help break through deflection defenses. The purpose of such techniques when the group includes predominantly pathological gamblers is not so much to generate activity—this is hardly ever necessary—as to focus it.

Individual therapy and counseling certainly have their place in the treatment of the pathological gambler. In some cases the therapy can be short term with the goal of assisting the gambler in modifying certain aspects of his personality to make them more confluent with the recovery process. An example here would be the case of the overcontrolled pathological gambler who needs to modify, even if slightly, the degree to which he expresses emotion, particularly anger at the moment that the anger-producing event occurs. In this same example, the gambler might be helped to increase the amount of personal sharing that he does with intimate significant others. Longer-term therapy might be called for in other cases. One example of this need might be with the seriously depressed or avoidant gambler who requires considerable work in increasing his self-worth and in beginning to recognize his own internal responsibility both for the negative things that occur and for the positive successes he achieves. Such long-term therapy can be of assistance with the pathological gambler who, on assessment, clearly has a large gulf between his own expectations for himself and his own achievements. This gulf most often needs to be bridged through both a decrease, toward a more rational level, of his own expectations and more willingness to recognize his assets and accomplishments.

As noted in our literature review, psychoanalytic therapists have reported success with the individual treatment of the gambler. This is consistent with the assertions (e.g., Refs. 42, 43) that narcissism is a treatable personality disorder. The reader is particularly referred to the writings of Rosenthal (44) and Bergler (7).

Long-term supportive counseling may be called for in the case of the pathological gambler who has very little self-control and who does not have available to him, because of geographical and situational factors, a good GA sponsor or group to provide the constant external feedback necessary to maintain the recovery process. In this case counseling will not be aimed toward personality change as much as toward coping with reality issues and providing the gambler with early warning when he begins to slip.

Values Clarification

It is often helpful in the treatment of the pathological gambler to explicitly deal in a therapeutic manner with his value system. Particular needs for values clarification should be uncovered in the assessment process. It is especially important to consider values regarding competition and money, which, when central, underline the externalized nature of the gambler's value system. The gambler who is obsessed with competition tends to be constantly looking outward for direction, often because he has no real internalized personal set of values. Money, and all the externals it can buy, take on special value. The gambler needs to be helped to understand that for many individuals work, for example, can be more than just a means for obtaining money; it can actually be an end in itself and carry other satisfactions. During the values clarification process, the gambler can be helped to discover the historical source of his value system. Often this source is full of conflict, such as a parent with whom the gambler had a negative relationship. Modifying or instilling an internalized value system is a difficult, long process. The therapist may, at least, raise the gambler's awareness of the need and help him begin the process.

Pharmacological Treatment

Because of the tendency for many gamblers to either have a history of or be susceptible to other addictions, particularly substance abuse, the use of psychotropic medication should be judicious. While it is usually advisable to wait and determine if depression will lift with other therapeutic techniques, in selected cases, particularly where the assessment indicates long-standing depression which seems to either precede or cycle with the pathological gambling, antidepressants may be worth a trial. In the case of the severely hyperactive pathological gambler, lithium may be of significant assistance in slowing the gambler down to enable him to better engage in the therapeutic process and to deal, step by step, with the issues at hand (45). Again, a careful assessment is necessary to differentiate the usual high activity level associated with high-stimulation gambling from a bipolar process. Anxiolytics are, in our opinion, seldom called for and should be used sparingly, if at all.

Gambling, as is the case with other addictions, can easily occur in conjunction with other serious psychopathology. The psychotic gambler presents special treatment dilemmas. The assessment process must be thorough enough to carefully differentiate the misbeliefs of many gamblers from actual delusions. When a psychotic gambler does present, major tranquilizers are indicated.

Special Treatment Issues

Involvement of the spouse and family in treatment, and in the assessment process, is highly advised. The family are often involved in "buying the gambler out of his problem." When they do so, they implicitly support the gambler's belief that money is the solution. As is the case with the gambler, the family needs to be given a clearer understanding that the gambling behavior is the problem, not the lack of money that results from this behavior. They need to understand that the gambling is a deepening cycle that will not merely pass in time. Having accepted the reality of the seriousness of the gambler's problem, the family can be effectively integrated into the treatment process. Depending on the stability of the family member, they can be effective in providing ongoing monitoring for the pathological gambler outside of the therapeutic milieu. It is often necessary to deal in marital or family therapy with deep-seeded issues of anger and abandonment. The family also needs to look at their own set of values, since very often the family feeds into the gambler's belief that he is only highly regarded when he can bring home monetary gifts.

For many pathological gamblers, changes in life-style are advisable which go beyond a change in the family structure or family value system. For example, many pathological gamblers have moved toward vocations that involve high commissions rather than stable base salaries. Their vocational earnings then parallel in many ways the excitement of the gambling process. It is difficult for a gambler to maintain absence when he is still engaged in this vocational life-style. The gambler will also have to consider altering or supplementing his recreational life. The gambler's recreational life will have generally centered around competitive games and sports. Events of a more serene nature are often either alien or untried by the pathological gambler. The therapist can be of assistance in urging the gambler to at least experiment with other recreational options.

SUMMARY

In summary, we have attempted, within space limitations, to emphasize the importance of pathological gambling as a clinical entity in modern society. The problem is certainly growing, and if clinicians are alert, the number of identified cases will continue to rise. Specialized treatment programs have many advantages, although at this time they are few in number. They are generally able to provide for the networking of the gambler with community and peer group resources. Staff in established programs, which usually includes recovering individuals who serve as peer counselors, have considerable experience with the pathological gambler. Nevertheless, most pathological gamblers will continue to require treatment from sources outside of the established treatment programs. The clinician, especially the clinician who has some experience with addictive disorders in general, can provide effective and useful treatment. Such treatment must be based on a thorough assessment. We have attempted to highlight major areas that the assessment needs to cover. Treatment can then be designed differentially for the pathological gambler, focusing on the dimensions assessed. While many of our statements have by necessity been general in nature, it is important to reemphasize that pathological gamblers differ significantly from one another. The dimensions we have highlighted can help the clinician to identify clinically meaningful subtypes of pathological gamblers.

REFERENCES

1. American Psychiatric Association (1987). *Diagnostic and statistical manual of mental disorders* (third edition-revised). Washington, DC: Author.
2. Commission on the Review of the National Policy Toward Gambling (1976). *Gambling in America*. Washington, DC: Government Printing Office.
3. NADLER, L. B. (1985). The epidemiology of pathological gambling. *J. Gambling Behav.*, *1*, 35–50.
4. McCORMICK, R. A., RUSSO, A. M., RAMIREZ, L. F., & TABER, J. I. (1984). Affective disorders among pathological gamblers seeking treatment. *Am. J. Psychiatry*, *141*, 215–218.
5. RAMIREZ, L. F., McCORMICK, R. A., RUSSO, A. M., & TABER, J. I. (1983). Patterns of substance abuse in pathological gamblers undergoing treatment. *Addict. Behav.*, *8*, 425–428.
6. FREUD, S. (1975). Dostoevsky and parricide. In J. Halliday & P. Fuller (Eds.), *The psychology of gambling*. New York: Harper & Row. (Original work published 1928.)
7. BERGLER, E. (1958). *The psychology of gambling*. New York: International Universities Press.
8. FULLER, P. (1974). Gambling: A secular "religion" for the obsessional neurotic. In J. Halliday & P. Fuller (Eds.), *The psychology of gambling*. New York: Harper & Row.

9. FENICHEL, O. (1945). *The psychoanalytic theory of neurosis*. New York: Norton.
10. TABER, J. I., McCORMICK, R. A., & RAMIREZ, L. F. (1987). The prevalence and impact of major life stressors among pathological gamblers. *Int. J. Addict.*, *22*(1), 77–79.
11. GLEN, A. M. (1979, September). Personality research on pathological gamblers. Paper presented to the American Psychological Association, New York.
12. ROSTON, R. (1961). Some personality characteristics of male compulsive gamblers. Unpublished doctoral dissertation, University of California, Los Angeles.
13. LOWENFELD, B. H. (1979). Personality dimensions of a pathological gambler. Unpublished doctoral dissertation, Kent State University, Kent, OH.
14. MORAVEC, J. D., & MUNLEY, P. H. (1983). Psychological test findings on pathological gamblers. *Int. J. Addict.*, *18*, 1003–1009.
15. DELL, L. J., RYZICKA, M. F., & PALISI, A. T. (1981). Personality and other factors associated with the gambling addiction. *Int. J. Addict.*, *16*, 149–156.
16. ADLER, M., & GOLEMAN, D. (1969). Gambling and alcoholism: Symptom substitution and functional equivalents. *Q. J. Stud. Alcohol*, *30*, 733–736.
17. MORAN, E. (1975). Pathological gambling. *Br. J. Psychiatry*, *9*, 416–428.
18. LESIEUR, H. R. (1977). *The chase*. New York: Doubleday.
19. GOORNEY, A. B. (1968). The treatment of a compulsive horse race gambler by aversion therapy. *Br. J. Psychiatry*, *114*, 329–333.
20. SEAGER, C. P., POKORNY, N. R., & BLACK, D. (1968). Aversion therapy for compulsive gamblers. *Lancet*, *1*, 546.
21. McCONAGHY, N., ARMSSTRONG, M. S., BLASZCZYNSKI, A., & ALLCOCK, C. (1983). Controlled comparison of aversive therapy and imaginal desensitization in compulsive gambling. *Br. J. Psychiatry*, *141*, 366–372.
22. GREENBERG, A., & RANKIN, H. (1982). Compulsive gamblers in treatment. *Br. J. Psychiatry*, *140*, 364–366.
23. RUSSO, A. M., TABER, J. I., McCORMICK, R. A., & RAMIREZ, L. F. (1984). An outcome study of an inpatient treatment program for pathological gamblers. *Hosp. Commun. Psychiatry*, *36*, 823–827.
24. BLACKMAN, S., SIMONE, R. V., & THOMAS, D. R. (1986, April). Treatment of gamblers. (Letter to the editor). *Hosp. Commun. Psychiatry*, *37*(4), 404.
25. CLAYTON, P. J. (1981). The epidemiology of bipolar affective disorders. *Comp. Psychiatry*, *22*, 31–43.
26. POTTENGER, M., McKERNON, J., PATRIE, L. E., et al. (1978). The frequency and persistence of depressive symptoms in the alcohol abuser. *J. Nerv. Ment. Dis.*, *166*, 562–569.
27. ROUNSAVILLE, B. J., WEISSMAN, M., CRITS-CHRISTOPH, K., et al. (1982). Diagnosis and symptoms of depression in opiate addicts. *Arch. Gen. Psychiatry*, *39*, 151–156.
28. WINOKUR, G., REICH, T., RIMMER, J., et al. (1970). Alcoholism: III. Diagnosis and familial psychiatric illness in 259 alcoholic probands. *Arch. Gen. Psychiatry*, *23*, 104–111.
29. MERIKANGAS, K. R., WEISSMAN, M. M., PRUSOFF, B. A., et al. (1985). Depressives with secondary alcoholism; psychiatric disorders in offspring. *J. Stud. Alcohol*, *46*, 199–204.
30. VAN PRAAG, H. M. (1982, December). Neurotransmitters and CNS disease: Depression. *Lancet*, *II*(8310), 1259–1264.
31. SIEVER, J. L., UHDE, T. W., & MURPHY, D. L. (1984). Strategies for assessment of noradrenergic receptor function in patients with affective disorders. In R. M. Post & J. C. Ballenger (Eds.), *Neurobiology of mood disorders*. Baltimore: Williams & Wilkins.
32. ZUCKERMAN, M. (1985). Sensation seeking, mania, and monoamines. *Neuropsychobiology*, *13*, 121–128.
33. BROWN, G. L., GOODWIN, F. K., BALLENGER, J. C., et al. (1979). Aggression in humans correlates with cerebrospinal fluid amine metabolites. *Psychiatr. Res.*, *1*, 131–139.
34. CUSTER, R. L. (1982). Profile of the pathological gambler. *J. Clin. Psychiatry*, *45*, 35–38.

35. RAVI, S. D., DORUS, W., NAM, P. Y., et al. (1984). The dexamethasone suppression test and depression symptoms in early and late withdrawal from alcohol. *Am. J. Psychiatry, 141,* 1445–1448.
36. SWARTZ, C. M., & DUNNER, F. J. (1982). Dexamethasone suppression testing of alcoholics. *Arch. Gen. Psychiatry, 39,* 1309–1312.
37. SOLOMON, R. S. (1982). Validity of the MMPI narcissistic personality disorder scale. *Psychol. Rep., 50,* 463–466.
38. RASKIN, R. N., & HALL, C. S. (1979). A narcissistic personality inventory. *Psychol. Rep., 45,* 590.
39. ADKINS, B. J., TABER, J. I., & RUSSO, A. M. (1985). The spoken autobiography: A powerful tool in group psychotherapy. *Social Work, 30,* 435–439.
40. HOLMES, T. H., & RAHE, R. H. (1967). The Social Readjustment Rating Scale. *J. Psychosom. Res., 11,* 213–218.
41. TABER, J. I. (1981). Group psychotherapy with pathological gamblers. In W. R. Eadington (Ed.), *The gambling papers: Proceedings of the 1981 conference on gambling.* Reno, NV: University of Nevada, Reno.
42. HORWITZ, L. (1980). Group psychotherapy for borderline and narcissistic patients. *Bull. Menninger Clin., 44*(2), 181–200.
43. KERNBERG, O. (1982). Narcissism. In S. L. Gilman (Ed.), *Introducing psychoanalytic theory.* New York: Brunner/Mazel.
44. ROSENTHAL, R. J. (1986). The psychodynamics of pathological gambling. *J. Gambling Behav., 2*(2), 108–120.
45. MOSKOWITZ, J. A. (1980). Lithium and lady luck. *NY State J. Med., 5,* 785–788.

9

HOMICIDE

KENNETH TARDIFF, M.D., M.P.H.

Associate Professor of Psychiatry and of Public Health,
Cornell University Medical College–The New York Hospital,
New York, New York

Homicide is among the most serious public as well as psychiatric concerns. Rates of homicide in the countries of the world differ greatly: for example, from 63.0 per hundred thousand population in Guatemala to 0.7 in Greece and Ireland in 1980, according to World Health Organization statistics (1). However, caution should be exercised in comparing homicide rates from different countries because of differences in reporting methods as well as a number of other socioeconomic factors. For purposes of discussing determinants and patterns of homicide in this chapter, the author will focus primarily on homicide in the United States. Although the United States had the highest absolute number of homicides in 1980 (23,967 persons), it was not the highest in terms of rates, with a rate of 10.5 per hundred thousand population.

According to the Federal Bureau of Investigation Uniform Crime Reports, 39% of the homicides involved friends or acquaintances, 18% were within families, 18% were between strangers, and 25% involved persons with the relationship unknown. The latter homicides were probably committed by strangers (2). Some people are more likely to be killed than others. Men are four times more likely to be victims of homicide and nonwhites have been 8 to 15 times more likely to be murdered than whites. In both sexes persons aged 25 to 34 are most likely to be victims of homicide, followed by those aged 35 to 44 and then by those aged 15 to 24 (3).

The preceding studies have used aggregate national statistics in the United States. A number of studies since 1950 have taken a more in-depth view of homicide in a number of cities in the United States, for example Philadelphia, Chicago, St. Louis, Cleveland, and Allegheny County in

Pennsylvania (4–9). These studies have generally found that nonwhites, the young, and men are most likely to be victims of homicide. None of these studies delineated Hispanics as a separate group; however, a study of homicides during 1981 in Manhattan by the author and his colleagues found that Hispanics as well as blacks have higher rates of homicide than other groups. It concurred with other studies in terms of higher rates among men and the young, but found that the percentage of homicides related to disputes was less than the national experience. Rather, drug-related activities, robbery, and other criminal activities account for a large proportion of homicides in that large metropolitan area and probably in other large cities in the United States (10). Thus it is important not to consider homicide as one homogeneous phenomenon but rather a number of subtypes, namely those resulting from disputes, from drug-related activities, from robbery and other criminal activities, and from mass and serial murderers. This chapter will focus on aspects of homicide relevant to clinical practice, but one must take into consideration the environment in which homicides occur since homicide and human violence, like any other aspect of human behavior, involve many factors. The interaction of environmental factors impinges on the individual, who in turn has a unique set of internal or innate factors operating to increase or decrease the risk of violence for that particular individual.

SOCIAL FACTORS

Early studies have pointed to an association of violence and major social factors. The high rates of homicide and other types of violence in the South suggested that violence is part of the southern culture and tradition. An alternative explanation was that poor economic conditions in the southern states accounted for their higher rates of violence. Others have explained that there are greater numbers of blacks in the South, who have higher crime rates than whites. Criminal violence in black ghettos has been explained in terms of the necessity to fight rather than being able to achieve through verbal or legitimate means. Added to this is the breakup of families, alienation, discrimination, and frustration. Thus some have hypothesized that blacks live in a violent subculture (11–13). Others have found that for domestic violence, there is no difference between blacks and whites if socioeconomic status is controlled in the analysis (14).

In a study of large metropolitan areas that compared rates of violent crime including homicide as reported by the FBI, Blau and Blau (15) found that racial inequality and stress were associated with rates of homicide and that the increased rates of violent crime for blacks and for southern regions of the country were both based on economic inequality. Economic inequality was not merely poverty, but rather relative income differences between individuals. Thus violence occurs because of hostility in one person who perceives he is disadvantaged relative to other persons (16). Some studies have found that economic inequality is not related to violence but that absolute poverty is — for example, the percentage of persons below the poverty line of the U.S. Social Security Administration (17, 18).

The contradictory results are probably due to the use of large metropolitan areas (SMSAs) as units of analysis, and these areas are often heterogeneous. A recent study by Messner and the author used neighborhoods as smaller units of analysis, which were more homogeneous, and found that economic inequality and race were not related to homicide, but rather the prime determinants were absolute poverty and marital disruption. There is probably a cycle in terms of inability to have basic necessities of life, disruption of marriages, single-parent families, unemployment, and further difficulty in maintaining interpersonal ties, family structure, and social control (19).

ENVIRONMENTAL FACTORS

There is evidence that social control of crime by members of society other than law enforcement officials may deter violence and other crime. Shotland and Goodstein (20) have found that the number of bystanders available for surveillance and intervention may prevent the commission of crime, and in a cyclical way, fear of crime may reduce the number of bystanders available for surveillance. The social control of crime is based on the relative balance between the offenders' fear of surveillance and the bystanders' fear of crime, and the relative strength of each of these forces determines whether a neighborhood will be either safe or a hostile and dangerous setting in terms of violence. This was confirmed in a later study by Messner and the author (21) which analyzed homicide patterns in New York City in relation to a routine activities approach.

Physical crowding may be related to homicide and violent crime, yet there are conflicting studies as to whether density, defined by the number of buildings in a geographical area or the number of inhabitants in a building, is related to violent crime. Some contend that there is increased contact, decreased defensible space, and increased violence in high-density areas, while others argue that increased density is related to increased social control and decreased violent crime (22, 23). Bell and Baron (24)

have reviewed a number of studies that correlated the ambient temperature of the environment with violent crime and riots. They concluded that
there is a relationship between heat and aggression in that moderately
uncomfortable ambient temperatures produce an increase of aggression
while extremely hot temperatures decrease aggression.

FIREARMS

Firearms are important since they probably turn what would have been
an assault into homicide. Nationally, Jason et al. (25) found that over two
thirds of homicides in the period from 1976 to 1979 involved firearms, and
there has been a significant increase in the number of homicides associated
with firearms particularly since 1960. Determining whether this increase
is due to increased availability of firearms is complex. Some measures of
availability have included information about the manufacture, import,
and sales of guns, but imports are not measured accurately and there is
little available information on exports and the rate at which all guns are
removed from circulation. In addition to difficulty in quantifying availability of guns, the overall availability of guns may not reveal much about
the relationship of firearms to violence (26, 27).

Other researchers have turned to evaluation of the impact of gun control
legislation, but findings concerning state gun control legislation are not
consistent. The Gun Control Act of 1968 was found to have no effect on
homicide in New York and Boston (28), but both the Bartley-Fox Amend-
ment and the District of Columbia's Firearms Control Act of 1975 have
been shown to be related to a decrease of homicides involving firearms (29,
30). We do not know the availability of guns for criminals in the illegitimate market and whether their use in homicide-related crimes would be
decreased by gun control legislation. We do know that keeping a firearm in
the home is not advisable since this usually results in death of the inhabitants more often than of intruders (31).

DEVELOPMENTAL FACTORS

Some factors impact on the development of the child and increase that
individual's propensity for violence as an adult. Kempe and Helfer (32)
have reported that being abused as a child is related to becoming a physically abusive adult, that is, a child abuser or otherwise violent adult.
Furthermore, child abuse is not infrequent and there are reports that 1%
of children are physically abused each year (33). This rate reflects actual

reports of child abuse, and since only serious physical abuse is reported, the real incidence of child abuse is probably higher than this. There is evidence not only that being abused as a child is related to adult violence, but also that witnessing intrafamily violence, for example spouse abuse, is related to increased problems with violence among children, especially boys (34). There are indications that domestic violence directed toward spouses is a common problem in the United States; for example, of 492 male and female patients interviewed in a general-hospital emergency room, 22% reported being pushed around, hit, or hurt by their spouses or boy/girlfriends (35). Thus we see that child and spouse abuse are significant problems and that being abused as a child or being in a family where a spouse is abused may tip the balance toward being violent as an adult. Physicians should be familiar with guidelines for the identification and management of child and spouse abuse and other domestic violence so as to prevent these from becoming homicide cases (36, 37).

EFFECTS OF MASS MEDIA

Television viewing and other mass media have been suspected as factors in violence. A recent report by the National Institute of Mental Health focused on entertainment programming and reviewed approximately 2,500 studies since 1970. It concluded that most of these studies demonstrated a relationship between televised violence and later aggressive behavior (38). Freedman (39) criticized this report, pointing out that few of the studies reviewed have been concerned with the relatively long-term effects of television and that they have not involved natural settings. He concluded that there is a consistent small correlation between television violence and aggressiveness, but that there is little convincing evidence in natural settings that viewing television violence causes people to be more aggressive. Not addressed is the role of news reports depicting violence, assassinations and other murders, motion pictures, and other forms of mass media on the production of violence in society.

PSYCHOPATHOLOGY

As Dietz has pointed out, there are no adequate diagnostic studies of a representative group of homicide offenders in that most do not use standardized diagnostic criteria and that the groups studied may not be representative of murderers in general for they had been referred for psychiatric evaluation (40). It is this author's impression, however, that if one excludes alcohol and drug abuse, overall psychiatric patients constitute a small percentage of murderers despite the fact that they receive a great amount of publicity in newspapers and on television. There has been controversy as to whether psychiatric patients were more likely to commit crimes including homicides; a number of studies have been reviewed by Rabkin (41). Data support the concern that certain types of psychiatric patients, particularly patients with alcohol and drug abuse problems, are more likely than the general population to be arrested for violent crime. There is evidence that schizophrenic patients are also at higher risk of violent behavior than the general population. A study of a nonurban area in New York State found that there was an increase in homicides by persons found not guilty by reason of insanity which was correlated with discharging of mental patients into the community. In geographical areas such as this where homicide rates are low, murders by psychotic or severely disturbed mental patients may be disproportionately high (42). In larger urban areas, as has been discussed, a greater proportion of homicides may be a function of socioeconomic determinants rather than severe psychopathology.

Schizophrenia

On the other hand, given that some psychiatric patients are violent, it should be of interest to clinicians as to which diagnostic groups have an increased risk of violent behavior. Krakowski and his colleagues have reviewed many clinical studies of a large number of patients in terms of patterns of violence. They concluded that overall, schizophrenics were at a higher risk of behavior problems than other types of patients (43). This author has found that the risk in relation to types of schizophrenia differs in terms of the course of the treatment; in other words, violent patients presenting to hospitals for admission are increased in both paranoid and nonparanoid types of schizophrenia (44, 45), whereas violent patients who have resided in hospital for long periods of time are relatively overrepresented in the nonparanoid schizophrenic category and not in the paranoid schizophrenic category (46). This suggests that paranoid schizophrenics may be more amenable to treatment with neuroleptics in the acute phase of hospitalization and that those paranoid schizophrenics continuing to reside in hospital may be better able to control violent behavior. In fact, the author found that among psychiatric patients residing in hospital for a long period of time, paranoid schizophrenic patients were more likely than other violent patients to be deemed ready for community placement (47).

However, once these patients are discharged, problems arise in terms of noncompliance, especially for paranoid schizophrenics, who are prone to discontinue medication. This results in a reemergence of delusional thinking, loss of control, and subsequent likelihood of assaultive and homicidal behavior. Programs of mandatory aftercare for patients who were violent have been implemented with varying success throughout the United States. Problems have arisen in implementing these laws because mental health professionals do not view themselves as police pursuing patients who refuse treatment; also, they have realistic concerns about approaching patients who may be homicidal and armed.

Another diagnostic category associated with increased risk of violent behavior is psychotic organic mental disorders (44–46). In fact, psychosis of any type increases the risk of violent behavior, as was confirmed in a study by Taylor, who examined over 200 male prisoners and found that 46% were driven to commit violent offenses by their psychotic symptoms; if indirect consequences of the psychosis are taken into account, 83% of the offenses were probably attributable to the illnesses (48).

Alcohol

In terms of other organic mental disorders, alcohol consumption is frequently associated with homicide. This association has been known since the early study by Wolfgang where drinking occurred in 72% of homicides by stabbing and 45% of homicides by other means. In addition, alcohol related homicides were more likely to occur on the weekend (70%) as opposed to weekdays (50%) (5). Later studies continued to find a high degree of association of alcohol and homicide. Hollis found that 86% of offenders and 75% of victims were drinking at the time of the homicide. In fact, in 80% of the cases both the offenders and the victims were drinking (49). In his study, as in a number of other studies, the interval between injury and death was not taken into consideration. Since a blood alcohol level of 0.03% is metabolized in two hours, it is possible that victims surviving injuries for even a few hours would have metabolized alcohol, and thus, his data may underestimate the use of alcohol by homicide victims. Constantino et al. attempted to take metabolism of the alcohol into consideration by declaring that all victims dying more than 12 hours after injury would be classified in an undetermined alcohol category. In fact, they should have taken the actual blood alcohol level into consideration in their calculations. Nevertheless, they found that 42% of victims had positive blood alcohol levels, which again is probably an underestimate of the true prevalence in the population studied (50).

Voss and Hepburn found differences by race in terms of the presence of alcohol in that 56% of nonwhite and 46% of white victims had positive blood alcohol levels. There was a slight increase of alcohol in the blood of female compared to male victims (6). Whether increased alcohol levels in nonwhites are related to the phenomenon of homicide or to other aspects of being nonwhite is not apparent; however, Harper has indicated that, in general, alcohol is a major health problem of blacks in the United States. Alcohol as a cause of death is three times as frequent for blacks as whites in the United States (51).

Virkkunen, in Finland, found that 66% of murderers and 68% of victims had positive blood alcohol levels at the time of the homicide. Of particular interest is his finding that the victims were just as likely as perpetrators to have initiated aggression or quarreling prior to the homicide (52). Although this theory of the role of alcohol in homicide has never been tested, one can speculate that there is decreased inhibition in both victim and murderer. As a result, the victim becomes verbally or physically abusive and provocative. The murderer also, secondary to a loss of inhibition, acts rather than restraining himself or talking in response to this provocation. Often in men this provocation involves jealousy, undermining of the masculine image, or even homosexual advances. One would predict that alcohol has its greatest effect in the midrange of blood alcohol levels or, conversely, that there is little effect at low blood alcohol levels and a greater degree of incapacitation of the potential murderer at very high blood alcohol levels. Two recent studies confirm that alcohol use plays an important part in homicide. The author and his colleagues, in his Manhattan study, found that 38% of male and 36% of female victims were found to have brain alcohol levels of .01 per cent or more and an additional 8% of males and 4% of females had no alcohol but died more than one hour after injury, so that alcohol could have been metabolized in the interval between injury and death (10). Goodman and his colleagues, in their Los Angeles study, found that 40% of victims had alcohol in their bodies (53). Both studies found that victims with alcohol in their bodies were more likely than those without alcohol to die in disputes, usually with friends, acquaintances, or family members.

Although there is general agreement that alcohol abuse is common among murderers as well as their victims, there is a scarcity of data as to how abuse of alcohol in homicide compares to abuse in society in general.

Lester analyzed states' consumption of alcohol in relation to their homicide rates and did not find a statistically significant association (54). No doubt the use of this gross measure in relation to an event that occurs for 1% of the population, in addition to numerous other variables affecting homicide in individual states may have accounted for a lack of association between general consumption of alcohol and homicide rates. On the other hand, Langven et al. conducted a controlled study in which they compared murderers to nonviolent offenders seen for psychiatric assessment in a forensic setting. Murderers (36%) were more likely than nonviolent offenders (5%) to use alcohol as well as drugs at the time of their offenses. Furthermore, 40% of the murderers indicated that they "drink too much," in comparison to 15% of the nonviolent offenders (55). Although one should be cautious about generalizing beyond this prison population, there are indications that alcohol is more likely to be associated with homicide and violent crimes rather than nonviolent crimes.

Drug Abuse

Drug abuse is related directly to homicide for some drugs, e.g., amphetamines, phencyclidine, sedatives, and minor tranquilizers, and indirectly to homicide for other drugs, such as narcotics, mainly in terms of drug-seeking behavior.

Abuse of amphetamines has been found to be associated with violence (56). The role of amphetamines in homicide has been explored by Ellinwood, who found that amphetamine-related homicides involved increasing paranoid delusions in the murderers followed by their obtaining weapons and further amphetamine abuse until the homicide occurred (57). Fauman and Fauman have found phencyclidine to be directly related to violence, including homicide. In the cases they reviewed phencyclidine abuse was usually chronic and associated with a past history of violence. Often there was abuse of other drugs and alcohol (58). Sedatives and minor tranquilizers, probably related to decreased inhibition and impairment of judgment, have also been associated with violent behavior (56, 59). Methaqualone abuse has been increasing in popularity and has been found to be associated with violent death, including homicides, accidents, and suicides. Over a 10-year period ending in 1981 Wetli found 31 homicide victims with methaqualone in their blood. From his report it was not possible to calculate the percentage of homicides this represented. He did indicate that deaths for these homicide victims were usually associated with their committing crimes (60).

Opioid drug abuse is related to homicide indirectly, not in terms of a primary effect on violence. Langven et al. found only a slight increase of narcotics abuse among homicidal versus nonviolent offenders (55). Rather, narcotics play a key role in many homicides because of activities aimed at obtaining these drugs. Furthermore, the author found that in Manhattan, 30% of male and 20% of female victims had one or more drugs in their bodies, narcotics being the most common type. These narcotics included not only morphine, the metabolic product of heroin, but also methadone, cocaine, and in many cases combinations of morphine with methadone or cocaine. A better indication of the importance of drugs is the fact that homicides were preceded by drug-related activities in one-third of the cases involving male victims (10).

Neurophysiological Dysfunction

In terms of other organic factors, neurophysiological dysfunction has been associated with homicide and other violence. In 1970 Mark and Ervin (61) and Monroe (62) pointed to the role of temporal-lobe epilepsy and other forms of limbic ictus and episodic dyscontrol in the production of violent behavior. Recently, Devinsky and Baer (63) have continued to emphasize the role of temporal-lobe epilepsy in violence. They did not address, however, the prevalence of violent behavior among temporal-lobe epileptic patients compared to the general epileptic population or the general nonepileptic population. Instead, they used a number of case histories to emphasize their point. Likewise, Monroe (64) has continued to maintain that episodic dyscontrol is often associated with limbic ictus that is not detected because the surface EEG is an insensitive measure of subcortical activity. He supports his theory by pointing out that a number of these individuals respond to anticonvulsant medications.

On the other hand, a large international collaborative study found that violence was rare among epileptic patients (65). Another review of 500 cases referred to a neurologist found that of the 17 patients referred for temper tantrums, none had organic factors such as epilepsy or episodic dyscontrol syndrome (66). Hermann and Whitman (67) reviewed 64 studies since 1962 that assessed whether there was a relationship between temporal-lobe epilepsy and aggression and concluded that controlled investigations showed no overall difference in the level of violence between persons with or without epilepsy. Among individuals with epilepsy other factors were found to be associated with violence, including low socioeconomic status, sex, age, and earlier developmental problems.

In terms of more severe or gross physiological impairment, Lewis and her colleagues studied 15 death row inmates and found that all had histories of severe head injury and that five had major neurological impairment and seven had less serious neurological problems such as blackouts or other soft neurological signs. Psychoeducational testing provided further evidence of central nervous system dysfunction. It should be noted that eight of these murderers had schizophrenia or affective illness (68). The role of epilepsy and other neurophysiological dysfunction and violence is unsettled. There are probably some persons with temporal-lobe epilepsy who manifest hostility and violence in the interictal period as well as nonpurposeful violence during their seizures. However, their number is probably small among persons with epilepsy and very small in relation to homicide and violence in general. Gross neurophysiological dysfunction may be associated with poor impulse control independent of seizure activity, thus producing violent behavior.

Genetics

Other biological factors have been studied in terms of violent behavior. Recent studies of twins have found that there is more criminal behavior among monozygotic twins than dizygotic twins (69). Since twins share the same environment as well as genetic material, researchers have turned to the study of adoptees. Two studies in Scandinavia found no support for a direct genetic basis for homicide but some support for a genetic association in terms of crime involving property. Thus criminality may be linked with genetics through economic factors (70, 71). There has been a great amount of research in the past two decades on the XYY chromosomal abnormality, especially looking at prison populations. Yet according to a recent review (72), there is no evidence for a relationship between violence and the XYY complement in the population at large.

Hormones

Other studies of biological determinants have explored the role of hormones in violent behavior. Many have not found a significant relationship between testosterone levels and aggressive behavior among prison populations (73–76). The role of the premenstrual period has recently become the focus of attention because it has been accepted as a contributing factor in manslaughter, arson, and assault cases in England and France. Dalton (77) and d'Orban and Dalton (78) found that among women charged with crimes of violence, 44% committed the offense during their premenstrual period. Critics of their research argue that their methodologies are flawed and that recommendations that progesterone be used for treatment do not take into account other factors in treatment, such as recommendations to avoid alcohol and to maintain a stable diet, as well as personality of the individual (79). Another hormonal disturbance, namely hypoglycemia, has been implicated in violent behavior in that habitually violent offenders were found to have reactive hypoglycemia to a greater degree than a controlled population (80).

Neurotransmitters

Earlier studies of neurotransmitters have found increased levels of norepinephrine and dopamine in aggressive behavior (81). However, the most promising work has involved the serotonergic system. Brown and his colleagues have conducted two studies of men with a history of aggressive behavior, excluding those with a history of primary affective disorders, schizophrenia, or severe brain syndromes, as well as those ingesting drugs or alcohol 10 days preceding the study. They found a history of aggressive behavior and a history of suicidal behavior were both related to decreased cerebral spinal fluid 5-hydroxyindolacetic acid (5-HIAA) levels (82, 83). Lidberg and his colleagues studied the CSF 5-HIAA levels in a group of men convicted of criminal homicide and a group of men who attempted suicide and found that these groups had lower levels of 5-HIAA in spinal fluid than did male controls (84). Linnolia et al. studied violent offenders excluding schizophrenics or those with major affective disorders, but not alcoholics. All of the subjects had killed or attempted to kill with unusual cruelty. They found that impulsive offenders had significantly lower CSF 5-HIAA concentrations than nonimpulsive offenders, the latter group being defined as those who had premeditated their crime. They concluded that low CSF 5-HIAA concentration may be a marker of impulsivity rather than a specific type of violence, that is, suicide or externally directed aggression (85).

Personality Disorders

If one looks at the setting of outpatient clinic rather than the inpatient psychiatry unit or prison, psychiatric patients with increased rates of assault are not in the psychotic and/or organic groups, but rather have personality or childhood and adolescent disorders (86–89).

Persons with personality disorders or nonpsychotic, nonorganic disorders can be classified into four categories: intermittent explosive disorders, antisocial personalities, borderline personalities, and isolated explosive disorders. The intermittent explosive disorder is characterized by several discrete episodes of loss of control with violence toward others. There is little apparent precipitation, violence may last from minutes to hours, and following the violent episode there is usually remorse, for example in a man having beaten his wife or child. As indicated earlier, some researchers believe that this problem with impulse control may be related to either neurophysiological dysfunction or abnormal neurotransmitter metabolism.

The second category is the antisocial personality where there is violence and other antisocial behavior on an ongoing basis — in essence, violence is a way of attaining one's goals in life. The third category is the borderline personality with a broad pervasive instability of interpersonal relationships, mood, and identity when violent behavior is just one of many impulsive behaviors, others being excessive sexual behavior, overspending, overeating, and suicidal behaviors. The isolated explosive disorder involves one unexpected episode of profound violence, for example, mass murder. Often there is no history of prior violence or of psychiatric treatment. Usually the perpetrators of mass killings appeared normal to neighbors or have led very isolated lives. Examples of such slayings are those of Sherrill, who killed 14 people in Oklahoma in 1986, Huberty, who killed 20 people in California in 1984, and Whitman, who killed 14 people in Texas in 1966. All three of these murderers were obsessed by firearms and militaristic themes.

Another category of mass murder which is done in a serial fashion has been noted by Dietz (40). Often these murderers kill 10 or more victims in separate incidents. Examples of these include Bundy, Kemper, Gacy, and Williams. Often these murderers are preoccupied with sexual themes and fantasies which often motivate the murders.

PSYCHIATRIC PATIENTS AS VICTIMS

The attention given to psychiatric patients in this chapter is not based on the frequency with which they kill other people, but rather on the assumed focus of interest of the readers. The author would be remiss if he were not to point out that psychiatric patients are at greater risk than the general population in terms of being victims of homicides. For example, Hillard followed over 5,000 psychiatric patients presenting to an emergency room and found that the rate of homicidal death of these patients was nearly twice the expected rate and the rates of accidental deaths were two and a half times the rate of the general population. Furthermore, psychiatric patients are at risk of being killed or assaulted within psychiatric hospitals, as has been described most notably in terms of homicides committed by psychotic patients in a hospital in the United States (90) as well as in Switzerland (91).

REFERENCES

1. ROSENBERG, M. L., & MERCY, J. A. (1986). Homicide: Epidemiologic analysis at the national level. *Bull. NY Acad. Med.*, *62*, 376.
2. US Dept. of Justice (1985). *Crime in the United States, 1980.* Uniform Crime Reports. Washington, DC: Govt. Print. Office.
3. FARLEY, R. (1980). Homicide trends in the United States. *Demography*, *17*, 177.
4. HOLINGER, P. C. (1980). Violent deaths as a leading cause of mortality: An epidemiological study of suicide, homicide, and accidents. *Am. J. Psychiatry*, *137*, 472.
5. WOLFGANG, M. E. (1958). *Patterns in criminal homicide.* New York: Wiley.
6. VOSS, H. L., & HEPBURN, J. R. (1968). Patterns in criminal homicide in Chicago. *J. Crim. Law Criminol. Police Sci.*, *59*, 499.
7. BLOCK, B., & ZIMRING, R. E. (1973). Homicide in Chicago. *J. Res. Crime Delinquency*, *10*, 1.
8. HERJANIC, M., & MEYERS, D. A. (1976). Notes on epidemiology of homicide in an urban area. *Forensic Sci.*, *8*, 235.
9. RUSHFORTH, N. B., FORD, A. B., HIRSCH, L. S., et al. (1977). Violent death in a metropolitan county. *N. Engl. J. Med.*, *297*, 531.
10. TARDIFF, K., GROSS, E., & MESSNER, S. (1986). A study of homicide in Manhattan. *Am. J. Public Health*, *76*, 139.
11. SILBERMAN, C. E. (1980). *Criminal violence, criminal justice.* New York: Vintage.
12. WOLFGANG, M. E., & FERRACUTI, F. (1967). *The subculture of violence: Toward an integrated theory in criminology.* New York: Methuen.
13. WOLFGANG, M. E. (1981). Sociocultural overview of criminal violence. In J. R. Hays, T. K. Roberts, & K. S. Solway (Eds.), *Violence and the violent individual.* New York: S. P. Medical and Scientific Publishers.
14. CENTERWALL, B. S. (1984). Race, socioeconomic status and domestic homicide: Atlanta, 1971–72. *Am. J. Public Health*, *74*, 813.
15. BLAU, J. R., & BLAU, P. M. (1982). The cost of inequality: Metropolitan structure and violent crime. *Am. Sociol. Rev.*, *47*, 114.
16. VOLD, G. V. (1979). *Theoretical criminology.* New York: Oxford University Press.
17. DEFRONZO, J. (1983). Economic assistance to impoverished Americans: Relationship to incidence of crime. *Criminology*, *21*, 119.
18. WILLIAMS, K. (1984). Economic sources of homicide: Reestimating the effects of poverty and inequality. *Am. Sociol. Rev.*, *49*, 283.
19. MESSNER, S., & TARDIFF, K. (1986). Economic inequality and levels of homicide: An analysis of urban neighborhoods. *Criminology*, *24*, 297.
20. SHOTLAND, R. L., & GOODSTEIN, L. I. (1984). The role of bystanders in crime control. *J. Soc. Issues*, *40*, 9.

21. Messner, S., & Tardiff, K. (1985). The social ecology of urban homicide: An application of the "routine activities" approach. *Criminology*, *23*, 241.
22. Anderson, A. C. (1982). Environmental factors and aggressive behavior. *J. Clin. Psychiatry*, *43*, 280.
23. Sampson, R. J. (1983). Structural density and criminal victimization. *Criminology*, *21*, 276.
24. Bell, P. A., & Baron, R. A. (1981). Ambient temperature and human violence. In P. F. Brain & D. Benton (Eds.), *Multidisciplinary approaches to aggression research*. Amsterdam: Elsevier, Holland Biomedical Press.
25. Jason, J., Strauss, L. T., & Tyler, C. W. (1983). A comparison of primary and secondary homicides in the United States. *Am. J. Epidemiol.*, *117*, 309.
26. Kleck, G. (1979). Capital punishment, gun ownership and homicide. *Am. J. Sociol.*, *84*, 882.
27. Cook, P. J. (1982). The role of firearms in violent crime: An interpretive review of the literature. In M. E. Wolfgang & N. A. Weiner (Eds.), *Criminal violence*. Beverly Hills, CA: Sage.
28. Zimring, F. (1975). Firearms and federal law: The Gun Control Act of 1958. *J. Legal Studies*, *4*, 133.
29. Deutsch, S. J. (1980). Intervention modeling: Analysis of changes in crime rates. In *Frontiers in quantitative criminology*. New York: Academic Press.
30. Jones, E. D. (1981). The District of Columbia's Firearms Control Regulations Act of 1975: The toughest handgun control law in the United States — Or is it? *Ann. Am. Acad. Political Social Sci.*, *5*, 135.
31. Kellerman, A. L., & Reay, D. T. (1986). Protection or peril? An analysis of firearm-related deaths in the home. *N. Engl. J. Med.*, *314*, 1557.
32. Kempe, C. H., & Helfer, R. (Eds.) (1980). *The battered child syndrome* (3rd ed.). Chicago: University of Chicago Press.
33. Heins, M. (1984). The "battered child" revisited. *JAMA*, *251*, 3295.
34. Jaffe, P., Wolfe, D., & Wilson, S. K. (1986). Family violence and child adjustment: A comparative analysis of girls' and boys' behavioral symptoms. *Am. J. Psychiatry*, *143*, 74.
35. Goldberg, W. G., & Tomlanovich, M. C. (1984). Domestic violence victims in the emergency room: New findings. *JAMA*, *251*, 3259.
36. Council on Scientific Affairs (1985). A.M.A. diagnostic and treatment guidelines concerning child abuse and neglect. *JAMA*, *254*, 976.
37. Straus, M. A. (1986). Domestic violence and homicide antecedents. *Bull. NY Acad. Med.*, *62*, 446.
38. NIMH (1982). Television and behavior: 10 years of scientific progress and implications for the eighties. Washington, DC: US Govt. Prntg. House.
39. Freedman, J. L. (1984). Effect of television violence on aggressiveness. *Psychol. Bull.*, *96*, 227.
40. Dietz, P. E. (1987). Patterns of human violence. *American Psychiatric Association Annual Review* (Vol. 6). Washington, DC: American Psychiatric Press.
41. Rabkin, J. G. (1979). Criminal behavior of discharged mental patients: A critical appraisal of research. *Psychol. Bull.*, *86*, 1.
42. Grunberg, F., Klinger, B. I., & Grumet, B. R. (1978). Homicide and community-based psychiatry. *J. Nerv. Ment. Dis.*, *166*, 868.
43. Krakowski, M., Volavka, J., and Brizer, D. (1986). Psychopathology and violence: A review of literature. *Comp. Psychiatry*, *27*, 131.
44. Tardiff, K., & Sweillam, A. (1980). Assault, suicide and mental illness. *Arch. Gen. Psychiatry*, *37*, 164.
45. Tardiff, K. (1984). Characteristics of assaultive patients in private psychiatric hospitals. *Am. J. Psychiatry*, *141*, 1232.

46. TARDIFF, K., & SWEILLAM, A. (1982). The occurrence of assaultive behavior among chronic psychiatric inpatients. *Am. J. Psychiatry, 139,* 212.

47. TARDIFF, K., & SWEILLAM, A. (1979). Characteristics of violent patients admitted to public hospitals. *Bull. Am. Acad. Psychiatry Law, 7,* 11.

48. TAYLOR, P. J. (1985). Motives for offending among violent and psychotic men. *Br. J. Psychiatry, 147,* 491.

49. HOLLIS, W. S. (1974). On the etiology of criminal homicides — The alcohol factor. *J. Police Sci. Admin., 2,* 50.

50. CONSTANTINO, J. P., KULLER, L. H., PERPER, J. A., et al. (1977). An epidemiological study of homicides in Allegheny County, Pennsylvania. *Am. J. Epidemiol., 106,* 314.

51. HARPER, F. D. (1976). *Alcohol abuse and black America.* Alexandria, VA: Douglas Publishers.

52. VIRKKUNEN, M. (1974). Alcohol as a factor precipitating aggression and conflict behavior leading to homicide. *Br. J. Addict., 69,* 149.

53. GOODMAN, R. A., MERCY, J. A., & LOYA, F. (1986). Alcohol use and interpersonal violence: Alcohol detected in homicide victims. *Am. J. Public Health, 76,* 144.

54. LESTER, D. (1980). Alcohol and suicide and homicide. *J. Stud. Alcohol, 41,* 1220.

55. LANGVEN, R., PAITICH, D., ORCHARD, B., et al. (1982). The role of alcohol, drugs, suicide attempts and situational strains in homicide committed by offenders seen for psychiatric assessment: A controlled study. *Acta Psychiatr. Scand., 66,* 229.

56. MOYER, K. E. (1976). *The psychobiology of aggression.* New York: Harper & Row.

57. ELLINWOOD, E. H. (1971). Assault and homicide associated with amphetamine abuse. *Am. J. Psychiatry, 127,* 1170.

58. FAUMAN, M. A., & FAUMAN, B. J. (1979). Violence associated with phencyclidine abuse. *Am. J. Psychiatry, 136,* 1584.

59. TINKLENBERG, J. R., MURPHY, P. L., MURPHY, P., et al. (1974). Drug involvement in criminal assaults by adolescents. *Arch. Gen. Psychiatry, 30,* 685.

60. WETLI, C. U. (1983). Changing patterns of methaqualone abuse: A survey of 246 fatalities. *JAMA, 249,* 621.

61. MARK, V. H., & ERVIN, F. R. (1970). *Violence and the brain.* New York: Harper & Row.

62. MONROE, R. R. (1970). *Episodic behavioral disorders.* Cambridge, MA: Harvard University Press.

63. DEVINSKY, O., & BAER, D. (1984). Varieties of aggressive behavior in temporal lobe epilepsy. *Am. J. Psychiatry, 141,* 651.

64. MONROE, R. R. (1985). Episodic behavioral disorders and limbic ictus. *Comp. Psychiatry, 26,* 466.

65. DELGADO-ESCUETA, A. V., MATTSON, R. H., & KING, L. (1981). The nature of aggression during epileptic seizures. *N. Engl. J. Med., 305,* 711.

66. LEICESTER, J. (1982). Temper tantrums, epilepsy and episodic dyscontrol. *Br. J. Psychiatry, 141,* 262.

67. HERMANN, B. P., & WHITMAN, S. (1984). Behavioral and personality correlates of epilepsy: A review, methodological critique and conceptual model. *Psychol. Bull., 95,* 451.

68. LEWIS, D. O., PINCUS, J. H., & SHANOK, S. S. (1986). Psychiatric, neurological and psychoeducational characteristics of 15 death row inmates in the United States. *Am. J. Psychiatry, 143,* 838.

69. MEDNICK, S. A., & VOLAVKA, J. (1980). Biology and crime. In N. Morris & M. Touny (Eds.), *Crime and justice: An annual review of research* (Vol. II). Chicago: University of Chicago Press.

70. BOHMAN, M. (1978). Some genetic aspects of alcoholism and criminality. *Arch Gen. Psychiatry, 35,* 269.

71. HUTCHINGS, B., & MEDNICK, S. A. (1977). Criminality in adoptees and their biological parents: A pilot study. In S. A. Mednick & K. O. Christiansen (Eds.), *Biosocial bases of criminal behavior.* New York: Gardner.

72. SCHIAVI, R. C., THEILGAARD, A., OWEN, D. R., et al. (1984). Sex chromosome abnormalities, hormones and aggressivity. *Arch. Gen. Psychiatry, 41*, 93.
73. EHRENKRANZ, J., BLISS, E., & SHEARD, M. H. (1974). Plasma testosterone: Correlation with aggressive behavior and social dominance in man. *Psychosom. Med., 36*, 469.
74. KREUZ, I. E., & ROSE, R. M. (1972). Assessment of aggressive behavior and plasma testosterone in a young criminal population. *Psychosom. Med., 34*, 321.
75. MATTHEWS, R. (1979). Testosterone levels in aggressive offenders. In M. Sandler (Ed.), *Psychopharmacology of aggression.* New York: Raven Press.
76. MATTSSON, A., SCHALLING, D., OLWENS, D., et al. (1980). Plasma testosterone, aggressive behavior, and personality dimensions in young male delinquents. *J. Am. Acad. Child Psychiatry, 19*, 476.
77. DALTON, K. (1980). Cyclical criminal acts in premenstrual syndrome. *Lancet, 2*, 1070.
78. D'ORBAN, P. T., & DALTON, J. (1980). Violent crime and the menstrual cycle. *Psychol. Med., 10*, 353.
79. REID, R. L., & YEN, S. S. C. (1981). Premenstrual syndrome. *Am. J. Obstet. Gynecol., 139*, 85.
80. VIRKKUNEN, M. (1982). Reactive hypoglycemia tendency among habitually violent offenders: A further study by means of the glucose tolerance test. *Neuropsychobiology, 8*, 35.
81. EICHELMAN, B., ELLIOTT, G. R., & BARCHAS, J. (1981). Biochemical, pharmacological and genetic aspects of aggression. In D. A. Hamburg & M. B. Trudeau (Eds.), *Biobehavioral aspects of aggression.* New York: Alan Liss.
82. BROWN, G. L., GOODWIN, F. K., BALLENGER, J. C., et al. (1979). Aggression in humans correlates with cerebrospinal fluid amine metabolites. *Psychol. Res., 1*, 131.
83. BROWN, G. L., EBERT, M. H., GOYER, P. F., et al. (1982). Aggression, suicide and serotonin: Relationship to CSF amine metabolites. *Am. J. Psychiatry, 136*, 741.
84. LIDBERG, L., TUCK, J. R., ASBERG, M., et al. (1985). Homicide, suicide and CSF 5-HIAA. *Acta Psychiatr. Scand., 71*, 230.
85. LINNOLIA, M., VIRKKUNEN, M., SCHEININ, M., et al. (1983). Low cerebrospinal fluid 5-hydroxyindoleacetic acid concentration differentiates impulsive from nonimpulsive violent behavior. *Life Sci., 33*, 2609.
86. TARDIFF, K., & KOENIGSBERG, H. W. (1985). Assaultive behavior among psychiatric outpatients. *Am. J. Psychiatry, 142*, 960.
87. MENUCK, M. (1983). Clinical aspects of dangerous behavior. *J. Psychiatry Law, 11*, 277.
88. LION, J. R., & TARDIFF, K. (1987). The long term treatment of the violent patient. In R. E. Hales & A. J. Frances (Eds.), *The American Psychiatric Association annual review* (Vol. 6). Washington, DC: American Psychiatric Press.
89. REID, W. H., & BALIS, G. U. (1987). Evaluation of the violent patient. In R. E. Hales & A. J. Frances (Eds.), *The American Psychiatric Association annual review* (Vol. 6). Washington, DC: American Psychiatric Press.
90. COURNOS, F. (1985). Staff reaction to an inpatient homicide. *Hosp. Commun. Psychiatry, 36*, 664.
91. MODESTIN, J., & BOKER, W. (1985). Homicide in a psychiatric institution. *Br. J. Psychiatry, 146*, 321.

10

MUNCHAUSEN SYNDROME

MICHEL R. LOUVAIN, M.D.

Assistant Professor, Loyola University of Chicago,
Chicago, Illinois

The Baron of Munchausen was a German Officer in the Russian Army. His name would have been forgotten if he had not become famous for the fantastic military stories that he made up for his comrades, and if John Kendrick Bangs (3), a British writer, had not related the Baron's fantastic exploits in the book, *Mr. Munchausen: An Account of Some of His Recent Adventures.*

The modern Munchausen "barons" and "baronesses" elaborate factitious medical exploits; they make up signs and symptoms, they simulate surgical diseases.

According to the DSM-III-R (1), the group of factitious disorders includes: factitious disorder with psychological symptoms, factitious disorder with physical symptoms, and factitious disorder not otherwise specified (includes both psychological and physical symptoms). Their common characteristic is that they appear to be under the individual's voluntary control. The somatoform disorders, somatization disorders, conversion disorders, and psychogenic pain disorders do not include such voluntary control in their criteria, but are very close symptomatically. Depending on the patients' medical knowledge and observation skills, they will simulate medical, psychiatric, or surgical illnesses.

The term Munchausen syndrome, introduced by Asher (2) and Williams (19) in 1951 is reserved for those individuals who do not hesitate to compete with surgeons. However, this classification, necessary for diagnostic purposes, is somewhat irrelevant. The same individual will fit the different criteria at different times.

The personality structure is complex. Factitious disorders can be compared to an addiction, and as in any addiction, two elements are necessary: the potential addict and the drugs. The potential addict is the patient, impatient to be treated. The drugs are the physician, the psychiatrist, and, in the case of Munchausen, the surgeon.

HISTORY

The first writings indicate a tendency for some patients to look for surgical mutilations, which was described by Charcot (8) as mania operativa passiva. This is opposed to the mania operativa activa of surgeons (9), either individually or as a historical fashion, like hysterectomy, circumcision, tonsillectomy, appendectomy, total extraction of the teeth, and possibly, now, bypass surgery.

Literature is filled with these patients (10). Paul Bourget coined the word pathomimy (imitation of a disease), used by Dieulafoy to describe this entity at the beginning of the century.

TYPICAL PRESENTATION

An individual arrives at the emergency room usually with challenging symptoms. There is a long history of multiple diseases and multiple surgeries. Typically the patient cooperates very well and gives a good medical, surgical, and psychiatric history, indicates the names of numerous physicians and the names of the surgeries, but claims a total ignorance of anatomy. For example, one patient had three types of bladder surgeries — urethroplasty, meatotomy, and Marshall-Marchetti — and was able to give the technical names of the surgeries with amazing accuracy. When I indicated surprise at the fact the patient had had a splenectomy in "passing" during one of these bladder surgeries, considering how far apart these two organs are, she replied with a sweet smile, "I do not even know where the spleen is." This ignorance is even more surprising when we learn that the patient has had some involvement with the medical field, such as lab technician, nurse's aide, or secretary to a physician.

We also observe two features or characteristics which usually emerge during the interview. First is the total detachment from the sacrificed organs. One patient indicated that the appendix was lost along the road; the spleen decided to rupture during a bladder surgery. Each organ or function seems to be an alien that has to be taken out. The second characteristic is the incredible extent of the lies: A patient was born four months prematurely, the weight at birth was two ounces; twenty-three tablets of lithium carbonate a day not only are inefficient, but they do not even produce any side effects; formed green stools come out of the ureterostomy stoma. The list is endless.

One should become suspicious of this disorder when a patient refuses to sign the consent form for release of information on past admissions and the reason for the refusal is unclear.

Admitted to the unit, the patient will be a model patient at first, and no test will be too uncomfortable or too painful. The patient cooperates, with the alleged goal of better understanding her disease. To help with the diagnosis, the patient suggests multiple consultations. While in the hospital, other symptoms appear, usually linked to the urogenital sphere or abdominal emergencies. One of my patients even went to the trouble of calling the consultations herself, impersonating the resident, and she was even convincing enough to obtain an appendectomy on an appendix that was long gone; this occurred two hours after I had seen her in stable condition during a session where she had complained only of slight vaginal discharges.

Then one of the following occurs: Either the patient obtains the surgery he or she was longing for, to "get over all these problems," followed by a temporary reduction or occasionally by disappearance of the symptoms, or, especially if there was no surgical involvement, new symptoms appear with less credibility until the fraud is discovered and the patient signs out AMA (against medical advice) hastily, rushing to another emergency room. At this time the thoughtful physician understands why the patient so strongly refused to sign the release of medical information that would have made it possible to arrive at the proper diagnosis earlier.

VARIABILITY OF DIAGNOSTIC CATEGORY

In a very dramatic case, one of my patients was out of hospitals only 13 days of a whole year. When I encountered this patient, she presented a clinical picture that fitted the diagnostic criteria for atypical psychosis. She had been admitted to the psychiatric floor with the major complaint of visual hallucinations of her father surrounded by flames coming to haunt her in her bed. The following year she was readmitted with a diagnosis of adjustment reaction with depressed mood. She had just spent five months in a hospital in one of the southern states (migration is part of the clinical picture [6, 11]) with the diagnosis of multiple sclerosis, and prior to that admission, she had had surgery on one knee and a hysterectomy.

When she was readmitted for depression secondary to multiple sclerosis, a neurological consultation was requested. When the findings were negative, the patient immediately signed herself out AMA, and the diagnosis was corrected to factitious disorder with physical symptoms. This diagnosis should be suspected whenever a patient presents an exuberant medico-surgical history. The gridiron abdomen is the hallmark of Munchausen syndrome. But the Munchausen syndrome can also be designated, "Munchausen syndrome by proxy." In this case the child presents sicknesses usually determined (inflicted) by the mother (7, 17, 18).

LET'S WONDER . . .

Modern medicine has become "scientific." Some researchers are still doing double-blind studies to learn whether chlorpromazine, discovered in 1952, and amitriptyline, synthesized in 1960, are superior to placebos, as if the emptying of state psychiatric facilities was not evidence enough. All physicians have been trained to diagnose diseases by identifying a cluster of symptoms, ordering the proper laboratory tests, and prescribing the right treatment.

It is mind-boggling to try to understand how a young, attractive woman involved in a car accident with a closed trauma of the right elbow should end up having a disarticulation of the shoulder after multiple surgeries for burns—"I made a mistake, I poured the tea on the stump instead of in the cup"—cutaneous infection with *Escherichia-coli* and other fecal germs, and finally osteomyelitis. On the other hand, is it not surprising to find a surgeon performing bladder surgery on an 18-year-old woman who suddenly starts being incontinent without any other neurological findings? Once the first step has been taken, it is less surprising to find the same woman with a ureterostomy five years later.

PSYCHOPATHOLOGY

It is difficult to understand why some individuals, consciously or not, should induce surgeons to inflict such mutilations on them. It is even more difficult to understand why these patients think they have to pay such a sacrificial price and derive such a childish pride in their mutilations. There is a masochistic quality to this behavior. What is the basic need—one could even say the basic fault—that demands payment of such a high price?

It is relatively easy to determine what the factitious disorders are not, in terms of psychopathology; it is more complicated to have an idea of what they are, especially since, at one or more points in their lives, these patients do present psychiatric disorders.

A schizophrenic etiology has been entertained. This hypothesis of schizophrenia, as it has been described by Kraepelin, defined by Bleuler in 1911, more recently classified by DSM-III-R, and reevaluated by Andreasen with her studies of the negative symptoms, is not realistic. Schizophrenics are primarily withdrawn. They do not put any energy into convincing others that they are sick and need surgery. Occasionally, they may present somatic delusions, but as in any false fixed belief, these delusions never present the variability, ubiquity, and exuberance of the classical Munchausen patient.

Affective disorders are also unlikely (16). These patients occasionally present depressive episodes between surgical highlights. They may also exhibit episodes of rage or pseudomanic episodes if they are not taken seriously enough, especially by the spouse, the insurance agent, or the physician, but these episodes should be considered a side issue. One patient's severe depression and visual hallucinations disappeared as soon as she fell in her room (without witnesses), reportedly broke a toe, and obtained a cast. These patients are usually discharged to surgery, or if discharged home, they refuse psychiatric follow-up or miss their appointments because of new medicosurgical problems and do not relapse; they switch to another syndrome or disease.

To be successful, a Munchausen baron needs to be determined, convincing, and most of all, needs to be involved in challenging situations. "How high can I throw this weight?" Munchausen asks himself, as if he were in an amusement park.

This need, to be involved in a challenge, has the deep meaning of wanting to be understood, but medical schools do not teach how to understand humans and the meaning of their diseases. They teach how to classify syndromes and give treatment. Understanding the deep significance of a disease is of no importance anymore. A new term has even been recently created: the nonresponder. A depressed patient who does not improve with antidepressants is a nonresponder. There is no need anymore to understand why this patient is depressed.

A woman with abdominal pain (13) will be treated by laparoscopy, ovariectomy, and hysterectomy. She will have further surgeries for adhesions and only later will be referred to a psychiatrist for somatization disorder, though at that time she indeed has good reason to have persistent pain. What questions were asked about the symptom "abdominal pain"? Was surgery necessary? What would have been the evolution of the heroine of the book *Les Mots pour le Dire (The Words to Express It)*, by Marie Cardinal (4), if, after a thorough gynecological workup for her persistent vaginal bleeding, she had been sent to a surgeon instead of a psycho-analyst?

Hysteria (12, 14, 15) has disappeared from the DSM-III, but unlike Hydra of Lerna, the monster with regrowing heads Hercules finally slew, crossing hysteria out of the nomenclature does not make it disappear from hospital beds and doctors' offices, and undoubtedly Munchausen syn-drome has an hysterical flavor. It has been said that hysteria is at the forefront of medical research. It is hysteria that made Charcot famous, that introduced Freud to psychoanalysis, that prodded Babinski to discover his famous sign. It is no more elaborate to simulate multiple sclerosis than grand mal seizures, as was the case 100 years ago. But at that time, hysteria was safe, medicine was unarmed, and perhaps now we need a hand knife control law.

Incidentally, it is worth mentioning that management of the increased number of Munchausen cases has been facilitated by the safety of surgery and the increased efficacy of antibiotics.

Lucien Israel (14), a French psychoanalyst of the Lacanian school, has named the Munchausen syndrome "*neurosis beyond recall.*" He has switched the responsibility away from the patient, who becomes the victim of "iatro-genia." As soon as the scream of distress of the human being has been answered by surgery, the wound has solidified the scream. From there on, there is no other way to communicate but to continue to offer new physical symptoms covering up, over and over again, the initial unanswered need that will never be fulfilled. It is because there is an awareness of something missing in themselves that humans speak. In the case of Munchausen this confused awareness of an undefined and unknown need has been replaced by a real vacuum of which nothing more can be said. This emptiness cannot be filled by any object, and even the desire itself is dead. The person is condemned to continue to appeal to those who thought that a psycholog-ical need could be satisfied by a surgical act.

TREATMENT

It is difficult for physicians to understand their responsibility in the etiology of this syndrome. Initially there is a fortuitous disease that could have been treated differently, and the addiction starts there, like a ball pushed down a slope, like an innocent snort of cocaine at a party.

These patients usually refuse psychiatric treatment. Occasionally, there may be a kind of equilibrium, reached through a variety of means, foreign to the patient's wishes: insurance running out, fear on the part of the surgeons to operate further; but the rule is the progressive worsening of the physical condition with complete scotomization of the psychological needs. Like the burned-out alcoholic, whose brain has become worthless, the burned-out Munchausen has nothing left to offer: his body is worthless for further surgeries. For the physician, it is extremely difficult to guide these patients toward other alternatives. They have become unable to communicate. Each medical act is engraved within as a message fixed forever.

The most useful attitude is to avoid any medical or surgical treatment that aims at suppressing a symptom when the origin of that symptom is psychological. Any medical or surgical procedure not necessitated by the patient's condition is professional misconduct. Therapeutic abstention should be the "Golden Rule."

Human beings speak only because they feel a need, a lack within themselves. Often communication is achieved through symptoms offered to physicians. If this way of communication did not exist, 80% of the medical profession would be out of business. But when medicine chooses the Alexandrian way, shutting off the discourse by cutting the Gordian knot of the symptoms, instead of trying to unravel and understand it, nothing is left to the hysterics but to keep dead silent and continue to offer their mutilated bodies, instead of their scream of distress.

VIDEOTAPES

Louvain, M. (1985). Munchausen syndrome. Aesculape Productions presented at 138th A.P.A. Convention, Dallas, 1985.

REFERENCES

1. American Psychiatric Association (1987). *Diagnostic and statistical manual of mental disorders* (3rd edition-revised). Washington, DC: American Psychiatric Association.
2. Asher, R. (1951). Munchausen's syndrome. *Lancet, 1*, 339–341.
3. Bangs, J. K. (1901). *Mr. Munchausen: An Account of Some of His Recent Adventures.* Salem, NH: Ayer.
4. Cardinal, M. (1970). *Les mots pour le dire.* Paris, France: Grasset.
5. Carlson, R. J. (1985). Factitious psychiatric disorders: Diagnostic and etiologic considerations. *Psychiatry Med., 2*, 383–388.
6. Chapman, J. S. (1957). Peregrinating problem patients, Munchausen's syndrome. *JAMA, 165*, 927–933.
7. Clark, G. D., Key, J. D., & Rutherford, P. (1984). Munchausen's syndrome by proxy (child abuse) presenting as apparent autoerythrocyte sensitization syndrome: An unusual presentation of Polle syndrome. *Pediatrics, 74*(6), 1100–1102.
8. Charcot, J. M. (1889). *Clinical Lectures, Diseases of the Nervous System*, Vol. 3 (p. 319). London: New Sydenham Society.

9. CHERTOK, L. (1972). Mania operativa: Surgical addiction. *Psychiatry Med.*, *3*, 105–118.
10. DELAHOUSSE, J., MILLE, C., & PEDINIELLI, J. L. (1986). *Lasthenie de Ferjol, Le Baron de Munchausen, Les Desordres Factices du DSM III*. Congres de Psychiatrie et de Neurologie de langue francaise (pp. 212–225). Paris, France: Masson.
11. FIALKOV, M. J. (1984). Peregrination in the problem pediatric patient. The pediatric Munchausen syndrome. *Clin. Pediatr.*, *13*(10), 571–575.
12. FORD, C. V. (1973). The Munchausen syndrome: A report of four new cases and a review of psychodynamic considerations. *Int. J. Psychiatry Med.*, *4*, 31–45.
13. HUSTEAD, R. M., LEE, R. A., & MARUTA, T. (1982). Factitious illness in gynecology. *Obstet Gynecol.*, *59*(2), 214–219.
14. ISRAEL, L. (1977). *L'Hysterique, le sexe et le medicin*. Paris: Masson.
15. JUSTUS, P. G., KREUTZIGER, S. S., & KITCHENS, C. S. (1980). Probing the dynamics of Munchausen's syndrome. Detailed analysis of a case. *Ann. Intern. Med.*, *93*(1), 120–127.
16. LAZARUS, A. (1986). Factitious disorder in a manic patient: Case report and treatment considerations. *Int. J. Psychiatry Med.*, *15*(4), 365–369.
17. MEADOW, R. (1982). Munchausen syndrome by proxy and pseudo-epilepsy (letter). *Arch. Dis. Child*, *57*(10), 811–812.
18. MEADOW, R. (1984). Munchausen by proxy or Polle syndrome: Which term is correct? *Pediatrics*, *74*(4), 554–556.
19. WILLIAMS, B. (1951). Munchausen's syndrome. *Lancet*, *1*, 527.

11

AGORAPHOBIA

MICHAEL J. GARVEY, M.D.

Associate Professor,
Department of Psychiatry,
University of Iowa College of Medicine,
Iowa City, Iowa

and

RUSSELL NOYES, JR., M.D.

Professor, Department of Psychiatry,
University of Iowa College of Medicine,
Iowa City, Iowa

During the past several years there has been increased interest in anxiety disorders generally and agoraphobia more specifically. Agoraphobia will at sometime affect approximately 5% of all adults. It is a disorder that is seen in both psychiatric and general practice settings. Treatment with certain medications or specific behavioral therapies can be quite effective. This chapter will assist the clinician with an update and review of longitudinal course, clinical features, genetics, differential diagnosis, theories of pathogenicity, and treatments.

CLINICAL PICTURE

Agoraphobia is characterized by a marked fear of being alone or of being in public places from which escape might be difficult. These fears lead to the avoidance of such places and bring about a constriction of daily activities. The diagnostic criteria for agoraphobia are detailed in Table 1.

Panic attacks — sudden surges of anxiety lasting for minutes to part of an hour — frequently accompany agoraphobia. These attacks are characterized by difficulty breathing, choking, palpitations, chest discomfort, dizzi-

Table 1
Diagnostic Criteria for Agoraphobia*

Agoraphobia

Fear of being in places or situations from which escape might be difficult (or embarrassing) or in which help might not be available in the event of a panic attack. (Include cases in which persistent avoidance behavior originated during an active phase of Panic Disorder, even if the person does not attribute the avoidance behavior to fear of having a panic attack.) As a result of this fear, the person either restricts travel or needs a companion when away from home, or else endures agoraphobic situations despite intense anxiety. Common agoraphobic situations include being outside the home alone, being in a crowd or standing in a line, being on a bridge, and traveling in a bus, train, or car.

---

*Reprinted with permission from Diagnostic and Statistical Manual of Mental Disorders. Third Edition, Revised. Copyright 1987 American Psychiatric Association.

ness, paresthesias, trembling, sweating, feelings of unreality, and fears of going crazy or dying. When such attacks occur frequently and are not secondary to another major psychiatric disorder, the patient is given the diagnosis of panic disorder. The criteria for panic disorder are listed in Table 2.

Agoraphobia is almost always associated with panic attacks (1–4). Some researchers believe that agoraphobia may not be a distinct psychiatric disorder, but rather a variant of panic disorder (5–7). The notion that panic attacks are the primary disturbance and agoraphobia a complicating second feature is reflected in a revision of the third edition of the *Diagnostic and Statistical Manual of Mental Disorders* (DSM-III-R) (8).

Patients with agoraphobia often report that their panic attacks precede or coincide with the onset of their phobic avoidance behavior (4). Initial panic attacks may occur in a variety of situations. Some are associated with stressful life events (9, 10), whereas others come "out of the blue." Patients experiencing panic attacks often fear a major medical calamity and patients with recurrent attacks often develop a syndrome of anticipatory anxiety (11, 12). This anxiety occurs between attacks and has several characteristics of generalized anxiety, such as motor tension, autonomic hyperactivity, hypervigilance, and apprehensive expectation.

Some patients become fearful of having panic attacks in certain situations and begin to avoid these situations. These avoidant or agoraphobic behaviors may develop gradually or, at times, quite rapidly. Commonly avoided situations include cars, planes, and crowded or confined places,

Table 2
Diagnostic Criteria for Panic Disorder*

A. At some time during the disturbance, one or more panic attacks (discrete periods of intense fear or discomfort) have occurred that were (1) unexpected, i.e., did not occur immediately before or on exposure to a situation that almost always caused anxiety, and (2) not triggered by situations in which the person was the focus of others' attention.

B. Either four attacks, as defined in criterion A, have occurred within a four-week period, or one or more attacks have been followed by a period of at least a month of persistent fear of having another attack.

C. At least four of the following symptoms developed during at least one of the attacks:
  (1) shortness of breath (dyspnea) or smothering sensations
  (2) dizziness, unsteady feelings, or faintness
  (3) palpitations or accelerated heart rate (tachycardia)
  (4) trembling or shaking
  (5) sweating
  (6) choking
  (7) nausea or abdominal distress
  (8) depersonalization or derealization
  (9) numbness or tingling sensations (paresthesias)
  (10) flushes (hot flashes) or chills
  (11) chest pain or discomfort
  (12) fear of dying
  (13) fear of going crazy or of doing something uncontrolled

  Note: Attacks involving four or more symptoms are panic attacks; attacks involving fewer than four symptoms are limited symptom attacks

D. During at least some of the attacks, at least four of the C symptoms developed suddenly and increased in intensity within ten minutes of the beginning of the first C symptom noticed in the attack.

E. It cannot be established that an organic factor initiated and maintained the disturbance, e.g., Amphetamine or Caffeine Intoxication, hyperthyroidism.

*Reprinted with permission from *Diagnostic and Statistical Manual of Mental Disorders. Third Edition, Revised.* Copyright 1987 American Psychiatric Association.

such as shopping malls, theaters, and elevators. Agoraphobic patients also avoid situations in which they are alone. In severe cases patients are reluctant or unwilling to go out to do ordinary tasks, such as shopping, recreational activities, or visits to friends, and are said to be housebound.

Case History

Mrs. A., a 27-year-old married physical-education teacher, was in good health prior to the onset of her agoraphobia. After playing softball one evening, she experienced the sudden onset of palpitations, chest discomfort, shortness of breath, dizziness, trembling, and the sense of impending doom. She feared she was having a heart attack and presented herself to a hospital emergency room. Serum laboratory tests, a physical examination, and an electrocardiogram were all normal. Two weeks later she experienced a second panic attack at work. During the next two months the frequency of the attacks gradually increased to an average of two per day. Repeat visits to her family doctor proved frustrating; she was told there was "nothing physically wrong" with her.

Within the first several weeks of the onset of the panic attacks Mrs. A. developed the feeling that the panic attacks were associated with certain situations such as shopping, visiting friends, or attending church services. Consequently she began to limit or discontinue such activities in the belief that by reducing her contact with those situations she might reduce the number of attacks and the level of her generalized anxiety. However, her attacks and generalized anxiety continued unchanged with the result that she restricted her activities even further. During the fourth month of her illness a friend told her about a television program describing agoraphobia. The symptoms recounted in the report were similar to those experienced by the patient. This prompted Mrs. A. to seek an evaluation appointment at an anxiety disorders clinic of a nearby university. Mrs. A.'s condition was diagnosed as agoraphobia, and she was started on imipramine. Within three weeks there was a noticeable reduction in Mrs. A.'s panic attacks. Her avoidant behavior was little changed during the first month of treatment. By the second month of treatment she no longer had the attacks. Within a short time after the cessation of attacks the avoidant behavior gradually diminished and eventually disappeared. By the third month of treatment the patient noticed very mild somatic sensations, which she called "muted" panic attacks. These occurred once or twice a week and caused little distress.

EPIDEMIOLOGY

A large community survey of psychiatric disorders called the Epidemiological Catchment Area (ECA) program was conducted in the early 1980s (13). Structured psychiatric interviews were administered to several thousand randomly selected individuals from several communities. The results of this study suggest that the lifetime prevalence of agoraphobia is approximately 5% (14). If agoraphobia and panic disorder are combined, the figure rises to 7.5%. Previous community surveys of the prevalence of agoraphobia ranged from .6% to 26% (15, 16). These earlier studies suffered from methodological problems, including the lack of an agreed-upon definition for agoraphobia and lack of standardized interviews that would permit surveys of large populations by trained raters.

The ECA Survey (14) indicates that agoraphobia is approximately three times more common in women than men. There was a slightly increased lifetime prevalence of agoraphobia in black individuals when compared to nonblack individuals. Agoraphobia was twice as prevalent in persons not graduating from college as in college graduates.

Genetics

Family and twin studies suggest that panic disorder and agoraphobia have a genetic basis. A study of first-degree relatives of patients with agoraphobia revealed an increased age-adjusted morbidity risk of both agoraphobia (11.6%) and panic disorder (8.3%) compared to nonill controls (4.2% and 4.2%, respectively) (17). The morbidity risk of first-degree relatives of panic-disordered patients was 17.3% for panic disorders, but only 1.9% for agoraphobia. Adding the morbidity risk for agoraphobia and panic disorder for the two sets of first-degree relatives produces very similar results, 19.9% versus 19.2%. These data are consistent with the hypothesis that agoraphobia is a more severe variant of panic disorder and may be produced by a similar set of genetic and environmental disturbances.

Another research method used to establish the genetic nature of a psychiatric illness is to compare the concordance of monozygotic (MZ) and dizygotic (DZ) twins. Concordance is a measure of how often a twin with an illness has a cotwin with the same illness. If there is a significant genetic component to an illness, then one would expect the concordance between MZ twins to be greater than that between DZ twins. There are no twin studies for agoraphobia, but a study of panic disorder suggested an MZ concordance of 15% for panic disorder, 31% for panic attacks, and 46% for any anxiety disorder (2). DZ twins had a concordance of 25% for any anxiety disorder and 0% for panic disorders and panic attacks.

ETIOLOGICAL THEORIES

If agoraphobia is a severe variant of panic disorder (17), then pathogenic theories need to consider the genesis of both the panic attacks and the avoidant behaviors. There are several theories for the etiology of panic attacks, including overactivity of the locus ceruleus, metabolic abnormalities of the neurotransmitters, norepinephrine or serotonin, or their receptors, psychological disturbances such as early childhood separation, stressful life events, and faulty learning.

Biological Theories

Several lines of evidence raise the possibility that overactivity of the locus ceruleus may be responsible for panic attacks. The locus ceruleus (LC) is a nucleus located in the pons which sends afferent projections to many brain areas (18). Electrical stimulation of the LC in animals produced a fear or anxiety response that is not present after surgical abalation of the LC (19). Other investigators have disputed some of these findings (20). Drugs, such as yohimbine, that stimulate LC neuronal firing have produced anxiety reactions in both healthy controls and psychiatric patients (21, 22). Conversely, drugs that decrease LC firing, such as beta blockers, benzodiazepines, tricyclic antidepressants, and clonidine, also block spontaneous panic attacks in some patients (23–25).

Another pathogenic mechanism proposed for panic attacks is that there is a relative excess of certain neurotransmitters or their receptors. One such neurotransmitter is norepinephrine. A variety of evidence suggests that anxiety may be associated with increased turnover of norepinephrine and that this is reflected in increased urine or plasma levels of the norepinephrine metabolite 3-methoxy-4-hydroxyphenylglycol (MHPG). Elevations in urinary MHPG have been reported to be associated with increases in state anxiety in healthy controls (26–28). Plasma levels of MHPG were positively correlated with anxiety levels in phobic patients experiencing panic attacks (29). Similarly, anxiety induced by yohimbine in panic disorder patients was associated with rises in plasma MHPG (30). However, not all studies have found an association between anxiety and MHPG (31–34).

Another theory about the etiology of panic attacks involves the hypothesis that there is an increased number or increased sensitivity of beta-adrenergic receptors. Isoproterenol, a beta-receptor-stimulating drug, has been shown to produce panic attacks in some patients with panic disorder (35). In these same patients improvement in spontaneous panic attacks was noted after treatment with a beta blocker. Another group of investigators demonstrated a greater increase in heart rate with intravenous isoproterenol in panic disorder patients than in healthy controls (36). However, other investigators have not been able to replicate these findings (37, 38).

Another neurotransmitter postulated to play a role in anxiety disorders is gamma-aminobutyric acid (GABA). The GABA receptor is part of a macromolecule that includes a benzodiazepine receptor. Benzodiazepines and GABA appear to work in concert with each other to reduce the excitability of some neuronal cells. GABA coexists in some neurons with neuropeptides that may serve as cotransmitters (39). These cotransmitters are natural substances that interact with the benzodiazepine receptor. Possibly in anxiety-disordered patients there is some kind of defect in the cotransmitter system. This point is illustrated by the disruption of normal neurotransmission caused by a benzodiazepine antagonist, beta-carboline. It produced anxiety when given to rhesus monkeys (12). The natural occurrence of a similar antagonist could lead to anxiety symptoms that are relieved when the antagonist is displaced by exogenously administered benzodiazepine (40, 41).

Psychological Theories

Some investigators postulate that developmental factors such as childhood separations may predispose a person to panic disorder or agoraphobia in adulthood (42). An analysis of life events experienced at the time of onset of agoraphobia suggested these patients had encountered an excess of negative events (43). However, in another study a specific search for traumatic life events occurring prior to the onset of agoraphobia showed that the majority of patients had not experienced such events (44). Even if an association between life events and agoraphobia could be demonstrated, it would not by itself prove causality. In fact, prodromal symptoms of the disorder might cause or contribute to the life events.

According to learning theories, panic attacks and avoidant behaviors are conditioned responses. A problem with such theories is that many agoraphobic patients experience panic attacks spontaneously. Such attacks are not in response to a stimulus. While learning theories may not explain the occurrence of panic attacks, they may provide useful insights into the avoidant behaviors that subsequently develop. It is not uncommon for agoraphobic patients to avoid situations or places where they have experienced an attack. Since the panic attacks are usually spontaneous, they occur in various situations. Over time the agoraphobic patient "learns" to avoid more and more situations. In severe cases significant restriction of activity ensues.

NATURAL HISTORY

Onset of Illness

The onset of agoraphobia usually occurs in the mid- to late twenties (44–47). Most patients experience the onset of their agoraphobia between ages 15 and 35 (10). Very few patients have the onset of agoraphobia after age 40.

Several authors have suggested that initial panic attacks are precipitated by a stressful life event (9, 43, 48, 49). In some instances these life events are specific, such as choking on a piece of meat, being stung by a man-o'-war, experiencing sex for the first time, or being exposed to high altitude (9). For other patients, however, the stressful life events were recalled as being less specific and more of a general nature, e.g., conflict with spouse, job dissatisfaction (44).

Studies examining the relationship of onset of anxiety symptoms to stressful life events have the problem of eliciting such information months or even years after the events in question have occurred (9, 43, 48, 49). Whether such time lapses would tend to lead to an underestimate or an overestimate of the association between life events and the onset of panic attacks and agoraphobia is not clear. Some authors have suggested that stressful events in childhood, specifically separation from a parent, may predispose a child to agoraphobia in adolescence or adulthood (42). The evidence for such an association is presently not very strong (48).

Course of Illness

Ascertaining the natural history of agoraphobia is difficult for the following reasons. Many studies examining the longitudinal course of agoraphobia were performed before the current definitions of anxiety disorders were promulgated. Often patients with various anxiety and phobic disorders were studied together. Current evidence suggests that many of the broad categories of anxiety disorders are heterogeneous with respect to course of illness. In addition, patients in these studies received various forms of treatment that may have altered the "natural" course. Another problem with ascertainment of the natural history of agoraphobia is that patients with short-lived episodes are probably underrepresented in most studies.

In spite of these shortcomings, a tentative picture of the natural history of agoraphobia can be put forth. Ignoring those patients who may have had short-lived episodes and therefore were not included in follow-up studies, it appears that agoraphobia follows a relatively chronic course. Complete and total remissions appear to be an exception (9, 50–57). However, a substantial percentage of agoraphobics have symptom-free intervals lasting for months or longer. Forty percent of agoraphobics in one study claimed to have one or more symptom-free periods (17). Similar periods of improvement have been noted in some studies (44, 45, 58) but not in others (59, 60).

The duration of illness appears to be predictive of the longitudinal course. Most anxiety-disordered patients, including agoraphobics, demonstrate a more chronic course of illness if symptoms have been continuously present for three years or more. A much better prognosis was noted in patients with symptom duration of less than one year (17).

Complications

Patients with anxiety disorders, including agoraphobia, may develop secondary depression and alcohol abuse. Depression develops in half or more of the patients with agoraphobia or panic disorder (17, 61–69). Those patients who experience secondary depression tend to have a more chronic and severe anxiety disorder (63, 70). This complication may explain, in part, the increased risk of suicide in panic disorder (71).

One problem with diagnosing a secondary depression in a patient with agoraphobia is that several of the symptoms of the two disorders overlap. For example, in addition to panic attacks and agoraphobic symptoms, an agoraphobic may experience such problems as initial insomnia, guilt, loss of interest, decreased sexual drive, fatigue, and difficulty concentrating. All these symptoms may be the result of an uncomplicated anxiety disorder. However, this list of symptoms was chosen from the DSM-III–R criteria for major depressive disorder to illustrate the overlap between the two disorders. If such an agoraphobic patient were also experiencing dysphoria, he would technically meet criteria for major depression. This raises the question of whether such a patient has a separate new illness (secondary depression) or whether he has only one illness, namely agoraphobia to which the single symptom dysphoria has been added.

A second major psychiatric complication of agoraphobia is alcoholism. For some agoraphobic patients excessive use of alcohol may be an attempt to self-medicate their anxiety symptoms (72). Alcoholism has been noted in approximately 30% of patients with agoraphobia (17). Examining this issue from another perspective, one group of investigators have reported that a substantial minority of patients diagnosed as alcoholic have a variety of anxiety disorders (73, 74). In many of these patients it appears that the anxiety disorder preceded the alcoholism.

Agoraphobia is associated with varying degrees of social and occupational impairment. For much of their illness agoraphobics seem to experience subjective distress but show little in the way of outward signs of it (9, 50). During times of frequent panic attacks and pronounced avoidance, many patients will reduce outside contacts and activities. During such times patients can usually continue with their jobs, but find work burdensome and difficult. In extreme cases of agoraphobia patients may become housebound and stop working. Most agoraphobics do not experience this degree of impairment.

Mortality

A 35-year follow-up of 113 former inpatients with panic attacks (both with and without agoraphobia) revealed an excess of deaths due to unnatural causes (71). Twenty percent of these patients had committed suicide. This is comparable to the rate seen in unipolar depression. There was also an excess of deaths in males secondary to cardiovascular disorders. A separate follow-up study of patients diagnosed by a cardiologist 20 years earlier as "neurocirculatory asthenia" revealed no increases in mortality (50).

DIFFERENTIAL DIAGNOSIS

The differential diagnosis for agoraphobia includes generalized anxiety disorder, social and simple phobias, major depressive disorder, and somatoform disorders. A variety of medical illnesses can simulate the symptom picture of agoraphobia. Examples of these illnesses are pheochromocytoma, hyperthyroidism, cardiac arrhythmias, mitral valve prolapse, and withdrawal from certain sedative medications.

Psychiatric Illnesses

Generalized anxiety disorder is characterized by (1) motor tension, such as jitteriness, restlessness, fatigability; (2) autonomic hyperactivity, manifested by sweating, palpitations, dizziness, nausea, frequent urination, and increased respiratory rate; (3) apprehensive expectation, including worry, fear, rumination; and (4) vigilance, illustrated by distractibility, irritability, insomnia, and concentration difficulties. Patients with agoraphobia often have generalized anxiety symptoms. However, patients with agoraphobia also have avoidant behavior and almost always have panic attacks. Generalized anxiety disorder patients do not, by definition, have these additional symptoms.

Social phobia involves the irrational fear of and the compelling desire to avoid any situation that may expose the individual to the scrutiny of others with the potential for embarrassment or humiliation. Simple phobia is the irrational fear of and the compelling desire to avoid a specific object or situation, such as an animal, heights, or closed spaces. Agoraphobic avoidance is not limited to social situations or to one specific object.

Major depressive disorder is ordinarily not difficult to differentiate from agoraphobia unless panic attacks are present, as they may be in approximately one-third of depressed patients (75). If the panic attacks are prominent and withdrawal and isolation are associated with the depression, such patients may be misdiagnosed as agoraphobic. In such patients the depressive symptoms, such as dysphoria, sleep changes, appetite changes, thoughts of death, fatigue, anhedonia, and cognitive slowing, should help differentiate major depression from agoraphobia.

Patients with agoraphobia may exhibit significant somatic features (76, 77). If these somatic complaints are prominent, differentiation between somatoform disorders and agoraphobia may be necessary. Somatoform disorder often has associated anxiety symptoms, multiple somatic complaints involving many organ systems, an onset in late adolescence or early adulthood, a preponderance of females, and a chronic course of illness. Panic attacks and avoidant behavior are not usually a prominent part of the somatoform syndrome. The somatic complaints of the agoraphobic, when present, usually concern worry over symptoms that are related to panic attacks. For example, agoraphobics will seek cardiac evaluation for palpitations or chest pain or neurological evaluation of their dizziness.

Physical Illness

Certain medical illnesses should be considered in the differential diagnosis of agoraphobia. Patients with hyperthyroidism experience tachycardia, tremor, excessive sweating, and nervousness, which may be confused with an anxiety disorder. They also have heat intolerance, warm skin, hyperreflexia, and at times exophthalmos. Thyroid laboratory tests enable the clinician to make the diagnosis of hyperthyroidism.

A pheochromocytoma may at times masquerade as an anxiety disorder, especially if the release of catecholamines from the adrenal gland is episodic. Symptoms include hypertension, nervousness, headache, sweating, tremor, dyspnea, nausea, weakness, chest pain, and dizziness. Urinary assays for catecholamines aid in the diagnosis.

Patients with certain cardiac arrythymias, such as paroxysmal atrial tachycardia, may present a syndrome similar to that of agoraphobia. Such patients may have acute episodes of palpitations, chest discomfort, dizziness, and shortness of breath. Although they may have apprehension about future attacks, they would not ordinarily develop the extensive avoidant behaviors of the agoraphobic. An electrocardiogram during the attack or continuous cardiac monitoring can often identify the presence of an arrhythmia.

The cardiac syndrome of mitral valve prolapse (MVP) is interesting in the differential diagnosis of agoraphobia. MVP is diagnosed by a mid systolic click followed by a mid- to late systolic apical murmur, with evidence of prolapse of one or both leaflets of the mitral valve on echocardiography (78). There are various similarities between MVP and panic disorder or agoraphobia with panic attacks. Both syndromes affect approximately 5% to 10% of the population, affect women more often than men, have a familial pattern of occurrence, and may have a similar symptom profile. Several, but not all, studies (79–85) have found an increased incidence of MVP in patients with panic disorder. Possibly the selection of patients and the criteria used to diagnose MVP account for the differences found between studies, but most have found that between a quarter and a third of panic-disordered patients have MVP (range from 0% to 50%) (78–85).

The differential diagnosis of agoraphobia includes anxiety syndromes that result from use of certain medications. Examples include agents such as ephedrine, phenylpropanolamine, amphetamine, methylphenidate, aminophylline, or thyroid replacements. Caffeine used in large enough quantities can cause an anxiety syndrome. Anxiety resulting from one of these substances tends to be generalized. However, peak levels of a drug may make such an iatrogenic anxiety syndrome appear to be more episodic in nature and therefore resemble agoraphobia. It is important to obtain an accurate medication history in patients with an anxiety syndrome.

Medication withdrawal also needs to be considered in the differential diagnosis of agoraphobia. Patients who intermittently misuse or abuse drugs, such as various pain medications or sedatives, may develop a syndrome of waxing and waning anxiety symptoms corresponding to their withdrawal from these drugs.

TREATMENT

Medications

Four classes of drugs are used in the treatment of agoraphobia: tricyclic antidepressants, monoamine oxidase inhibitors, beta blockers, and benzodiazepines. The efficacy of the tricyclic imipramine for panic attacks was first reported in 1962 (86). Since this report there have been several controlled studies demonstrating imipramine's superiority over placebo (40). The dose of imipramine used to treat panic attacks is similar to that used for major depressive disorder, namely, 150 mg to 300 mg per day. Some investigators have observed that approximately 15% of patients given imipramine become overly stimulated (87, 88). These patients feel restless, nervous, irritable, and may have difficulty sleeping. This syndrome can occur with very low dosages of imipramine. If tolerance to this side effect does not develop, a switch to another medication may be necessary.

Imipramine is of benefit to 70% to 80% of patients with panic attacks who receive adequate dosages for several weeks. For patients who improve it is uncertain how long treatment should be maintained. Some authors suggest tapering and discontinuing imipramine after six months of treatment (12). Thirty percent of one group of agoraphobic patients treated for six months relapsed after imipramine was discontinued (87). Other tricyclic antidepressants have not been evaluated as thoroughly as imipramine for the treatment of panic attacks or agoraphobia. Clomipramine has been reported to be effective in agoraphobia. Some clinicians have found other tricyclics to be efficacious for agoraphobia (89).

Monoamine oxidase inhibitors (MAOI) are also of benefit to patients with panic attacks or agoraphobic symptoms (40). One review of MAOI use in agoraphobia concluded that these medications have their effect after four weeks of use, may improve anxious symptoms more than avoidant symptoms, and may have a rather high relapse rate when the medication is discontinued (10). A study comparing imipramine with the MAOI phenelzine found the phenelzine to be slightly better (90). Dosages of MAOIs used to treat agoraphobia are similar to those used in the treatment of depression. It should be noted that the efficacy of the MAOIs or the tricyclics does not depend on the presence of depressive symptoms (11, 12). Patients taking MAOIs need to remain on a tyramine-free diet.

Benzodiazepines are effective in the treatment of panic attacks (41) as well as generalized anxiety symptoms (91). Diazepam in dosages of 10 mg to 40 mg reduces the frequency and severity of panic attacks in most panic-disordered or agoraphobic patients (40, 41). There is no evidence to date to suggest greater efficacy of one benzodiazepine over another in the treatment of anxiety disorders. There is a great deal of concern among professionals and lay persons alike that benzodiazepines lead to abuse and dependence. Studies that have examined this issue suggest that abuse of these medications is low (92–96). Because of the fear of addiction it is not unusual to see agoraphobic or panic-disordered patients decrease their benzodiazepine dose below that which was recommended for them. At times this leads to an increase in symptoms.

Beta-blocking drugs such as propranolol are effective in treating certain panic symptoms, including somatic manifestations of anxiety such as palpitations and tremor (97). Psychic manifestations of anxiety disorders seem to be less affected. There have not been extensive studies of beta blockers in agoraphobic patients. One study of beta blockers in anxious patients included three agoraphobics (98) none of whom responded to the drug. If a beta blocker is to be tried, a dosage equivalent to 80 mg to 240 mg of propranolol should be used. If lower dosages are not effective, a gradual increase over several weeks may be tried.

Various supportive measures can be of assistance in the medical management of agoraphobic patients. Educating the patient about his illness promotes a clearer understanding of agoraphobia and what can be expected from treatment. Books about agoraphobia that are written for lay persons often help in this educational process. The involvement of significant family members can be helpful in the treatment of agoraphobia. It is important for patients and family members to realize that medications have side effects, may take several weeks to be fully effective, may not completely alleviate all of the anxiety and avoidant symptoms, and may need to be used for months or longer. Repeat discussions about these issues during the initial treatment phase can reduce misunderstandings and poor compliance.

Behavioral Treatments

Behavioral treatments attempt through various mechanisms to expose the patient to the feared situation. A review of these treatments suggests they have passed through three phases during the past 20 years (10). The earliest of the treatments encouraged patients to enter the feared situation in a gradual manner. Graded rationing gave way in time to imaginal methods, such as systematic desensitization. Patients using this technique had a hierarchy of mental images ranging from neutral to those provoking significant anxiety. As the anxiety-evoking scenes were imagined, a tension reduction device such as muscle relaxation was employed. This technique was later to be used in the real-life fear situation. Comparisons of systematic desensitization to individual or group psychotherapy showed the imaginal technique produced better outcomes (99–101). By the late 1960s techniques were used in which the patient was "flooded" with images of the most feared situation. This led some investigators to employ actual or in vivo exposure of the patient to the feared situations. Patients individually or in groups would confront the feared situations, usually with the assistance of a therapist. Exposure techniques appear to be enhanced by the use of an antipanic drug such as imipramine (87). A review of behavioral therapy for agoraphobics concluded the following (10): Exposure to the actual feared situations is superior to imaginal exposure. Prolonged exposure is more effective than brief exposure. Anxiety level during the exposure does not seem to be crucial.

Psychotherapy

A review of traditional psychotherapies suggests the following (10): Treatments that place agoraphobic patients in a passive role do not appear helpful. Other forms of psychotherapy appear to have limited usefulness. However, supportive and educational therapy used in conjunction with medications and/or behavioral techniques may benefit some patients.

During the past decade a specific form of psychotherapy, cognitive therapy, has been utilized in the treatment of agoraphobic patients (102, 103). It is hypothesized that agoraphobic patients experience faulty cognitions that lead to their disorder. The therapist elicits these counterproductive thoughts and assists patients in reevaluating them and creating other ways of thinking about their fears. Cognitive therapy is useful in the treatment of some depressions and may be of benefit for some cases of agoraphobia.

REFERENCES

1. DeNardo, P. A., O'Brien, G. T., Barlow, D. H., et al. (1983). Reliability of DSM III anxiety disorder categories using a new structured interview. *Arch. Gen. Psychiatry*, 40, 1070.
2. Torgersen, S. (1983). Genetic factors in anxiety disorders. *Arch. Gen. Psychiatry*, 40, 1085.
3. Zitrin, C. M., Klein, D. F., Woerner, M. B., et al. (1983). Treatment of phobias. *Arch. Gen. Psychiatry*, 40, 125.
4. Garvey, M. J., & Tuason, V. B. (1984). Relationship of panic disorder to agoraphobia. *Comp. Psychiatry*, 25, 529.
5. Noyes, R., Crowe, R. R., Harris, E. L., Hamra, B. J., McChesney, C. M., & Chaudhry, D. R. (1986). Relationship between panic disorder and agoraphobia. *Arch. Gen. Psychiatry*, 43, 227.
6. Klein, D. F. (1980). Anxiety reconceptualized. *Comp. Psychiatry*, 21, 411.
7. Hallam, R. S. (1978). Agoraphobia: A critical review of the concept. *Br. J. Psychiatry*, 133, 314.
8. American Psychiatric Association. *Diagnostic and statistical manual of mental disorders* (DSM-III-R) (3rd ed., revised). (1987). Washington, DC.
9. Noyes, R., Jr., Clancy, J., Hoenk, P. R., & Slymen, D. J. (1980). The prognosis of anxiety neurosis. *Arch. Gen. Psychiatry*, 37, 173.
10. Mathews, A. M., Gelder, M. G., & Johnston, D. W. (1981). *Agoraphobia: Nature and treatment*. New York: Guilford Press.
11. Mandel, J. G. C., & Klein, D. F. (1969). Anxiety attacks with subsequent agoraphobia. *Compr. Psychiatry*, 10, 190.
12. Gorman, J. M., Liebowitz, M. R., & Klein, D. F. (1984). *Panic disorder and agoraphobia*. Kalamazoo, MI: Upjohn Company.
13. Regier, D. A., Myers, J. K., Kramer, M., et al. (1984). The NIMH epidemiologic catchment area program. *Arch. Gen. Psychiatry*, 41, 934.
14. Robins, L. N., Helzer, J. E., Weissman, M. M., Orvaschel, H., Greenberg, E., Burke, J. D., & Regier, D. A. (1984). Lifetime prevalence of specific psychiatric disorders in three sites. *Arch. Gen. Psychiatry*, 41, 949.
15. Agras, W. S., Sylvester, D., & Oliveau, D. (1969). The epidemiology of common fears and phobias. *Br. J. Psychiatry*, 10, 151.
16. Langer, T. S., & Michael, S. T. (1956). *Life stress and mental health*. New York: Macmillan.
17. Noyes, R., Jr., Crowe, R.R., Harris, E. L., McChesney, C., & Hamra, B. (1986). Relationship of panic disorder and agoraphobia: A family study. *Arch. Gen. Psychiatry*, 43, 227.
18. Grant, S., & Redmond, D. E., Jr. (1981). The neuroanatomy and pharmacology of the nucleus locus coeruleus. In H. Lal & S. Fielding (Eds.), *The psychopharmacology of clonidine*. New York: Alan R. Liss.
19. Redmond, D. E. (1979). New and old evidence for the involvement of a brain norephinephrine system in anxiety. In W. E. Fann, I. Karacan, A. D. Pokorny, et al. (Eds.), *Phenomenology and treatment of anxiety*. New York: SP Medical & Scientific Books.
20. Mason, S. T., & Fibiger, H. C. (1979). Current concepts I. Anxiety: The locus coeruleus disconnection. *Life Sci.*, 25, 2141.
21. Holmberg, G., & Gershon, S. (1961). Autonomic and psychic effects of yohimbine hydrochloride. *Psychopharmacologia*, 2, 93.
22. Garfield, S. L., Gershon, S., Sletten, I., et al. (1967). Chemically induced anxiety. *Int. J. Neuropsychiatry*, 3, 426.

23. LIEBOWITZ, M. R., FYER, A. J., McGRATH, P., et al. (1981). Clonidine treatment of panic disorder. *Psychopharmacol. Bull.*, *17*, 122.

24. HOEHN-SARIC, R., MERCHANT, A. F., KEYSER, M. L., et al. (1981). Effects of clonidine on anxiety disorders. *Arch. Gen. Psychiatry*, *38*, 1278.

25. NYBACK, H. V., WALTERS, J. R., AGHAJANIAN, G. K., et al. (1975). Tricyclic antidepressants: Effects on the firing rate of brain noradrenergic neurons. *Eur. J. Pharmacol.*, *32*, 302.

26. BUSHBAUM, M. S., MUSCETTOLA, G., & GOODWIN, F. K. (1981). Urinary MHPG, stress response, personality factors and somatosensory evoked potentials in normal subjects and patients with major affective disorders. *Neuropsychobiology*, *7*, 212.

27. FRANKENHAEUSER, M., VON WRIGHT, M. R., VON WRIGHT, J., SEDVALL, G., & SWAHN, C. (1978). Sex differences in psychoneuroendocrine reactions to examination stress. *Psychosom. Med.*, *40*, 334.

28. RUBIN, R. T., MILLER, R. G., CLARK, B. R., POLAND, R. E., & ARTHUR, R. J. (1970). The stress of aircraft carrier landings: 3-Methoxy-4-hydroxyphenylglycol excretion in naval aviators. *Psychosom. Med.*, *32*, 589.

29. KO, G. N., ELSWORTH, J. D., ROTH, R. H., RIFKIN, G. G., LEIGH, H., & REDMOND, E. (1983). Panic-induced elevation of plasma MHPG levels in phobic-anxious patients. *Arch. Gen. Psychiatry*, *40*, 425.

30. CHARNEY, D. S., HENINGER, G. R., & BREIER, A. (1984). Noradrenergic function in panic anxiety. *Arch. Gen. Psychiatry*, *41*, 751.

31. CHARNEY, D. S., HENINGER, G. R., & JATLOW, P. I. (1985). Increased anxiogenic effects of caffeine in panic disorders. *Arch. Gen. Psychiatry*, *42*, 233.

32. HAMLIN, C. L., LYDIARD, R. B., MARTIN, D., DACKIS, C. A., POTTASH, A. C., SWEENEY, D., & GOLD, M. A. (1983). Urinary excretion of nondrenaline metabolite decreased in panic disorder. *Lancet*, *2*, 740.

33. SHEEHAN, D. V., CARR, D. B., SURMAN, O. S., NOLAN, J. M., FISHER, J. F., & CLAYCOMB, J. B. (1984). Sodium lactate infusion as a model for biological investigation of panic. *Scientific Proceedings of the American Psychiatric Association 137th Annual Meeting*. May 5–11, Los Angeles.

34. UHDE, T. W., BANLENGER, J. P., SIEVER, L., VITTONE, B., JIMERSON, D. C., & POST, R. (1984). Panic disorder: Drug challenge strategies. *Scientific Proceedings of the American Psychiatric Association 137th Annual Meeting*. May 5–11, Los Angeles.

35. EASTON, J. D., & SHERMAN, D. G. (1976). Somatic anxiety attacks and propranolol. *Arch. Neurol.*, *33*, 689.

36. SCHMIDT, H. S., & ELIZABETH, J. I. (1982). Mitral valve prolapse: Relationship to panic attacks/anxiety disorders and beta-adrenergic hypersensitivity. Presented at the thirty-seventh annual meeting of the Society of Biological Psychiatry, Toronto.

37. GORMAN, J. M., LEVY, G. F., LIEBOWITZ, M. R., et al. (1983). Effect of acute beta-adrenergic blockade on lactate induced pain. *Arch. Gen. Psychiatry*, *40*, 1979.

38. NESSE, R., CAMERON, O., CURTIS, G., & McCANN, D. (1983). *Adrenergic function in panic disorder*. Presented at the 136th annual meeting of the American Psychiatric Association, New York City.

39. COSTA, E., CORDA, M. G., EPSTEIN, B., FORCHETTI, C., & GUIDOTTI, A. (1983). GABA-benzodiazepine interactions. In E. Costa (Ed.), *The benzodiazepines: From molecular biology to clinical practice*. New York: Raven Press.

40. NOYES, R., JR. (1983). Anxiety, phobic and obsessional disorders. In D. G. Graham-Smith, H. Hippius, & G. Winokur (Eds.), *Psychopharmacology review*, Vol. 1 (pp. 203–230). Amsterdam: Excerpta Medica.

41. NOYES, R., JR., ANDERSON, D. J., CLANCY, J., et al. (1984). Diazepam and propranolol in panic disorder and agoraphobia. *Arch. Gen. Psychiatry*, *41*, 287.

42. KLEIN, D. F. (1981). Anxiety reconceptualized. In D. F. Klein & J. G. Rabkin (Eds.), *Anxiety — New research and changing concepts*. New York: Raven Press.

43. SOLYOM, L., BECK, P., SOLYOM, C., & HUGEL, R. (1974). Some etiological factors in phobic neurosis. *Can. Psychiatr. Assoc. J., 19*, 69.
44. BUGLASS, D., CLARKE, J., HENDERSON, A. S., KREITMAN, N., & PRESLEY, A. S. (1977). A study of agoraphobic housewives. *Psychol. Med., 7*, 73.
45. BURNS, L. E., & THORPE, G. L. (1977). Fears and clinical phobias: Epidemiological aspects and the national survey of agoraphobics. *J. Intern. Med. Res., 17*, 243.
46. MARKS, I. M., & GELDER, M. D. (1965). A controlled retrospective study of behaviour therapy in phobic patients. *Br. J. Psychiatry, 111*, 561.
47. MARKS, I. M., & HERST, E. R. (1970). A survey of 1,200 agoraphobics in Britain. *Soc. Psychiatry, 5*, 16.
48. TEARNAN, B. H., TELCH, M. J., & KEEFE, P. (1984). Etiology and onset of agoraphobia: A critical review. *Compr. Psychiatry, 25*, 51.
49. SNAITH, R. A. (1968). A clinical investigation of phobias. *Br. J. Psychiatry, 114*, 673.
50. WHEELER, E. O., WHITE, P. D., REED, E. W., & COHEN, M. E. (1950). Neurocirculatory asthenia (anxiety neurosis, effort syndrome, neurasthenia), a twenty year follow-up study of one hundred and seventy-three patients. *JAMA, 142*, 878.
51. MILES, H. H. W., BANABEE, E. L., & FINESINGER, J. E. (1951). Evaluation of psychotherapy with a follow-up of 62 cases with anxiety neurosis. *Psychosom. Med., 13*, 83.
52. EITINGER, L. (1955). Studies in neuroses. *Acta Psychiatr. Scand., 101*, 5.
53. BLAIR, R., GILROY, J. M., & PILKINGTON, F. (1957). Some observations on outpatient psychotherapy with a follow-up of 235 cases. *Br. Med. J., 1*, 318.
54. ERNST, K. (1959). Die prognose der neurosen. *Monographon neurologn und psychiatry.* No. 85. Berlin: Springer.
55. GREER, S., & CRAWLEY, R. H. (1966). Some observations on the natural history of neurotic illness. *Archdall Medical Monograph No. 3.* Sydney: Australian Medical Publishing Co.
56. SCHAPIRA, K., ROTH, M., KERR, T. A., & GURNEY, C. (1972). Prognosis of affective disorders — The differentiation of anxiety states from depressive illness. *Br. J. Psychiatry, 121*, 175.
57. CORYELL, W., NOYES, R., JR., & CLANCY, J. (1983). Panic disorder and primary unipolar depression: A comparison of background and outcome. *J. Affect. Dis., 5*, 311.
58. FRIEDMAN, J. H. (1950). Short term psychotherapy of a "phobia of travel." *Am. J. Psychother., 4*, 259.
59. AGRAS, W. S., CHAPIN, H. N., & OLIVEAU, D. C. (1972). The natural history of phobia. *Arch. Gen. Psychiatry, 26*, 315.
60. ROBERTS, A. H. (1964). Housebound housewives — A follow-up study of a phobic anxiety state. *Br. J. Psychiatry, 110*, 191.
61. UHDE, T. W., BOULENGER, J., ROY-BYRNE, P. P., GERACI, M. F., VITTONE, B. J., & POST, R. M. (1985). Longitudinal course of panic disorder: Clinical and biological considerations. *Prog. Neuro-Psychopharmacol. Biol. Psychiatry, 9*, 39.
62. VANVALKENBURG, C., AKISKAL, H. S., PUZANTIAN, V., & ROSENTHAL, T. (1984). Anxious depressions: Clinical, family history, and naturalistic outcome — Comparisons with panic and major depressive disorders. *J. Affect. Dis., 6*, 67.
63. BREIER, A., CHARNEY, D. S., & HENINGER, G. R. (1984). Major depression in patients with agoraphobia and panic disorder. *Arch. Gen. Psychiatry, 41*, 1129.
64. RASKIN, M., PEEKE, H. V. S., DICKMAN, W., & PINSKER, H. (1982). Panic and generalized anxiety disorders. *Arch. Gen. Psychiatry, 39*, 687.
65. MUMJACK, D. J., & MOSS, H. B. (1981). Affective disorder and alcoholism in families of agoraphobics. *Arch. Gen. Psychiatry, 38*, 869.
66. DELAY, R. S., ISHIKI, D. M., AVERY, D. H., WILSON, L. G., & DUNNER, D. L. (1981). Secondary depression in anxiety disorders. *Compr. Psychiatry, 22*, 612.
67. CLONINGER, C. R., MARTIN, R. L., CLAYTON, P., & GUZE, S. B. (1981). A blind follow-up and family study of anxiety neurosis: Preliminary analyses of the St. Louis 500. In

D. F. Klein & J. Rabkin (Eds.) *Anxiety: New research and changing concepts.* New York: Raven Press.

68. BOWEN, R. C., & KOHOUT, J. (1979). The relationship between agoraphobia and primary affective disorders. *Can. J. Psychiatry, 24,* 317.

69. WOODRUFF, R. A., GUZE, S. B., & CLAYTON, P. J. (1972). Anxiety neurosis among psychiatric outpatients. *Compr. Psychiatry, 13,* 165.

70. CLANCY, J., NOYES, R., JR., HOENK, P. R., et al. (1979). Secondary depression in anxiety neurosis. *J. Nerv. Ment. Dis., 166,* 846.

71. CORYELL, W., NOYES, R., JR., & CLANCY, J. (1982). Excess mortality in panic disorder. *Arch. Gen. Psychiatry, 39,* 701.

72. QUITKIN, F. M., RIFKIN, A., KAPLAN, J., & KLEIN, D. F. (1972). Phobic anxiety syndrome complicated by drug dependence and addiction, a treatable form of drug abuse. *Arch. Gen. Psychiatry, 27,* 159.

73. SMAIL, P., STOCKWELL, T., CANTER, S., & HODGSON, R. (1984). Alcohol dependence and phobic states. I. A prevalence study. *Br. J. Psychiatry, 144,* 53.

74. WEISS, K. J., & ROSENBERG, D. J. (1985). Prevalence of anxiety disorders among alcoholics. *J. Clin. Psychiatry, 46,* 3.

75. LECKMAN, J. F., WEISSMAN, M. M., & MERIKANGAS, K. R. (1983). Panic disorder and major depression. *Arch. Gen. Psychiatry, 40,* 1055.

76. NOYES, R., JR., CLANCY, J., HOENK, P. R., et al. (1978). Physical illness in anxiety neurosis. *Compr. Psychiatry, 19,* 407.

77. NOYES, R., JR., REICH, J., CLANCY, J., & O'GORMAN, T. (1986). Reduction in hypochondriasis with treatment of panic disorder. *Br. J. Psychiatry, 149,* 631.

78. LIBERTHSON, R., SHEEHAN, D. V., KING, M. E., & WEYMAN, A. E. (1986). The prevalence of mitral valve prolapse in patients with panic disorders. *Am. J. Psychiatry, 143,* 511.

79. VENKATESH, A., PAULS, D. L., CROWE, R. R., et al. (1980). Mitral valve prolapse in anxiety neurosis (panic disorder). *Am. Heart J., 100,* 302.

80. PARISER, S. F., PINTA, E. R., & JONES, B. A. (1978). Mitral valve prolapse syndrome and anxiety neurosis/panic disorder. *Am. J. Psychiatry, 135,* 246.

81. KANTOR, J. S., ZITRIN, C. M., & ZELDIS, S. M. (1980). Mitral valve prolapse syndrome in agoraphobic patients. *Am. J. Psychiatry, 137,* 467.

82. GRUNHAAUS, L., GLOGER, S., REIN, A., et al. (1982). Mitral valve prolapse and panic attacks. *Isr. J. Med. Sci., 18,* 221.

83. MAVISSAKALIAN, M., SALERNI, R., THOMPSON, M. E., et al. (1983). Mitral valve prolapse and agoraphobia. *Am. J. Psychiatry, 140,* 1612.

84. HICKEY, A. J., ANDREWS, G., & WILCKEN, D. E. L. (1983). Independence of mitral valve prolapse and neurosis. *Br. Heart J., 50,* 333.

85. SHEAR, M. K., DEVEREUX, R. B., KRAMER-FOX, R., MANN, J. J., & ALLEN, F. (1974). Low prevalence of mitral valve prolapse in patients with panic disorder. *Am. J. Psychiatry, 141,* 302.

86. KLEIN, D. F., & FINK, M. (1962). Psychiatric reaction patterns to imipramine. *Am. J. Psychiatry, 119,* 432.

87. ZITRIN, C. M., KLEIN, D. F., & WOERNER, M. G. (1978). Behavior therapy, supportive psychotherapy, imipramine and phobias. *Arch. Gen. Psychiatry, 35,* 307.

88. MUSKIN, P. R., & FYER, A. J. (1981). Treatment of panic disorder. *J. Clin. Psychopharmacol., 1,* 81.

89. ZITRIN, C. M. (1981). Combined pharmacological and psychological treatment of phobias. In M. Mavissakalian & D. H. Barlow (Eds.), *Phobia: Psychological and pharmacological treatment.* New York: Guilford Press.

90. SHEEHAN, D. V., BALLENGER, J., & JACOBSEN, G. (1980). Treatment of exogenous anxiety with phobic, hysterical and hypochondriacal symptoms. *Arch. Gen. Psychiatry, 37,* 51.

91. RICKELS, K., CASE, W. G., DOWNING, R. W., & WINOKUR, A. (1983). Long-term diazepam therapy and clinical outcome. *JAMA, 250,* 767.
92. MARKS, J. (1978). *The benzodiazepines: Use, overuse, misuse, abuse.* Lancaster, England: MTP Press.
93. HOLISTER, L. E., CONLEY, F. K., BRITT, R. H. & SHUER, L. (1981). Long term use of diazepam. *JAMA, 246,* 1568.
94. RICKELS, K. (1981). Are benzodiazepines overused and abused? *Br. J. Clin. Pharmacol., 11,* 715.
95. HASDAY, J. D., & KARCH, F. E. (1981). Benzodiazepine prescribing in a family medicine center. *JAMA, 246,* 1321.
96. BOETHIUS, G., & WESTERHOLD, B.: Is the use of hypnotics, sedatives and minor tranquilizers really a major health problem? *Acta Med. Scand., 199,* 507.
97. NOYES, R., JR. (1983). Anxiety, phobic and obsessional disorders. In H. Hippius & G. Winokur (Eds.), *Psychopharmacology I; Part 2. Clinical psychopharmacology.* Princeton, NJ: Excerpta Medicine.
98. HEISER, J. F., & DEFRANCISCO, D. (1976). The treatment of pathological panic states with propranolol. *Am. J. Psychiatry, 133,* 1389.
99. GELDER, M. G., MARKS, I. M., & WOLFF, H. H. (1967). Desensitization and psychotherapy in the treatment of phobic states: A controlled clinical inquiry. *Br. J. Psychiatry, 113,* 53.
100. GELDER, M. G., & MARKS, I. M. (1968). Desensitisation and phobias: A crossover study. *Br. J. Psychiatry, 114,* 323.
101. GILLAN, P., & RACHMAN, S. (1974). An experimental investigation of desensitisation in phobic patients. *Br. J. Psychiatry, 124,* 392.
102. BECK, A. T., & EMERY, G. (1979). *Cognitive therapy of anxiety and phobic disorders.* Philadelphia: Center for Cognitive Therapy.
103. EMMELKAMP, P. M. G. (1982). *Phobic and obsessive-compulsive disorders: Theory, research, and practice.* New York: Plenum Press.

12
SOCIAL PHOBIA

Michael R. Liebowitz, M.D.

Director, Anxiety Disorders Clinic;
Associate Professor, Psychiatry,
College of Physicians & Surgeons, Columbia University,
New York, New York

and

Timothy J. Strauman, Ph.D.

Department of Psychology,
New York University,
New York, New York

Social phobia, until recently the most neglected of the anxiety disorders, has become the subject of increased attention. In contrast to the relative paucity of laboratory and clinical data available in the past, research is now beginning to appear regarding the prevalence, pathophysiology, and treatment of this disorder. In this chapter, we shall review these new developments as well as the continuing accumulation of knowledge regarding the classification, etiology, assessment, and treatment of social phobia.

DEFINITION

The original Marks and Gelder definition of social phobia (51) included patients with specific social fears, such as fear of speaking, signing a check, or eating in public, as well as those with more generalized forms of social anxiety (e.g., fears of initiating conversation or dating). The DSM-III description of social phobia also suggested a "broad" definition of the disorder. However, the examples given in the DSM-III description were all limited to specific social fears and involve anxiety about speaking or performing in public, using public lavatories, eating in public, and writing in the presence of others. Moreover, DSM-III asserted that social phobics generally have only one fear, implying that patients with multiple social fears or more generalized social anxiety are either rare or should be included in some other diagnostic category. Also, without empirical justification, DSM-III excluded patients whose social anxiety symptoms were due to avoidant personality disorder from the social phobia category.

A separate issue in defining social phobia is how to classify patients who develop spontaneous panic attacks leading to panic disorder or agoraphobia and then, as part of a larger syndrome, begin to avoid certain performance or social situations (*secondary* social phobics). In our view, primary social phobics fear *scrutiny* or *evaluation* by others, and their anxiety is generally confined to such situations or the anticipation of such situations. Secondary social phobics, on the other hand, also have panic attacks in a variety of nonsocial situations (e.g., subways, supermarkets, tunnels, bridges) and tend to fear or avoid any situations where easy or unobtrusive exit is difficult. Also, we have observed that patients with panic disorder are comforted by the presence of familiar figures when experiencing anxiety, while primary social phobics feel more comfortable if they can be alone (47).

DSM-III-R more clearly addresses the distinctions and concerns outlined here by recognizing discrete performance anxiety and generalized social fears as two subtypes of social phobia, and excluding social or performance anxiety due to spontaneous panic attacks from social phobia. In DSM-III-R, avoidant personality disorder can overlap with social phobia.

DISTINCTION FROM OTHER ANXIETY DISORDERS

Agoraphobia

Both demographic and clinical data support the distinction between social phobia and agoraphobia. Two studies have found age differences between the two phobic subtypes, indicating that social phobics seek treatment and report the onset of symptoms at an earlier age than agoraphobics (2, 49). Somatic anxiety symptoms reported by social phobics also appear to show differences from those of agoraphobics. Social phobics reported more blushing and muscle twitching and less limb weakness, breathing difficulty, dizziness or faintness, actual fainting, and buzzing or ringing in the ears than agoraphobics. These symptom differences suggest that agoraphobia and social phobia are pathophysiologically distinct. Social phobics also had lower extraversion scores on the Eysenck Personality Inventory than agoraphobics, whose scores were similar to those of a group of nonpsychiatric controls (2).

Panic Disorder

Findings from biological challenge and treatment studies have begun to clarify the distinction between social phobia and panic disorder (with or without agoraphobia). Patients with panic disorder show high rates of panic during infusion of sodium lactate (46, 68). Our finding (44) was that social phobics show a significantly lower rate of panic during lactate infusion than agoraphobics, a rate that appears equivalent to that of normal controls. Patients with spontaneous panic attacks are also highly responsive to the tricyclic imipramine (36, 80) and the monoamine oxidase inhibitor phenelzine sulfate (71). However, the responsiveness of social phobics to these medications is as yet unclear (see the "Treatment" section below).

Simple Phobias

Data also support the distinction between social phobia and the simple phobias, which consist of specific animal (birds, cats, insects) and environmental (heights, darkness, thunderstorms) fears. In terms of demographics, social phobics show a later age of onset than simple phobics, have a higher level of overt anxiety, and have higher neuroticism scores on the Maudsley Personality Inventory than animal phobics (49, 51). In clinical and laboratory settings, social phobics show more spontaneous fluctuation in galvanic skin response than animal phobics, but do not necessarily show comparable increases in self-reported anxiety or in heart rate during exposure to phobic stimuli (40, 78). At present, we lack the data to compare drug responsiveness of social and simple phobics. Simple phobics have been found unresponsive to tricyclics (36) and only weakly, if at all, responsive to beta-adrenergic blockers (6, 20).

Personality Disorders

Social phobics appear distinct from schizoid individuals in our view. Although both may avoid social interactions, social phobics desire social contact but are blocked by their anxiety while schizoid patients lack interest in social interaction. The relationship between social phobia and avoidant personality disorder, if any, has yet to be determined. Avoidant personalities manifest long-standing, pervasive withdrawal from social relationships due to hypersensitivity to potential rejection and humiliation. However, many social phobics are able to maintain relationships despite their anxiety in situations where evaluation or scrutiny seems likely. It is clear that demographic, family, treatment, and follow-up studies are needed to elucidate the degree of overlap between these two diagnostic categories.

MAGNITUDE OF THE PROBLEM

Prevalence

While epidemiological studies have indicated that phobic disorders in general may affect as much as 7% of the general population (1), the prevalence of social phobia is only now being clarified (10). Preliminary data from a multisite psychiatric epidemiological survey showed that the six-month prevalence of social phobia in two urban populations ranged from 0.9% to 1.7% for men and 1.5% to 2.6% for women (59). In a series of outpatients applying for treatment to one U.S. anxiety and phobic center, 8 (13%) of 60 were found to meet criteria for social phobia, which equaled the proportion with panic disorder and was exceeded only by the 38% with agoraphobia (15). In our Anxiety Disorders Clinic, social phobics represent the third most common anxiety disorder after panic disorder and agoraphobia. Moreover, some patients with panic disorder or agoraphobia have a history of social phobia that predates the onset and persists after successful treatment of their panic attacks.

Morbidity

Social phobia appears to begin early, characteristically between ages 15 and 20, and follow a chronic, unremitting course (2, 49, 51). The symptom pattern is typically consistent: of 11 patients meeting DSM-III criteria we recently studied, all complained of tachycardia, pounding heart, trembling, and sweating when in a performance and/or social situation. The associated disability, in terms of vocational and social impairment, is often significant. In our series, 2 of the 11 patients were unable to work, two dropped out of school, four had abused alcohol, one had abused tranquilizers, six were blocked from advancement at work, and five avoided almost all social interaction outside their immediate families.

Significant depressive symptoms are reported to be quite common in social phobics and were found in half of the patients in one large sample (2). In a similar series, one-third of the patients were found to have either a past or present depression (58). Aimes et al. (2) also found that 14 % of their social phobic patients had a history of "parasuicidal acts," which significantly exceeded the 2 % rate among agoraphobics. Social phobic symptoms are also frequently found among alcoholics, usually predating the drinking problem (57, 73).

PATHOPHYSIOLOGY AND ETIOLOGY

Pathophysiology

It is unclear whether normal and pathological social (or performance) anxiety lie on a continuum or are categorically distinct. A certain degree of social or performance anxiety is ubiquitous and may represent an evolutionary adaptive advantage by motivating preparation and rehearsal of important social events. In normals, however, such anxiety lessens with repeated exposure and usually attenuates over the course of any given performance or social encounter (14).

In contrast, our experience has been that social phobics often report their symptoms to be refractory to self-administered rehearsal or exposure. (Few have participated in formal desensitization or exposure programs.) Moreover, their anxiety does not seem to attenuate during the course of a social event or performance; they often report that their symptoms augment, as initial somatic disturbance becomes a further distraction and embarrassment for the already nervous individual, leading to further symptoms, which give rise to more distraction, and so on.

The symptoms that social phobic individuals suffer when they experience evaluation or scrutiny virtually always include tachycardia, sweating, blushing, and trembling, all of which suggest heightened autonomic arousal. Since normal individuals have been shown to experience brief twofold-to-threefold increases in plasma epinephrine levels during stressful public speaking (14), it is tempting to speculate that social phobics either experience greater or more sustained increases or are more sensitive to normal stress-mediated elevations in plasma catecholamine levels. These two possibilities have been examined experimentally in our laboratory by in vivo biochemical monitoring of social phobics in their feared situations and by challenges with infusions of epinephrine.

In one study, 11 social phobic patients were given intravenous infusions of epinephrine sufficient to raise plasma levels from an 85-to-125 pg/ml to the 850-to-1000 pg/ml range within 30 minutes. Epinephrine did not effectively provoke anxiety in these patients. Only 3 of the 11 individuals reported significant anxiety, while only one experienced the full naturally occurring symptom picture of social anxiety, and even this episode was for a briefer than usual duration (Papp et al., unpublished data).

In another study designed to investigate the pathophysiology of social anxiety during actual social stress, 22 social phobic patients and seven normal controls underwent a public-speaking simulation while facing a video camera and an audience of several staff members. During the procedure, heart rate and blood chemistry were continuously monitored. As expected, patients started and remained more anxious than normal controls; both patients and controls reported the procedure to be somewhat milder than challenging social situations in real life. The patient group reported significantly more anxiety symptoms and demonstrated significantly more behavioral impairment than the controls. More interestingly, however, 10 of the 22 patients had at least a 50% rise in serum epinephrine during the speech, while only one of the seven controls had a rise in epinephrine of this magnitude (Levin et al., unpublished data).

These two experiments suggest the following: (1) An increase in plasma epinephrine level is not sufficient to produce the full scope of social anxiety symptoms in social phobics. This implies that social phobia cannot be accounted for by a simple model of hypersensitivity to normal stress-related epinephrine elevation. (2) At least some social phobics produce greater epinephrine levels than normals during in vivo performance situations. If sustained, this finding would support the hypothesis that social phobic symptomatology is due in part to the excessive release of epinephrine.

The findings of both experiments point to the importance of psychological factors in social phobia, and specifically to the central role of the individual's perception that he or she is about to be scrutinized or embarrassed. All people are probably vulnerable to "social phobic" symptoms (e.g., autonomic arousal and a desire to flee) under sufficiently embarrassing conditions. What appears to distinguish the social phobic in this regard is the *range* of situations that trigger such reactions.

Etiology

Should a biological mediator of social phobia be found, questions will arise as to its inherited or acquired nature. To date, no family studies of social phobia have been conducted, so no genetic hypotheses can be evaluated at this point. There is evidence, though, that social anxiety may have an inheritable component. Torgersen (78) compared social fears among 95 monozygotic and dizygotic twin pairs chosen for the most part on a random basis from a Norwegian twin registry. The monozygotic twins were significantly more concordant for such social phobic symptoms as discomfort when eating with strangers, when being watched while working or writing, and trembling, suggesting a genetic contribution to social anxiety.

Among the postulated acquired causes of social phobia are social-skills deficits, traumatic early social or performance experiences, and "faulty cognitions" (16, 50). Other psychological antecedents and correlates of social anxiety have been outlined in Leary (42). There do not appear to be any psychological models of social phobia per se at present, although a great deal of research has been undertaken in areas that are more or less related (e.g., shyness, introversion, evaluation apprehension, public and private self-consciousness) (54). During the last decade, the simpler conditioning models of social anxiety found in the behavior therapy literature have begun to give way to more complex schemes that take into account the mediating role of cognitions (42). It remains to be demonstrated, however, that such "faulty" cognitions are causal antecedents of social phobia and not simply part of the typical symptom constellation. Also, many social phobics appear hypersensitive to rejection or criticism (61), which suggests an overlap with atypical depression or hysteroid dysphoria. The traditional psychoanalytic view that phobias represent the transformation of internal anxiety into external fear through displacement, and that the specific content of a phobia has some symbolic meaning (19), is also theoretically applicable to social phobia. This approach has not as yet been subjected to controlled investigation.

Nichols (61) has catalogued a variety of psychological and somatic traits observed in social phobic individuals. These included negative self-evaluation, an unrealistic tendency to experience others as critical or disapproving, rigid concepts of appropriate social behavior, negative fantasy-producing anticipatory anxiety, an increased awareness and fear of scrutiny by others, a fear of social situations from which it is difficult to leave unobtrusively, an exaggerated awareness of minimal somatic symptoms (such as blushing or feeling faint), a tendency to overreact with greater anxiety to such somatic arousal, and an exaggerated fear of others noticing that one is anxious. It is not clear, however, which among these or other factors are possible causes, which are consequences of, and which are not specifically related to social phobia.

Several controlled studies have also compared how adult social phobics, agoraphobics, simple phobics, and nonpsychiatric controls retrospectively rate their parents' child-rearing practices and attitudes. As a group, social phobics tended to perceive their parents as having been less caring, more lacking in emotional warmth, more rejecting, and more overprotective as compared with normal controls (4, 66). However, no contrasts were reported among the various phobic groups, so the specificity of these findings for social phobia is uncertain. These studies also suffer from the limitations inherent in retrospective self-report techniques.

ASSESSMENT

Investigators have employed subjective (both clinician ratings and self-assessments), biological, and performance measures to assess social phobia. Liebowitz et al. (47) reviewed the existing self-report instruments most frequently used to evaluate social anxiety and identified several shortcomings in such measures, particularly the lack of norms for these scales in social phobics diagnosed according to DSM-III criteria. Because no one measure has as yet demonstrated superiority for the assessment of social phobia, the authors recommended the use of a battery of self-rating and clinician-rating scales.

Biological monitoring of social phobics has typically involved measurement of heart rate, respiration, and skin conductance (31, 41, 78). In general, social phobics show considerable physiological responsivity (41, 78); in addition, heart rate, respiration rate, and subjective anxiety tend to be more highly correlated in social phobics than in other phobic groups (60). Biological measures not yet studied in social phobics include cardiac rhythm (to detect possible arrhythmias in individuals under stress) and in vivo biochemical monitoring of catecholamine levels, free-fatty-acid levels, cortisol levels, and so forth.

Performance evaluations can involve observation by professional or peer raters before and after treatment (7, 17), observation during role rehearsal in simulated situations in the clinic (7), or evaluation of patient responses in staged situations where the patient is unaware of the staging, such as when research assistants call patients and pretend to be intrusive, high-pressure salespeople (7). All have shown promise in analog studies but require further study with regard to their utility and reliability in social phobic samples.

TREATMENT

Two types of treatment for social phobia have been subjected to at least some controlled evaluation: pharmacotherapy and behavioral therapy.

Pharmacological Treatment

Social phobia has not been regarded as a discrete syndrome in need of independent study by pharmacologists. Instead, it has been viewed in at least three alternative ways: as a more severe form of a normal human trait (social anxiety), the treatment of which could be elucidated by analog instead of clinical studies (9, 13, 23, 27, 29, 30, 38, 39, 43, 60, 72); as a manifestation of one or more personality disorders that are *a priori* unresponsive to drug treatment (24); or as so closely related to agoraphobia (3, 5, 56, 67, 74, 75, 79) or the simple phobias (80) that the groups could be merged rather than studied independently. The unfortunate result has been that, with the exception of several small studies (18, 22, 45), to our knowledge no data on the drug responsiveness of a pure social phobic sample have been reported. The results of analog studies and clinical studies in mixed diagnostic groups, however, suggest the possible efficacy of MAOIs and beta-adrenergic blockers.

Monoamine oxidase studies. Several types of data suggest monoamine oxidase (MAOI) efficacy in social phobia. Four controlled studies found positive effects of phenelzine in patient samples that consisted of both agoraphobics and social phobics (56, 74, 75, 79). However, none reported response rates among the social phobics separately from the sample as a whole. Since agoraphobic patients also have been shown to benefit from MAOIs (18, 62), it is impossible to be sure that the social phobics in the mixed-patient studies benefited from MAOI therapy. Other limitations of those investigations were a lack of specified diagnostic criteria, relatively low dosages (45 mg/day or less of phenelzine sulfate in two of the trials), small sample sizes, and no information as to whether patients also suffered spontaneous panic attacks or associative depressive features.

Comparisons of MAOIs versus tricyclics in outpatient depressives have also suggested the efficacy of phenelzine in reducing social anxiety and discomfort (37). Liebowitz et al. (48) found phenelzine superior to both imipramine and placebo at six weeks on the interpersonal sensitivity (social discomfort) and paranoid ideation (touchiness, not psychosis) SCL-90 subscales in atypical depressives. Nies et al. (62) also found phenelzine superior to amitriptyline on the SCL-90 anxiety and interpersonal sensitivity scales in outpatient depressives. In both studies, interpersonal sensitivity was a better dimension than depression for distinguishing between the effects of MAOIs and tricyclics, suggesting a primary effect of phenelzine on social anxiety.

These findings are particularly interesting in light of Marks, Gray, and

Cohen's (52) assertion that antidepressants have efficacy in anxiety disorders only be relieving associated depressive or dysphoric symptoms. While some social phobics meet criteria for past or present major depression, atypical depression, or dysthymia, they appear to remain socially anxious during depression-free periods as well, indicating that in this population affective syndromes may be secondary when they occur. This is in contrast to patients who become socially avoidant only during affective episodes who do not meet DSM-III-R criteria for social phobia.

As a preliminary to embarking on controlled trials of MAOIs in social phobia, we conducted an open pilot study of phenelzine in 11 patients meeting DSM-III-R criteria for social phobia. Subjects were recruited from among outpatients presenting for treatment at an anxiety disorders research clinic. Phenelzine was administered in an open clinical fashion, starting at 30 mg/day for the first week and then increasing by 15 mg/day/week to a possible maximum of 90 mg/day. Seven of the eleven patients showed marked improvement on phenelzine, while the remaining four experienced moderate benefit. Response to treatment was typically manifest three to four weeks after starting the drug, at doses of 45 to 60 mg/day. Somatic symptoms of performance and/or social anxiety disappeared, and the patients reported being significantly more comfortable and outgoing in vocational and social settings. The optimal phenelzine dose was 45 mg/day or less for 6 of the 11 patients, with uncomfortable side effects such as insomnia, memory problems, irritability, sexual dysfunction overstimulation, and edema occurring at higher doses. The regimen was well tolerated by most of the patients, although two discontinued treatment despite benefit owing to the dietary restrictions and another because of side effects. Courses of therapy ranged from several weeks to seven months with no diminution of gains as long as the drug was continued.

Beta-adrenergic blockers. The only reported placebo-controlled study of beta-blockers in social phobics involved 16 patients, all of whom were concomitantly receiving social-skills training (71). Patients were randomized to propranolol hydrochloride or to placebo, and the propranolol dose was adjusted to lower resting heart rate to 60 beats/minute. No significant differences were noted between the six patients who received propranolol and the six patients who received placebo and who completed the trial. Limitations of this study include small sample size, lack of specific diagnostic criteria, lack of controls and blind ratings for social-skills training, and finally the fact that four of the patients had panic attacks.

Numerous analog studies have examined the effect of beta blockers on anxiety during observed performance in nonpatient samples. This paradigm shares many features with social anxiety among patient samples, including the pattern of typical symptoms and the situations that evoke them. Of a total of 11 controlled trials that we reviewed (9, 13, 23, 27, 29, 30, 38, 39, 43, 60, 72), eight found a beta blocker superior to placebo in reducing some aspect of performance anxiety, while three others found no overall difference. Since the majority of these studies involved administration of short-term doses prior to a performance situation, their results are most relevant for those social phobics who experience only occasional and predictable anxiety episodes, such as those with public-speaking or audition anxiety.

In addition, it should be noted that 10 of the 11 studies we reviewed involved nonselective beta blockers. The study by Neftel et al. (6), however, used atenolol, a cardioselective beta blocker that penetrates the central nervous system far less well than propranolol (79). In addition to the lower incidence of central nervous system side effects reported for atenolol, demonstration of efficacy in social phobia would constitute support for a model of peripheral rather than central autonomic mediation of symptoms.

To test the efficacy of continuance therapy with a cardioselective beta blocker, 10 patients meeting DSM-III criteria for social phobia were openly treated with atenolol up to 100 mg/day, by Gorman et al. (22). Both individuals with isolated performance fears and those with pervasive social anxiety were included; in all cases, social phobia led to significant functional impairment. Five of the patients abused alcohol and one had a history of polydrug abuse, including significant benzodiazepine abuse. In addition, five of the subjects had histories of at least one depressive episode.

Patients were started on 50 mg/day of atenolol in a single dose. They were instructed to monitor their pulse each day and to withhold medication and contact the clinic if their heart rate dropped below 50 beats/minute. If after one week there was no significant improvement in the patient's condition and the pulse rate was above 50, the dosage was raised to the maximum recommended dosage of 100 mg/day, also in a single dose. Patients were then followed for at least five more weeks at this dose level.

Of the 10 social phobic patients who completed at least six weeks of treatment, five were rated to have "marked" response to atenolol (virtually complete symptom remission), four were rated as having "moderate" response (substantial symptomatic and behavioral gains), and only one had no significant response to the treatment. Seven of the ten patients remained at 100 mg/day, although one of these developed bradycardia at the higher dose and was lowered to 50 mg/day. The other three individuals experienced improvement at the lower, 50-mg/day dose level. Side effects of atenolol were surprisingly minimal. Two subjects complained of fatigue and decreased energy, although not severe enough to impair their functioning and require a dose adjustment. One subject's pulse rate went below the 50 beats/minute level on 100 mg/day, requiring a decrease in dosage. In addition, one patient reported a "fainting spell" while on 50 mg/day, and the drug was discontinued. Both the patient with mild bradycardia and the one who reported a fainting spell showed improvement on atenolol.

Responses to beta blockers may discriminate between social phobia and panic disorder or agoraphobia with panic attacks. While beta-blocker therapy in the latter patient groups has only been assessed in a preliminary manner, the available evidence suggests a lack of efficacy (25, 28, 33, 63). In addition, acute intravenous treatment with propranolol, producing marked peripheral beta-adrenergic blockade, did not prevent either the anxiety or the tachycardia of lactate-induced panic attacks (21).

Other drugs. There is a paucity of studies evaluating the efficacy of tricyclics in social phobic individuals. Two open (5, 67) and one controlled (3) trials have reported that clomipramine was effective in mixed samples containing social phobics but did not report outcome for social phobics separately. In two recent MAOI versus tricyclic studies in nonendogenous depression, tricyclics appeared less effective than MAOIs in reducing social anxiety (46, 62). Klein (personal communication, 1984) also found no evidence of imipramine efficacy among the social phobics included in his group of simple phobics (80). To our knowledge, benzodiazepines have not been investigated in social phobic populations. In trials based on analog samples, the evidence for the efficacy of the benzodiazepines has been conflicting (13, 38).

Behavioral Treatment

The behavioral treatment of social anxiety and social phobia has been the subject of a number of recent reviews (3, 5, 7, 16, 18, 22, 34, 45, 52, 62, 66, 67, 76) and so will be only briefly summarized here. In general, the three forms of behavioral treatment that have been found useful in controlled studies are desensitization or exposure, social-skills training, and cognitive restructuring.

On the basis of an extensive review, Emmelkamp (16) concluded that although systematic desensitization had consistently been found effective in the treatment of social anxiety in analog populations, it was of limited value in clinical samples of social phobics. In contrast, a study by Shaw (70) comparing desensitization, flooding, and social-skills training found "useful therapeutic gains" for all three treatments in a clinical sample of social phobics. However, this study did not include a "placebo" therapy control group, so the contribution of nonspecific factors to therapeutically induced changes cannot be assessed.

Several controlled investigations have demonstrated the superiority of social-skills training over systematic desensitization for socially anxious individuals (16); others did not find such consistent differences (26, 53, 70). As noted by Brady (7, 8), controlled studies of social-skills techniques in psychiatric outpatients have usually involved loosely defined samples of individuals with "social inadequacy" or vaguely deficient social skills rather than rigorously classified patient groups such as social phobics. One notable exception is the previously mentioned study by Shaw (70) comparing the effects of desensitization, flooding, and social-skills training in a group of 30 social phobics that found no differences among treatments. Another is a study by Stravynski and Marks (77) that compared social-skills training and social skills plus cognitive modification in social phobics and found both helpful, with no differences between treatments. Again, since neither of these studies included an appropriate control group, the therapeutic gains reported cannot be conclusively attributed to the specific treatments under investigation.

Cognitive therapies have been found helpful in reducing social anxiety (69), test anxiety (55), and speech anxiety in analog populations. Studies of cognitive therapy in clinical populations of social phobics, however, are for the most part lacking. Cognitive restructuring was found superior to desensitization and to a "waiting-list" control condition in reducing symptoms in socially anxious community volunteers (32). Kendrick et al. (35) found cognitive therapy and behavioral rehearsal more effective than a similar control condition for severe musical performance anxiety assessed five weeks after treatment, although not at the conclusion of the treatment program itself. Butler et al. (11) recently found anxiety management training plus exposure superior to exposure plus a control "associative therapy" condition for social phobia, particularly on measures of distress caused by, and attitudes relating to, social interaction. The anxiety management training involved three techniques, namely relaxation, distraction, and rational self-talk. Butler has also recently discussed (12) the problems of applying exposure techniques to social phobics. In her view, supplemental anxiety management techniques are helpful in treating the cognitive aspects of social phobia, particularly fear of negative evaluation.

In general, it remains to be established whether behavioral techniques result in substantial or only modest therapeutic gains when administered to clinically diagnosed social phobics. It is also uncertain at this point whether the various behavioral techniques have specific or nonspecific effects (64, 65). In addition, no data exist as to how various behavioral therapies compare with, or interact with, pharmacological treatments. Once the response patterns of social phobics to drug and behavioral therapies are elucidated, the comparative and interactive effects of the two approaches will require careful assessment. Other forms of psychotherapy may also be of use, but these have not been systematically assessed in the treatment of social phobia.

CONCLUSION

Social phobia appears to be distinct from other phobic subtypes and anxiety disorders on the basis of demographic findings as well as clinical features. The disorder is not uncommon and tends to be both chronic and potentially disabling, with alcoholism and depression as commonly associated syndromes. Analog and open clinical studies have suggested that beta-adrenergic blockers may have efficacy for reducing social anxiety, while both open clinical trials and controlled studies have indicated that MAOIs may be of benefit. Open and controlled trials have also supported the efficacy of several forms of behavioral therapy, including desensitization/exposure, social-skills training, and cognitive techniques.

Major uncertainties exist, however, concerning the definition, classification, prevalence, etiology, pathophysiology, assessment, and treatment of social phobia. While the disorder has historically received some attention from British investigators, it has been until recently dramatically neglected in the U.S. mental health literature, with the exception of behavior therapists. Interest in social phobia among American clinicians and researchers is beginning to grow, however, as the specialized anxiety clinics now being established continue to proliferate. We believe that this offers a number of exciting opportunities for refined diagnostic and decisive therapeutic action, as well as fertile ground for research in the biological and psychological aspects of anxiety disorders.

REFERENCES

1. AGRAS, S., SYLVESTER, D., & OLIVEAU, D. (1969). The common fears and phobias. *Compr. Psychiatry*, *10*, 151.
2. AIMES, P., GELDER, M., & SHAW, P. (1983). Social phobia: A comparative clinical study. *Br. J. Psychiatry*, *142*, 174.
3. ALLSOPP, L., COOPER, G., & POLLE, P. (1984). Clomipramine and diazepam in the treatment of agoraphobia and social phobia in general practice. *Current Med. Red. Opinion*, *9*(1), 64.
4. APRINDELL, W., EMMELKAMP, P., MONSMA, A., & BRILMAN, E. (1983). The role of perceived parental rearing practices in the aetiology of phobic disorders: A controlled study. *Br. J. Psychiatry*, *143*, 183.
5. BEAUMONT, G. (1977). A large open multicenter trial of clomipramine (Anafranil) in the management of phobic disorders. *J. Int. Med. Res.*, *5*, 116.
6. BERNADT, M., SILVERSTONE, T., & SINGLETON, W. (1980). Behavioral and subjective effects of beta-adrenergic blockade in phobia subjects. *Br. J. Psychiatry*, *137*, 452.
7. BRADY, J. P. (1984). Social skills training for psychiatric patients: I. Concepts, methods and clinical results. *Am. J. Psychiatry*, *141*, 333.
8. BRADY, J. P. (1984). Social skills training for psychiatric patients: II. Clinical outcome studies. *Am. J. Psychiatry*, *141*, 491.
9. BRANTIGAN, C., BRANTIGAN, T., & JOSEPH, N. (1982). Effect of beta blockade and beta stimulation on stage fright. *Am. J. Med.*, *72*, 88.
10. BRYANT, B., & TROWER, P. (1974). Social difficulty in a student sample. *Br. J. Ed. Psychol.*, *44*, 13.
11. BUTLER, G., CULLINGTON, A., MUNBY, M., AMIES, P., & GELDER, M. (1984). Exposure and anxiety management in the treatment of social phobia. *J. Consult. Clin. Psychol.*, *52*, 642.
12. BUTLER, G. (1985). Exposure as a treatment for social phobia: Some instructive difficulties. *Behav. Res. Ther.*, *23*, 651.
13. DESAI, N., TAYLOR-DAVIES, A., & BARNETT, D. (1983). The effects of diazepam and oxprenolol on short term memory in individuals of high and low state anxiety. *Br. J. Clin. Pharm.*, *15*, 197.
14. DIMSDALE, J., & MOSS, J. (1974). Short-term catecholamine response to psychological stress. *Psychosom. Med.*, *42*, 493.
15. DiNARDO, P., O'BRIEN, G., BARLOW, D., WADDEL, M., & BLANCHARD, E. (1983). Reliability of DSM-III anxiety disorder categories using a new structured interview. *Arch. Gen. Psychiatry*, *40*, 1070.
16. EMMELKAMP, P. M. G. (1982). *Phobic and obsessive-compulsive disorder: Theory, research and practice.* New York: Plenum Press.
17. FALLOON, I. (1980). Psychiatric patients as raters of social behaviour. *J. Behav. Ther. Exp. Psychiatry*, *11*, 215.
18. FALLOON, I., LLOYD, G., & HARPIN, R. (1981). Real-life rehearsal with nonprofessional therapists. *J. Nerv. Ment. Dis.*, *169*, 180.
19. FREUD, S. (1957). *New introductory lectures on psychoanalysis* (pp. 110–113). London: Hogarth Press.
20. GAIND, R., SURI, A., & THOMPSON, J. (1975). Use of beta blockers as an adjunct in behavioral techniques. *Scot. Med. J.*, *20*, 284.
21. GORMAN, J., LEVY, G., LIEBOWITZ, M., McGRATH, P., APPLEBY, I., DILLON, D., DAVIES, S., & KLEIN, D. (1983). Effect of acute beta-adrenergic blockade on lactate-induced panic. *Arch. Gen. Psychiatry*, *40*, 1079.
22. GORMAN, J., LIEBOWITZ, M., FYER, A., CAMPEAS, R., & KLEIN, D. (1985). Treatment of social phobia with atenolol. *J. Clin. Psychopharmacol.*, *5*(5), 298.

23. GOTTSCHALK, L., STONE, W., & GLESER, C. (1974). Peripheral versus central mechanisms accounting for antianxiety effects of propanolol. *Psychosom. Med.*, *36*, 47.
24. GREENBERG, D., & STRAVYNSKI, A. (1983). Social phobia (letter). *Br. J. Psychiatry*, *143*, 526.
25. HAFNER, J., & MILTON, F. (1977). The influence of propanolol on the exposure in vivo of agoraphobics. *Psychol. Med.*, *7*, 419.
26. HALL, R., & GOLDBERG, D. (1977). The role of social anxiety in social interaction difficulties. *Br. J. Psychiatry*, *131*, 610.
27. HARTLEY, L, UNPAGEN, S., DAVIE, I., & SPENCER, D. (1983). The effect of beta-adrenergic blocking drugs on speaker's performance and memory. *Br. J. Psychiatry*, *142*, 512.
28. HEISER, J., & DEFRANCISCO, D. (1976). The treatment of pathological panic states with propranolol. *Arch. Gen. Psychiatry*, *133*, 1389.
29. JAMES, I., BURGOYNE, W., & SAVAGE, I. (1983). Effect of pindolol on stress-related disturbances of musical performance: Preliminary communication. *J. Roy. Soc. Med.*, *76*, 194.
30. JAMES, I., GRIFFITH, D., PEARSON, R., & NEWBY, P. (1977). Effect of oxprenolol on stage-fright in musicians. *Lancet*, *2*, 592.
31. JOHANSSON, J., & OST, L. (1982). Perception of autonomic reactions and actual heart rate in phobic patients. *J. Behav. Assessment*, *4*, 133.
32. KANTER, N., & GOLDFRIED, M. (1979). Relative effectiveness of rational restructuring and self-control desensitization in the reduction of interpersonal anxiety. *Behav. Res. Ther.*, *10*, 472.
33. KATHOL, R., NOYES, R., SLYMEN, D., CROWE, R., CLANCY, J., & KERBER, R. (1980). Propranolol in chronic anxiety disorders. A controlled study. *Arch. Gen. Psychiatry*, *37*, 1361.
34. KELLY, D., GUIRGUIS, W., FROMMER, E., MITCHELL-HEGGS, N., & SARGANT, W. (1970). Treatment of phobic states with antidepressants: A retrospective study of 246 patients. *Br. J. Psychiatry*, *116*, 387.
35. KENDRICK, M., CRAIG, K., LAWSON, D., & DAVIDSON, P. (1982). Cognitive and behavioral therapy for musical-performance anxiety. *J. Consult. Clin. Psychol.*, *50*, 353.
36. KLEIN, D. (1964). Delineation of two drug-responsive anxiety syndromes. *Psychopharmacology*, *5*, 397.
37. KLEIN, D., & DAVIS, J. (1969). *Diagnosis and drug treatment of psychiatric disorders.* Baltimore: Williams & Wilkins.
38. KRISHNAN, G. (1975). Oxprenolol in the treatment of examination nerves. *Scot. Med. J.*, *20*, 288.
39. KROPE, P., KOHRS, A., OTT, H., WAGNER, W., & FICHTS, K. (1982). Evaluating mepindolol in a test model of examination anxiety in students. *Pharmacopsychiatry*, *15*, 41.
40. LADER, M., GELDER, M., & MARKS, I. (1967). Palmar skin-conductance measures as predictors of response of desensitization. *J. Psychosom. Res.*, *11*, 283.
41. LANDE, S. (1982). Physiological and subjective measures of anxiety during flooding. *Behav. Res. Ther.*, *20*, 81.
42. LEARY, M. (1974). *Understanding social anxiety: Social, personality and clinical perspectives.* Beverly Hills, CA: Sage.
43. LIDEN, S., & GOTTFRIES, C. (1974). Beta-blocking agents in treatment of catecholamine-induced symptoms in musicians. *Lancet*, *2*, 529.
44. LIEBOWITZ, M., FYER, A., GORMAN, J., DILLON, D., DAVIES, S., STEIN, J., COHEN, B., & KLEIN, D. (1985). Specificity of lactate infusions in social phobia vs. panic disorders. *Am. J. Psychiatry*, *142*(8), 947.
45. LIEBOWITZ, M., FYER, A., GORMAN, J., CAMPEAS, R., & LEVIN, A. (1986). Phenelzine in social phobia. *J. Clin. Psychopharmacol.*, *6*(2), 93–98.
46. LIEBOWITZ, M. R., GORMAN, J., FYER, A., LEVITT, M., LEVY, G., APPLEBY, I., DILLON, D., PALIJ, M., DAVIES, S., & KLEIN, D. (1984). Lactate provocation of panic attacks: I. Clinical and behavioral findings. *Arch. Gen. Psychiatry*, *41*, 764.

47. LIEBOWITZ, M., GORMAN, J., FYER, A., & KLEIN, D. (1985). Social phobia: Review of a neglected anxiety disorder. *Arch. Gen. Psychiatry, 42*, 729.
48. LIEBOWITZ, M. QUITKIN, F., STEWART, J., McGRATH, P., HARRISON, W., RABKIN, J., TRICAMO, E., MARKOWITZ, J., & KLEIN, D.: Phenelzine versus imipramine in atypical depression: A preliminary report. *Arch. Gen. Psychiatry, 41*(7), 669.
49. MARKS, I. (1970). The classification of phobic disorders. *Br. J. Psychiatry, 116*, 377.
50. MARKS, I. (1981). *Cure and care of neuroses.* New York: Wiley.
51. MARKS, I., & GELDER, M. (1966). Different ages of onset in varieties of phobia. *Am. J. Psychiatry, 123*, 218.
52. MARKS, I., GRAY, S., & COHEN, S. (1983). Imipramine and brief therapist-aided exposure in agoraphobics having self-exposure homework: A controlled trial. *Arch. Gen. Psychiatry, 40*, 153.
53. MARZILLIER, J., LAMBERT, C., & KELLETT, J. (1976). A controlled evaluation of systematic desensitization and social skills training for socially inadequate psychiatric patients. *Behav. Res. Ther., 14*, 225.
54. McEWAN, K., & DEVINS, G. (1983). Is increased arousal in social anxiety noticed by others? *J. Abnorm. Psychol., 92*, 417.
55. MORRIS, L., & ENGLE, W. (1981). Assessing various coping strategies and their effects on test performance and anxiety. *J. Clin. Psychol., 37*, 165.
56. MOUNTJOY, C., ROTH, M., GARSIDE, R., & LEITCH, I. (1977). A clinical trial of phenelzine in anxiety depressive and phobic neuroses. *Br. J. Psychiatry, 131*, 486.
57. MULLANEY, J., & TRIPPETT, C. (1979). Alcohol dependence and phobias: Clinical description and relevance. *Br. J. Psychiatry, 135*, 563.
58. MUNJACK, D., & MOSS, H. (1981). Affective disorder and alcoholism in families of agoraphobics. *Arch. Gen. Psychiatry, 38*, 869.
59. MYERS, J., WEISSMAN, M., TISCHLER, G., HOLZER, C., LEAF, P., ORVASCHEL, H., ANTHONY, J., BOYD, J., BURKE, J., KRAMER, M., & STOLTZMAN, R. (1984). Six-month prevalence of psychiatric disorders in three communities: 1980–1982. *Arch. Gen. Psychiatry, 41*(10), 959.
60. NEFTEL, K., ADLER, R., KAPPELL, L., ROSSI, M., DOLDER, M., KASER, H., BRUGGESSER, H., & VORKAUF, H. (1982). Stage fright in musicians: A model illustrating the effect of beta blockers. *Psychosom. Med., 44*, 461.
61. NICHOLS, K. (1974). Severe social anxiety. *Br. J. Med. Psychol., 47*, 301.
62. NIES, A., HOWARD, D., & ROBINSON, D. (1982). Antianxiety effects of MAO inhibitors. In R. Mathew (Ed.), *The biology of anxiety* (pp. 123–133). New York: Brunner/Mazel.
63. NOYES, R., ANDERSON, D., CLANCY, J., CROWE, R., SLYMEN, D., GHONEIM, M., & HINRICHS, J. (1984). Diazepam and propranolol in panic disorder and agoraphobia. *Arch. Gen. Psychiatry, 41*, 287.
64. OST, L., & HUGDAHL, K. (1981). Acquisition of phobias and anxiety response patterns in clinical patients. *Behav. Res. Ther., 19*, 439.
65. OST, L., JERREMALM, A., & JOHANSSON, J. (1980). Individual response patterns and the effects of different behavioral methods in the treatment of social phobia. *Behav. Res. Ther., 19*, 1.
66. PARKER, G. (1979). Reported parental characteristics of agoraphobics and social phobics. *Br. J. Psychiatry, 135*, 555.
67. PECKNOLD, J., McCLURE, D., APPELTAUER, L., ALLAN, T., & WRZESINSKI, L. (1982). Does tryptophan potentiate clomipramine in the treatment of agoraphobic and social phobic patients? *Br. J. Psychiatry, 140*, 484.
68. PITTS, F., & McCLURE, J. (1967). Lactate metabolism in anxiety neurosis. *N. Engl. J. Med., 277*, 1326.
69. SCHELVER, S., & GUTSCH, K. (1982). The effects of self-administered cognitive therapy on social-evaluative anxiety. *J. Clin. Psychol., 39*, 1378.
70. SHAW, P. (1979). A comparison of three behaviour therapies in the treatment of social phobia. *Br. J. Psychiatry, 134*, 620.

71. SHEEHAN, D., BALLENGER, J., & JACOBSON, G. (1980). Treatment of endogenous anxiety with phobic hysterical and hypocondriacal symptoms. *Arch. Gen. Psychiatry, 37*, 51.
72. SITTONEN, L., & JANNE, J. (1976). Effect of beta-blockage during bowling competitions. *Ann. Clin. Res., 8*, 393.
73. SMAIL, P., STOCKWELL, T., CANTER, S., & HODGSON, R. (1984). Alcohol dependence and phobia anxiety states: I. A prevalence study. *Br. J. Psychiatry, 144*, 53.
74. SOLYOM, L., HESELTINE, G., McCLURE, D., SOLYOM, C., LEDWEDGE, B., & STEINBERG, G. (1973). Behaviour therapy vs. drug therapy in the treatment of phobic neurosis. *Can. Psychiatr. Assoc. J., 18*, 25.
75. SOLYOM, C., SOLYOM, L., LAPIERRE, Y., PECKHOLD, J., & MORTON, L. (1981). Phenelzine and exposure in the treatment of phobias. *Biol. Psychiatry, 16*, 239.
76. STRAVYNSKI, A., & SHAHAR, A. (1983). The treatment of social dysfunction in nonpsychotic outpatients: A review. *J. Nerv. Ment. Dis., 171*, 721.
77. STRAVYNSKI, A., & MARKS, I. (1982). Social skills problems in neurotic outpatients. *Arch. Gen. Psychiatry, 39*(12), 1378–1385.
78. TORGERSON, S. (1979). The nature and origin of common phobic fears. *Br. J. Psychiatry, 134*, 343.
79. TYRER, P., CANDY, J., & KELLY, D. (1973). A study of the clinical effects of phenelzine and placebo in the treatment of phobic anxiety. *Psychopharmacologia (Berlin), 32*, 237.
80. WEISSBERG, M. (1977). A comparison of direct and vicarious treatments of speech anxiety: Desensitization with coping imagery and cognitive modification. *Behav. There, 8*, 606.

13

THE HOMELESS MENTALLY ILL

H. Richard Lamb, M.D.

Professor of Psychiatry,
Department of Psychiatry and the Behavioral Sciences,
University of Southern California School of Medicine,
Los Angeles, California

Homelessness is not a new phenomenon. Large urban centers have always attracted vagabonds, derelicts, and hoboes, but until recently these unfortunate individuals tended to cluster in more or less circumscribed areas, often called skid rows. Today, however, we are experiencing a new phenomenon — one of unprecedented magnitude and complexity — and hardly a section of the country has escaped the ubiquitous presence of ragged, ill, and hallucinating human beings, wandering through our city streets, huddled in alleyways, or sleeping over vents.

This rapidly growing problem of homelessness has emerged as a major national tragedy and has recently commanded increasing attention from all segments of society, including the various levels of government, the media, and the public at large. The individuals affected are clearly the victims of massive societal neglect and ineptness.

It is now apparent that a substantial portion of the homeless are chronically and severely mentally ill men and women who in years past would have been long-term residents of state hospitals. They now have no place to live because of efforts to depopulate public hospitals coupled with the unavailability of suitable housing and supervised living arrangements in "the community," inadequate continuing medical-psychiatric care and other supportive services, and poorly thought-out changes in the laws governing involuntary treatment.

The population to which I refer in discussing the homeless mentally ill are those homeless persons disabled by chronic major mental illness. By major mental illness, I am referring to persons suffering from schizophrenia or major affective disorders. The most methodologically sound studies thus far indicate that, among the total population of homeless persons, there is a prevalence of about 40% with major mental illness (2). Another way of defining this population is those persons who would have lived out their lives in state hospitals prior to deinstitutionalization.

DEINSTITUTIONALIZATION AND HOMELESSNESS

Is deinstitutionalization the cause of homelessness? Some would say yes and send the chronically mentally ill back to the hospitals. A main thesis of this chapter, however, is that problems such as homelessness are not the result of deinstitutionalization per se, but rather of the way deinstitutionalization has been implemented. It is the purpose of this chapter to describe these problems of implementation and the related problem of a lack of a clear understanding of the needs of the chronically mentally ill in the community. The discussion then turns to some additional unintended results of these problems, such as criminalization of the mentally ill, which usually accompanies homelessness. The chapter concludes with some ways of resolving these problems.

To see and experience the appalling conditions under which the homeless mentally ill exist has a profound impact on us; our natural reaction is to want to rectify the horrors of what we see with a quick, bold stroke. But for the chronically mentally ill, homelessness is a complex problem with multiple causative factors; in our analysis of this problem we need to guard against settling for simplistic explanations and solutions. For instance, homelessness is closely linked with deinstitutionalization in the sense that three decades ago most of the chronically mentally ill had a home—the state hospital. Without deinstitutionalization it is unlikely there would be large numbers of homeless mentally ill. Thus, in countries where deinstitutionalization has barely begun, homelessness of the chronically mentally ill is not a significant problem. But that does not mean we can simply explain homelessness as a result of deinstitutionalization; we have to look at what conditions these mentally ill persons must face in the community, what needed resources are lacking, and the nature of mental illness itself.

With the mass exodus into the community, we are now faced with the need to understand the chronically mentally ill's reaction to and tolerance of the stresses of the community and determine what has become of them, and why, without the state hospitals. There is now evidence that very substantial numbers of the severely mentally ill are homeless nationwide at any given time (2, 5, 17). Some are homeless continuously and some inter-mittently (6). We need to understand what characteristics of society and the mentally ill themselves have interacted to produce such an unforeseen and grave problem as homelessness. Without that understanding, we will not be able to conceptualize and then implement what needs to be done to resolve the problems of homelessness.

With the advantage of hindsight we can see that the era of deinstitution-alization was ushered in with much naïveté and many simplistic notions as to what would become of the chronically and severely mentally ill. The importance of psychoactive medication and a stable source of financial support was perceived, but the importance of developing such fundamen-tal resources as supportive living arrangements was often not clearly seen, or at least not implemented. "Community treatment" was much discussed, but there was no clear idea as to what this should consist of, and it was not anticipated how resistant the community health centers would be to pro-viding services to the chronically mentally ill. Nor was it foreseen how reluctant many states would be to allocate funds for community-based services.

In the midst of very valid concerns about the shortcomings and anti-therapeutic aspects of state hospitals, it was not appreciated that the state hospitals fulfilled some crucial functions for the chronically and severely mentally ill. The term "asylum" was in many ways an appropriate one, for these imperfect institutions did provide asylum and sanctuary from the pressures of the world with which, in varying degrees, most of these pa-tients were unable to cope (14). Further, these institutions provided such services as medical care, patient monitoring, respite for the patient's fami-ly, a social network for the patient, as well as food and shelter and needed support and structure (3).

In the state hospitals the treatment and services that did exist were in one place and under one administration. In the community the situation is very different. Services and treatment are under various administrative jurisdictions and in various locations. Even the mentally healthy have difficulty dealing with a number of bureaucracies, both governmental and private, and getting their needs met. Further, patients can easily get lost in the community as compared to a hospital where they may have been neglected, but at least their whereabouts were known. It is these problems that have led to the recognition of the importance of case management. It is probable that many of the homeless mentally ill would not be on the streets if they were on the caseload of a professional or paraprofessional trained to deal with the problems of the chronically mentally ill, monitor them, with considerable persistence when necessary, and facilitate their receiving services.

In my experience (10) and that of others (4) the survival of long-term patients, let alone their rehabilitation, begins with an appropriately supportive and structured living arrangement. Other treatment and rehabilitation are of little avail until patients feel secure and are stabilized in their living situation. Deinstitutionalization means granting asylum in the community to a large marginal population, many of whom can cope to only a limited extent with the ordinary demands of life, have strong dependency needs, and are unable to live independently.

Moreover, that some patients might need to reside in a long-term, locked, intensively supervised community facility was a foreign thought to most who advocated return to the community in the early years of emptying the state hospitals. "Patients who need a secure environment can remain in the state hospital" was the rationale. But in those early years most people seemed to think that such patients were few and that community treatment and modern psychoactive medications would take care of most problems. More people are now recognizing that a number of severely disabled patients present major problems in management and can survive and have their basic needs met outside of state hospitals only if they have a sufficiently structured facility or other mechanism of providing controls in the community (8). Some of the homeless appear to be from this group. A function of the old state hospitals that is often given too little weight is that of providing structure. Without this structure, many of the chronically mentally ill feel lost and cast adrift in the community — however much they may deny it.

THE USE OF SHELTERS IN PERSPECTIVE

There is currently much emphasis on providing emergency shelter to the homeless, and certainly this must be done. But it is important to get this "shelter approach" into perspective; it is a necessary stopgap, symptomatic measure, but does not address the basic causes of homelessness. As a matter of fact, too much emphasis on shelters can only delay our coming to grips with the underlying problems that result in homelessness. This must be kept in mind even as we sharpen our techniques for working with mentally ill persons who are already homeless.

Most mental health professionals are disinclined to treat "street people" or "transients" (16). Moreover, in the case of many of the homeless, we are working with persons whose lack of trust and desire for autonomy causes them to give us fictitious names, to refuse to accept our services, and to move along because of their fear of closeness or fear of losing their autonomy, or their not wanting to acquire a mentally ill identity. Providing food and shelter with no strings attached, especially in a facility that has a close involvement with mental health professionals, a clear conception of the needs of the mentally ill, and the ready availability of other services, can be an opening wedge that ultimately will give us the opportunity to treat a few of this population.

At the same time we have learned that we must beware of simple solutions and recognize that this shelter approach is grossly insufficient as a definitive solution to the basic problems of the homeless mentally ill. It does not substitute for the array of measures that will be effective in both significantly reducing and preventing homelessness: a full range of residential placements; aggressive case management; changes in the legal system that will facilitate involuntary treatment; a stable source of income for each patient; access to acute hospitalization and other vitally needed community services.

Still another problem with the shelter approach is that many of the homeless mentally ill will accept shelter, but nothing more, and eventually return to a wretched and dangerous life on the streets.

What was not foreseen in the midst of the early optimism about returning the mentally ill to the community and restoring and rehabilitating them so they could take their places in the mainstream of society was what was actually to befall them. Certainly it was not anticipated that criminalization and homelessness would be the lot for many.

ASYLUM AND DEPENDENCY

I turn now to the concept of asylum, and to dependency. When we talk about the homeless mentally ill, we are of course talking primarily about the chronically mentally ill. And I see these issues as crucial to understanding the needs of the chronically mentally ill.

Because the old state hospitals were called asylums, the word asylum took on a bad, almost sinister, connotation. Only in recent years has the word again become a respectable part of our language. But the fact that the chronically mentally ill have been deinstitutionalized does not mean they no longer need social support and protection, and relief, either periodic or continuous, from the pressures of life. In short, they need asylum and sanctuary, in the community. These words are rich with meaning—for the chronically mentally ill and for all of us. After all, is it not a period of asylum that we seek when we take a vacation?

The disability of chronic mental illness includes social isolation, vocational inadequacy, and exaggerated dependency needs. While many can eventually attain high levels of social and vocational functioning, a sizable proportion of the chronically mentally ill find it difficult to meet even the simple demands of living. Many are unable to withstand pressure and are likely to develop incapacitating psychiatric symptoms when confronted with a common crisis of life. Programs can help patients develop social and vocational skills, but there are limits to what can be accomplished; inability to tolerate even minimal stress is a severely limiting characteristic.

For a number of the chronically mentally ill, too many demands — and for some any demands at all — will reactivate symptoms and perhaps necessitate a hospitalization. On the other hand, however, too few demands and too low expectations may result in regression.

Some consider it likely that many patients with chronic mental illness will lose their active symptoms more rapidly in a setting that is undemanding and permits them to limit involvement — in contrast to a setting that seeks to involve them in normal social intercourse and move them toward even partial independence. The chronically mentally ill have a limited tolerance for stress, and avoidance of stress is one way of attempting to survive outside the hospital. Medications and other community supports may also be required to ensure that patients are able to remain in the community.

Normalization of the patient's environment and rehabilitation to the greatest extent possible should be the goal of treatment. This environment should include the social milieu, the living situation, and the work situation. To the degree possible, the patient's condition should not be allowed to set him or her apart from other citizens in our society. This ideal of normalization (or mainstreaming), however, frequently cannot be achieved for a sizable proportion of chronically mentally ill persons. Every patient should be given every opportunity to reach normalization, but we need to realize that a number of our patients will fall short of it. If we persist in fruitless efforts to adjust people to a lifestyle beyond their ability, not only may we cause them anguish, but we run the risk of contributing to the emergence of manifest psychopathology. Moreover, we ourselves become frustrated and then angry at the patients. In the end we may reject them and find rationalizations to refer them elsewhere.

Many chronically mentally ill persons gravitate toward a lifestyle that will allow them to remain free from symptoms and dysphoric feelings. Is this bad? For some it may lead to unnecessary regression and serve as an impediment to increasing their level of social and vocational functioning; for those it should be discouraged. But I think a case can be made that this restricted lifestyle meets the needs of many others and helps them maintain community tenure. Mental health professionals and society at large need to consider the crippling limitations of mental illness that do not yield to current treatment methods; they need to be unambivalent, moreover, about providing adequate care for this vulnerable group. For those who can be restored only to a limited degree, we should provide reasonable comfort and an undemanding life with dignity.

It is important that the moral disapproval of dependency in our society and unrealistic expectations of the severely disabled not prevent us from providing long-term patients with whatever degree of treatment, support, and sanctuary they need to survive.

A major obstacle to understanding and addressing the problems of deinstitutionalization and the long-term patient has been a failure to recognize that there are many different kinds of long-term patients who vary greatly in their capacity for rehabilitation. Patients differ in ego strength (the ability to cope with stress) and in motivation. The severely disabled differ also in the kinds of stress and pressure they can handle. Some who are amenable to social rehabilitation cannot handle the stresses of vocational rehabilitation, and vice versa. What may appear to be, at first glance, a homogeneous group turns out to be a group that ranges from persons who can tolerate almost no stress at all to those who can, with some assistance, cope with most of life's demands. Thus, for some long-term patients, competitive employment, independent living, and a high level of social functioning are realistic goals; for others, just maintaining their present level of functioning should be considered a success. Recognizing patients' limitations as well as their strengths is one way of supporting and protecting them. This is in contrast to the world generally, which is less forgiving and understanding.

Likewise, in stressing a need for providing asylum, I want to avoid simplistic conceptions that suggest a homogeneous patient population. Consequently, asylum must mean different levels of social support and different types of protection for each patient. Simplistic notions that suggest a homogeneous patient population will repeat the same mistakes made so often with deinstitutionalization. In stressing the need for asylum and sanctuary, I am only stressing a principle that will have a different meaning, both qualitative and quantitative, for each patient.

There tends to be a basic moral disapproval in our society of a passive, inactive lifestyle, and of accepting public support instead of working. Such a moral reaction seems to occur in all of us. Although as a rule we try to deny our disapproval, our moral reaction confuses the issues and may interfere with the provision of appropriate care for the severely disabled. Our dissatisfaction with a primary role of gratifying chronic dependency needs and a more or less covert moral rejection of our patients' surrender to passivity are probably two impediments to our embracing the concept of asylum for the long-term mentally ill.

INVOLUNTARY TREATMENT

A major factor contributing to deinstitutionalization was sweeping changes in the commitment laws of the various states. In California, for instance, the Lanterman-Petris-Short Act of 1968 provided further impetus for the movement of patients out of hospitals. Behind this legislation was a concern for the civil rights of the psychiatric patient, much of it from civil-rights groups and individuals outside the mental health professions (15). The act made the involuntary commitment of psychiatric patients a much more complex process, and it became difficult to hold psychiatric patients indefinitely against their will in mental hospitals. Thus the initial stage of what had formerly been the career of the long-term hospitalized patient — namely, an involuntary, indefinite commitment — became a thing of the past.

Some clearly recognized that while many abuses needed to be corrected, this legislation went too far in the other direction and no longer safeguarded the welfare of the patient. But these were voices in the wilderness. We still have not found a way to help some mental health lawyers and patients'-rights advocates see that they have contributed heavily to the problem of homelessness — that patients' rights to freedom are not synonymous with releasing them to the streets where they cannot take care of themselves, are too disorganized or fearful to avail themselves of what help is available, and are easy prey for every predator.

THE TENDENCY TO DRIFT

Drifter is a word that strikes a chord in all those who have contact with the chronically mentally ill — mental health professionals, families, and the patients themselves. It is especially important to examine the phenomenon of drifting in the homeless mentally ill. The tendency is probably more pronounced in the young (18 to 35), though is by no means uncommon in the older age groups. Some drifters wander from community to community seeking a geographical solution to their problems; hoping to leave their problems behind, they find they have simply brought them to a new location. Others, who drift in the same community from one living situation to another, can best be described as drifting through life: they lead lives without goals, direction, or ties other than perhaps an intermittent hostile-dependent relationship with relatives or other caretakers (11).

Why do they drift? Apart from their desire to outrun their problems, their symptoms, and their failures, many have great difficulty achieving closeness and intimacy. A fantasy of finding closeness elsewhere encourages them to move on. Yet all too often, if they do stumble into an intimate relationship or find themselves in a residence where there is caring and closeness and sharing, the increased anxiety they experience creates a need to run.

They drift also in search of autonomy, as a way of denying their dependency and out of a desire for an isolated lifestyle. Lack of money often makes them unwelcome, and they may be evicted by family and friends. And they drift because of a reluctance to become involved in a mental health treatment program or a supportive out-of-home environment, such as a halfway house or board-and-care home, that would give them a mental patient identity and make them part of the mental health system: they do not want to see themselves as ill.

Those who move out from board-and-care homes tend to be young; they may be trying to escape the pull of dependency and may not be ready to come to terms with living in a sheltered, segregated, low-pressure environment (9). If they still have goals, they may find life there extremely depressing. Or they may want more freedom to drink or to use street drugs. Those who move on are more likely to have been hospitalized during the preceding year. Some may regard leaving their comparatively static milieu as a necessary part of the process of realizing their goals—but a process that exacts its price in terms of homelessness, crises, decompensation, and hospitalizations. Once out on their own, they will probably stop taking their medications and after a while lose touch with Social Security and no longer be able to receive their SSI checks. They may now be too disorganized to extricate themselves from living on the streets—except by exhibiting blatantly bizarre or disruptive behavior that leads to their being taken to a hospital or to jail.

GAINING THEIR LIBERTY

Perhaps one of the brightest spots in looking at the effects of deinstitutionalization is that the mentally ill have gained a greatly increased measure of liberty. There is often a tendency to underestimate the value and humanizing effects of ex-hospital patients simply having their liberty to the extent that they can handle it (even aside from the fact that it is their right) and of having free movement in the community. It is important to clarify that, even if these patients are unable to provide for their basic needs through employment or to live independently, these are separate issues from that of having one's freedom. Even if they live in miniinstitutions in the community, such as board-and-care homes, these are not locked, and the patients generally have free access to community resources.

This issue needs to be qualified. A small proportion of long-term, severely disabled psychiatric patients lack sufficient impulse control to handle living in an open setting such as a board-and-care home or with relatives (8). They need varying degrees of external structure and control to compensate for the inadequacy of their internal controls. They are usually reluctant to take psychotropic medications and often have problems with drugs and alcohol in addition to their mental illness. They tend not to remain in supportive living situations and often join the ranks of the homeless. The total number of such patients may not be great when compared to the total population of severely disabled patients. However, if placed in the community in living arrangements without sufficient structure, this group may require a large proportion of the time of mental health professionals, not to mention other agencies such as the police. More important, they may be impulsively self-destructive or sometimes present a physical danger to others.

Furthermore, many of this group refuse treatment services of any kind. For them, simple freedom can result in a life filled with intense anxiety, depression, and deprivation, and often a chaotic life on the streets. Thus, they are frequently found among the homeless when not in hospitals or jails. These persons often need ongoing involuntary treatment, sometimes in 24-hour settings such as California's locked skilled-nursing facilities with special programs for psychiatric patients (8) or, when more structure is needed, in hospitals. It should be emphasized that structure is more than just a locked door; other vital components are high staff-patient ratios and enough high-quality activities to structure most of the patient's day.

In my opinion, a large proportion of those in need of increasing structure and control can be relocated from the streets and live in open settings in the community, such as with family or in board-and-care homes, if they receive the assistance of such mechanisms as conservatorship, as is provided in California. But even those with a structured situation in the community, such as conservatorship or guardianship, have varying degrees of freedom and an identity as persons in the community.

CRIMINALIZATION

Deinstitutionalization has led to large numbers of mentally ill persons in the community. At the same time, there are a limited amount of community psychiatric resources, including hospital beds. Society has a limited tolerance of mentally disordered behavior, and the result is pressure to institutionalize persons needing 24-hour care wherever there is room, including jail. Indeed, several studies describe a "criminalization" of mentally disordered behavior (1, 7, 12, 18), that is, a shunting of mentally ill persons in need of treatment into the criminal justice system instead of the mental health system. Rather than hospitalization and psychiatric treatment, the mentally ill often tend to be subject to inappropriate arrest and incarceration. Legal restrictions placed on involuntary hospitalization also probably result in a diversion of some patients to the criminal justice system.

Studies of 203 county jail inmates, 102 men and 101 women, referred for psychiatric evaluation (12, 13) shed some light on the issues of both criminalization and homelessness. This population has had extensive experience with both the criminal justice and mental health systems, is characterized by severe acute and chronic mental illness, and generally functions at a low level. Homelessness is frequent; 39% had been living, at the point of arrest, on the streets, on the beach, in missions, or in cheap transient, skid row hotels. Clearly the problems of homelessness and criminalization are interrelated.

Almost half of those men and women charged with misdemeanors had been living on the streets or on the beach or in missions or in cheap transient hotels, compared with a fourth of those charged with felonies (chi-square, $p < .01$). One can speculate on some possible explanations of this finding. Persons living in such places obviously have a minimum of community supports. It is possible that the less serious misdemeanor offense is frequently a way of asking for help. Still another factor may be that many of this group of uncared-for mentally ill persons are being arrested for minor criminal acts that are really manifestations of their illness, their lack of treatment, and the lack of structure in their lives. Certainly, these were the clinical impressions of the investigators as they talked to these inmates and their families and read the police reports.

WHAT SHOULD BE DONE?

I believe that homelessness among the mentally ill is essentially a symptom of the basic underlying problems facing the chronically mentally ill generally in the community. Thus, to address the problems of the homeless mentally ill, a comprehensive and integrated system of care for the chronically mentally ill, with designated responsibility, with accountability, and with adequate fiscal resources, must be established (19). More specifically, a number of steps need to be taken.

An adequate number and ample range of graded, step-wise, supervised community housing settings must be established. While many of the homeless may benefit from temporary housing such as shelters and some small portion of the severely and chronically mentally ill can graduate to independent living, for the vast majority neither shelters nor mainstream low-cost housing is appropriate. Most housing settings that require people to manage by themselves are beyond the capabilities of the chronically mentally ill. Instead, there must be settings offering different levels of supervision, both more and less intensive, including quarter-way and halfway houses, board-and-care homes, satellite housing, foster or family care, and crisis or temporary hostels.

Adequate, comprehensive, and accessible psychiatric and rehabilitative services must be available and must be assertively provided through outreach services when necessary. First, there must be an adequate number of direct psychiatric services, including on the streets and in the shelters when appropriate, that provide: outreach contact with the mentally ill in the community; psychiatric assessment and evaluation; crisis intervention, including hospitalization; individualized treatment plans; psychotropic medication and other somatic therapies; and psychosocial treatment. Second, there must be an adequate number of rehabilitative services, providing socialization experiences, training in the skills of everyday living, and social rehabilitation. Third, both treatment and rehabilitative services must be provided assertively — for instance, by going out to patients' living settings if they do not or cannot come to a centralized program. And fourth, the difficulty of working with some of these patients must not be underestimated.

General medical assessment and care must be available. Since we know that the chronically mentally ill have a considerably greater morbidity and mortality than their counterparts of the same age in the general population, and the homeless have even higher rates, the ready availability of general medical care is essential and critical.

Crisis services, both inpatient and outpatient, must be available and accessible to both the chronically mentally ill homeless and the chronically mentally ill in general.

A system of responsibility for the chronically mentally ill living in the community must be established, with the goal of ensuring that ultimately each patient has one mental health professional or paraprofessional (a case manager) responsible for his or her care. In such a case management system, each patient would have a case manager who would have the appropriate psychiatric and medical assessments carried out, would formulate, together with the patient, an individualized treatment and rehabilitation plan, including the proper pharmacotherapy, and would monitor the patient and assist the patient in receiving services. Clearly the shift of psychiatric care from institutional to community settings does not in any way eliminate the need to continue the provision of comprehensive services to mentally ill persons. As a result, society must declare a public policy of responsibility for the mentally ill who are unable to meet their own needs; governments must designate programs in each region or locale as core agencies responsible and accountable for the care of the chronically mentally ill living there; and the staff of these agencies must be assigned individual patients for whom they are responsible. The ultimate goal must be to ensure that every chronically mentally ill person has one person — such as a case manager — who is responsible for his or her treatment and care.

For the more than 50 % of the chronically ill population living at home or for those with positive ongoing relationships with their families, programs and respite care must be provided to enhance the family's ability to provide a support system. Where the use of family systems is not feasible, the patient must be linked up with a formal community support system. In any case, the entire burden of deinstitutionalization must not be allowed to fall on families.

Basic changes must be made in legal and administrative procedures to ensure continuing community care for the chronically mentally ill. In the 1960s and 1970s more stringent commitment laws and patients'-rights advocacy remedied some very serious abuses in public hospital care, but at the same time these changes neglected patients' right to high-quality, comprehensive outpatient care as well as the rights of families and society. New laws and procedures must be developed to ensure provision of psychiatric care in the community — that is, to guarantee a right to treatment in the community.

It must become easier to obtain conservatorship status for outpatients who are so gravely disabled and/or have such impaired judgment that they cannot care for themselves in the community without legally sanctioned supervision. Involuntary commitment laws must be made more humane to permit prompt return to active inpatient treatment for patients when acute exacerbations of their illnesses make their lives in the community chaotic and unbearable. Involuntary treatment laws should be revised to allow the option of outpatient civil commitment; in states that already have provisions for such treatment, that mechanism should be more widely used. Finally, advocacy efforts should be focused on the availability of competent care in the community.

A system of coordination among funding sources and implementation agencies must be established. Because the problems of the mentally ill homeless must be addressed by multiple public and private authorities, coordination, so lacking in the deinstitutionalization process, must become a primary goal. The ultimate objective must be a true system of care rather than a loose network of services, and an ease of communication among different types of agencies (for example, psychiatric, social, vocational, and housing) as well as up and down the governmental ladder, from local through federal.

An adequate number of professionals and paraprofessionals must be trained for community care of the chronically ill. Among the additional specially trained workers needed, four groups are particularly important for this population: psychiatrists who are skilled in, and interested in, working with the chronically mentally ill; outreach workers who can engage the homeless mentally ill on the streets; case managers, preferably with sufficient training to provide therapeutic interventions themselves; and conservators, to act for patients too disabled to make clinically and economically sound decisions.

General social services must be provided. Besides the need for specialized social services such as socialization experiences and training in the skills of everyday living, there is also a pressing need for generic social services. Such services include arranging for escort services to agencies and potential residential placements, help with applications to entitlement programs, and assistance in mobilizing the resources of the family.

Ongoing asylum and sanctuary should be available for that small proportion of the chronically mentally ill who do not respond to current methods of treatment and rehabilitation. Some patients, even with high-quality treatment and rehabilitation efforts, remain dangerous or gravely disabled. For these patients, there is a pressing need for ongoing asylum in long-term settings, whether in hospitals or in facilities such as California's locked skilled-nursing facilities that have special programs for the mentally ill.

Research into the causes and treatment of both chronic mental illness and homelessness needs to be expanded. Further, more accurate epidemiological data need to be gathered and analyzed. For instance, estimates of the total number of homeless persons in the United States range from 250,000 to 3,000,000. Currently the research findings or incidence of mental illness among homeless groups are also highly variable, ranging up to 91%; these differences depend largely on such methodological issues as where the sample is taken, whether standardized scales or comparable criteria of illness are used, and theoretical biases. Better data, using recognized diagnostic criteria, need to be acquired.

Finally, additional monies must be expended for long-term solutions for the chronically mentally ill. Adequate new monies and better use of existing monies are needed to finance the system of care envisioned here, which incorporates supervised living arrangements, assertive case management, and an array of other services. In addition, financial support from existing entitlement programs such as Supplemental Security Income and Medicaid must be ensured.

In summary, the solutions to the problems of the mentally ill homeless, and the chronically mentally ill generally, are as manifold as the problems they seek to remedy. However, only with comprehensive short- and long-term solutions will the plight of this neglected population be addressed.

REFERENCES

1. ABRAMSON, M. F. (1972). The criminalization of mentally disordered behavior. *Hosp. Commun. Psychiatry, 23,* 101.
2. ARCE, A. A., & VERGARE, M. J. (1984). Identifying and characterizing the mentally ill among the homeless. In H. R. Lamb (Ed.), *The homeless mentally ill.* Washington, DC: American Psychiatric Association.
3. BACHRACH, L. L. (1984). Asylum and chronically ill psychiatric patients. *Am. J. Psychiatry, 141,* 975.
4. BAXTER, E., & HOPPER, K. (1982). The new mendicancy: Homeless in New York City. *Am. J. Orthopsychiatry, 52,* 393.
5. BAXTER, E., & HOPPER, K. (1984). Troubled on the streets: The mentally disabled homeless poor. In J. A. Talbott (Ed.), *The chronic mental patient: Five years later.* New York: Grune & Stratton.
6. GOLDFINGER, S. M., & CHAFETZ, L. (1984). Developing a better service delivery system for the homeless mentally ill. In H. R. Lamb (Ed.), *The homeless mentally ill.* Washington, DC: American Psychiatric Association.
7. GRUNBERG, F., KLINGER, B. I., & GRUMENT, B. R. (1977). Homicide and the deinstitutionalization of the mentally ill. *Am. J. Psychiatry, 134,* 685.
8. LAMB, H. R. (1980). Structure: The neglected ingredient of community treatment. *Arch. Gen. Psychiatry, 37,* 1224.
9. LAMB, H. R. (1980). Board and care home wanderers. *Arch. Gen. Psychiatry, 37,* 136.
10. LAMB, H. R. (1981). What did we really expect from deinstitutionalization? *Hosp. & Commun. Psychiatry, 32,* 105.
11. LAMB, H. R. (1982). Young adult chronic patients: The new drifters. *Hosp. Commun. Psychiatry, 33,* 465.

12. Lamb, H. R., & Grant, R. W. (1982). The mentally ill in an urban county jail. *Arch. Gen. Psychiatry, 39,* 17.
13. Lamb, H. R., & Grant, R. W. (1983). Mentally ill women in a county jail. *Arch. Gen. Psychiatry, 40,* 363.
14. Lamb, R. H., & Peele, R. (1984). The need for continuing asylum and sanctuary. *Hosp. Commun. Psychiatry, 35,* 798.
15. Lamb, H. R., & Mills, M. J. (1986). Needed changes in law and procedure for the chronically mentally ill. *Hosp. Commun. Psychiatry, 37,* 475.
16. Larew, B. I. (1980). Strange strangers: Serving transients. *Social Casework, 63,* 107.
17. Lipton, F. R., Sabatini, A., & Katz, S. E. (1983). Down and out in the city: The homeless mentally ill. *Hosp. Commun. Psychiatry, 34,* 817.
18. Sosowsky, L. (1978). Crime and violence among mental patients reconsidered in view of the new legal relationship between the state and the mentally ill. *Am. J. Psychiatry, 135,* 33.
19. Talbott, J. A., & Lamb, H. (1984). Summary and recommendations. In H. R. Lamb (Ed.), *The homeless mentally ill.* Washington, DC: The American Psychiatric Association.

14

THE DUAL-CAREER FAMILY

CAROL C. NADELSON, M.D.

and

THEODORE NADELSON, M.D.

Department of Psychiatry,
New England Medical Center, Inc.,
Boston, Massachusetts

The past two decades have brought increasing numbers of dual-career couples, representing a major shift from traditional social patterns. Although they are no longer perceived to be aberrant, an ideal attitude or mythology that the "natural" state of couples is "man at work/woman at home"—or at least "man as head of household"—persists for dual-career families. Partners work more hours than usual, have greater commitment to fulfill responsibilities, and devote more time and energy to their jobs.

The observation that any marriage can really be separated into two marriages—his and hers—adds complexity to the dual-career marriage and may at times give the undertaking the dimensions of a corporate merger. Dual careers dictate a necessity for organization, trust, and integration in order to keep paths parallel, without collision at intersections. Husband and wife often have different career goals; but they usually do want the marriage to support the difficulty of this high-level, energy-depleting, and sometimes emotionally intensive work. They both want the marriage to sustain their individual careers. Marriage, however, is not necessarily the best institution for such maintenance.

G. B. Shaw (15), the inveterate misogynist, constructs a cynical foundation for marriage:

> . . . I said nothing about a woman's whole mind. I spoke of her view of Man as a separate sex. It is no more cynical than her view of herself

as above all things a mother. Sexually, Woman is Nature's contrivance for perpetuating its highest achievement. Sexually, Man is Woman's contrivance to carry out Nature's behest in the most economical way. She knows by instinct that far back in the evolutionary process she invented him, differentiated him, created him in order to produce something better than the single-sex process can produce. While he fulfills the purpose for which she made him, he is welcome to his dreams, his follies, his ideals, his heroisms, provided that the keystone of them all is the worship of Woman, of motherhood, of the family, of the hearth.

Marriage, set in motion by nature and powered by woman (as Shaw presents it), however, serves the individual woman poorly. Despite the shift toward idealization of the benefits of the dual-career marriage among professionals, Bernard (1) points to the fact that the nature of marriage requires that wives make greater adaptations and sacrifices than their husbands. Even in 1987, women generally continue to view their husbands' careers as more important than their own and they tend to relegate their own careers to second place. This dynamic often reverberates with their earlier socialization to regard their effect on a larger environment as less valued and less valuable. For men, it similarly supports the view that even career women are less serious about their work than are men in comparable fields.

Early in the 1960s warnings were expressed that changes in roles might prove difficult for men, who would have to cope with new demands and expectations of them as their wives extended their interest beyond "kinder and kuchen." While the evidence is not all in, it is clear that there are important effects on both men and women, as well as their children.

Women employed outside the home have been reported to be in better physical and mental health, with more positive attitudes toward marriage than their housewife sisters. Data from the Framingham coronary heart disease study (5), over a 10-year period, indicated that the incidence rates for coronary heart disease were generally higher for men than for women. Women in high-status occupations, however, had lower rates of heart disease. Work does appear to have a beneficial effect on mental and physical health for both men and women (2, 18).

Women with paid jobs also appear to be more satisfied with their lives than are housewives. Jobs can be a source of self-esteem, independent status, a social network enhancement, as well as income. Employed women also appear to have more positive coping strategies than women not employed outside of their homes (3, 17). The husbands of these employed women, however, have been reported to be in poorer health and more discontent with their marriages than the husbands of housewives. It has been suggested that the price to be paid within marriage for women's excursion into the world outside the home is exacted from their husbands.

Most of the studies that have been done, however, looked at nonrepresentative samples; moreover, the data were often collected very early in the history of the dual-career phenomenon, so that families were "societal deviants," not 20 % of the married population, as they are currently. Many studies were also influenced by social and political value systems (2). More recent evidence is neither consistent nor confirmatory of the outcomes previously reported.

Attempts at replication suggest, for example, that husbands of employed wives have no greater evidence for negative stress consequences than do husbands of housewives, when other variables are taken into account.

HOW DOES THE DUAL-CAREER RELATIONSHIP WORK?

Despite television commercials that promise that you can "have it all," it is difficult to work out the complexities of dual-career relationships. Even the question of *who* is the "spouse" is no longer simple; it often depends on whose office event one is at, or what form is being filled out. In dual-career families it is necessary, not only reasonable and equitable, that partners expect to make compromises and changes that are often unanticipated.

A balance of power and responsibility, with implicit or explicit guidelines and rules, must exist, and flexibility is essential for viability. There is always the danger of overadministration; that is when both partners must know their own and each others' schedules and household responsibilities in order to be able to take over. It is difficult, as in any organization or business, to have a perfectly run household when the household is not in the hands of a single-minded domestic executive.

If one partner travels a great deal, mundane issues like dental appointments for children and taking out the garbage cannot be the sole responsibility of the traveling partner. Even without travel, there are necessary daily decisions, such as who makes arrangements for transporting children, who waits for the plumber, and so forth. Despite the reality of the large numbers of two-income families, the assumption on the part of children's schools, other professionals, and those who are in the repair services is that there is always a "wife" at home who can wait — all day, or into the next.

Dual-career couples live with each other in delicate balance. They must implicitly trust each other, yet competition, anger, and tension about sex roles may remain active, even if not explicit. Attitudes and behaviors are often slow to change, despite commitment and love. Shared affection and respect tend to smooth the rough edges. It is not unusual, even in 1987, for a husband, his family, and even friends to perceive the wife with a career as too aggressive or, with some tutoring from peers and colleagues, as "castrating." With time, a husband must learn to understand that the smart lawyer he married would not be successful if she weren't aggressive, just as he must be. Some marriages cannot tolerate this strain. Even the couple who go into it with eyes open must learn to tolerate unexpected and unexplained feelings of frustration, resentment, and jealousy.

That women continue to bear the major responsibility for family and home, despite their career obligations, is well documented.

A chief executive officer in a medium-sized company still indicates that she makes all of the family preparations for holidays by herself. She feels she ought to do this; she indicates that she is uncomfortable if she does not. Despite the fact that she is squeezed by major scheduling difficulties, she still shops for all family gifts, makes preparations for the children's Christmas homecoming, and does most of the food preparation. Sleep and time for relaxation are sacrificed. For her, holidays are often drudgery rather than pleasure.

It is not an uncommon complaint of married women professionals that they fall asleep in the evenings over journals, books, and papers while their husbands still seem wide awake. As one distinguished woman professor said to her equally distinguished husband, "How often do you suddenly think in the midst of lecturing to a class, 'My God, we have no toilet paper! I'd better stop on the way home and pick some up'?"

Methods of allocation of household responsibilities are varied. Some couples use "household on-duty" scheduling with three months on, three months off; others find a parceling out of such responsibilities to work better: "you take care of worrying about groceries, I'll be responsible for the cars." There is usually a lack of symmetry in such assignments, and the male partner often presents a self-congratulatory image to the world and is rewarded with accolades for his "helpfulness." The fact that he is participating in household concerns (other than furnace and cars) is seen by him to be the equivalent of membership in a feminist strike force. Women, on the other hand, take on the executive responsibility of running the household as an expectation. In fact, if they don't sail through with grace, they often feel themselves to be failures, and those around them, including family, will support that conclusion. Partners generally conclude that they both need "a good wife."

Reports about changing roles in marriage are more often based on projections rather than reality. One national study of university freshmen reported that 39% of the males expressed a preference for an egalitarian marriage (compared with 69% of the females), but these attitudes do not necessarily reflect later behaviors, especially after there are children (10). The real crunch for dual-career couples does appear to occur when children enter the picture, bringing new demands and priorities. Day-to-day activities require coordination, and when there are emergencies or unexpected events, plans must be made and implemented regardless of other obligations. When a child is ill or needs extra attention, there seems an almost reflexive response on the part of most couples (despite other compelling duties) for the wife to assume the main task of finding medical care and taking time to stay home.

There is evidence that there has been some change. In addition to the recent election of a young man as the first male president of the Future Homemakers of America, many husbands now assume that they will take a major part in child rearing, and they are making career modifications in order to do so. There may be consequences for them, however, when traditional roles are changed. Osherson and Dill (13) found that egalitarian husbands felt they achieved less success at work, but did have greater career flexibility. They reported being able to pursue their own choice of activities rather than focusing primarily on job-related activities and found greater expression for their own self-development.

The data continue to show that within most two-income families there is gender differentiation in occupational behavior (11). Men on the average do work more hours than women; however, both men and women in higher-prestige occupations work more hours than those of the same sex in less prestigious occupations. Both men and women in dual-career couples work longer hours when their spouses also work longer hours. In general, then, when occupational status is high, there is greater equality of occupational involvement. When there is inequality of occupational status, there is lower occupational involvement of the spouse with lower status, and that is, usually, the woman. She is paid less and is less satisfied with her job than her husband is with his. She is more likely to be discriminated against by employers, and there are informal antinepotism regulations that make getting a job in the same company more difficult for her. She is more likely to interrupt her career than is her husband and she spends more hours in domestic activities and child care. Tryon and Tryon (16) believe that the reasons for these inequities stem mainly from spouses and employers, who endorse traditional gender roles.

From the sample of 127 dual-career families in a midwestern U.S. city, however, Sekaran (14) reported that there were no major gender differences in how work and family roles were perceived, how absorbed husbands and wives were with both roles, or how they set their priorities. Women did report that they perceived greater stress and higher expectations at work. The author suggests that greater sharing and support at home would be helpful for these families.

IS THERE CHANGE?

There have been some changes in the past decade. Public attitudes do appear to be catching up with the reality of such large numbers of women in the workplace. In the United States, well over 60% of married women with young children work outside of the home (19). These younger women represent an emerging population that will, most likely, continue to be employed.

The dual-career couple in the mid-1980s exists as a mutually interdependent system with strong attachment to ideals of companionship, communication, and sharing. That these are difficult to achieve is reflected by high divorce rates in most Western nations.

Young people are deeply affected by these marital disappointments and they are cautious about marriage. In 1970, one study reported that 5% of the college students surveyed indicated that they would not marry; by 1980, 40% responded negatively. Most of those students who negated marriage will, of course, subsequently marry; however, the survey was directed toward understanding social attitudes rather than prediction with regard to marital status. In any event, marriage has come to be viewed more as a choice, and the single life not taken as a visible sign of defect. Ninety-five percent of Americans still do marry, no matter what they say earlier in their lives. What choices today's young people will eventually make are still unknown, but it is a good guess that an overwhelming percent will also marry. Likewise, we do not know how many will divorce, but if current trends continue, the number will be high.

There has been a quantum leap with regard to husbands' attitudes about their wives working outside of the home. Currently the majority of men prefer this arrangement. In 1938 only 19% of husbands approved of a wife working; almost 50 years later the figure approached 80%. Moreover, 80% of college students believe that career and family are compatible for women.

Interestingly, a 1983 study reported that about 20% of women in professional and managerial occupations, or with postgraduate education, plan to have no children (12). Only 7% of women who never completed high school expect that they will not have children. Highly educated women have an average expectation of fewer children than those women who do not complete high school.

The decision to remain employed during early childbearing years leads to a greater probability that a woman will continue to work and achieve in her profession (19). Regardless of their employment status, however, women continued to spend considerably more time alone with their children than their husbands do. The shift toward more traditional role assignments, after having children, comes as a surprise to many couples and can lead to role dissatisfaction (4).

Of the 20% of U.S. couples who live as dual-career families, husbands most often earn more than their wives. There continues to be considerable ambivalence on the part of husbands about a wife earning more than they do, particularly if the wife is in a male-dominated field. The income gap between men and women continues to exist, although there has been some narrowing. Women earn about 60% of what men earn for the same jobs. As noted, even within most dual-career families wives have lower salaries, work fewer hours, and tend to adjust their schedules to a greater degree than their husbands. Generally in these couples the income differential decreases as the number of years of work increases. The dual-worker characteristics of those in lower socioeconomic groups have been less researched than of those who function at a higher socioeconomic level.

Less than 1% of dual-career couples in the United States (about 1 million) live a commuter life, where a partner works at such distance from home that going to work and returning home every night is not possible. There also continue to be differences between the willingness of wives and husbands to take positions in other cities, if the partner does not have an offer: 68% of the wives expressed reluctance to do so, while 40% of the husbands stated their willingness to do it; 26% of women would not expect their husbands to relocate if they did not have a job as well. Kilpatrick (9), however, reported that 35% of male candidates who were finalists for positions requiring relocation would not negotiate further unless a proposed move also met the wife's needs. This represents a substantial change over a decade.

DIVORCE

Those social commentators who see nothing ahead but dark days predicted by any social change cite rising divorce rates as an indication that there is an erosion within our social framework. These same commentators often compare the real against the idealized template. The idealization includes the belief that families in the past always stayed together, and that divorce was an occasional aberrant phenomenon within the expected framework. We must place the figures in perspective and consider other variables. With increased longevity there is an expectation that marriages will last through what used to be two lifetimes. Less than a century ago, death due to childbirth, occupational hazard, or infection was common enough to severely limit the numbers of adults who reached middle and old age. Thus, marriages often lasted little more than a decade before the death of one partner. As the death rate has decreased, the "decay of the American family" has become a greater concern than when death (rather than divorce) dissolved the partnership. Projections suggest that as many as 60% of the marriages today will last until the death of one partner.

Divorce rates are reported to be higher in dual-career couples, and when the female partner earns more than $15,000 per year there is three times the likelihood that divorce will occur, compared with women earning less than $3,000 a year. It is further computed that for every $1,000 increase in earnings by the wife, the divorce rate will go up by 2% (7). Hiller and Philliber (6) suggest that tension is created when wives take occupational positions that enable them to exceed the achievements of their husbands. They are at higher risk for divorce or negative job change. For those social commentators with more optimistic outlook and greater comfort with social change, that particular statistic does not necessarily have as negative a valence. Certainly, women who earn a higher salary have more choice and can leave an unrewarding marriage. It may be that marriages at lower economic levels stay together because of the wife's financial dependence on the husband. More divorced men than women remarry and women are far more likely to experience severe economic hardships than do men, following a divorce. It has been reported that in the first year following a divorce, men's income rose 73%, whereas women's fell by 43% (19).

CONCLUSION

That attitudes persist despite reality is reflected in the dynamics of relationships as well as in the world at large. There are still headlines which say "GRANDMOTHER RECEIVES NOBEL PRIZE" (referring to scientist Rosalyn Yalow) or "MOTHER OF TWO HEADS PSYCHIA-TRISTS" (referring to a coauthor of this chapter). Women continue to be viewed within the background or framework of motherhood. Although the alliance with such a position is less often expressed, it still remains a marker of "normality" for women. Women continue to be a projective screen for others' mythology and beliefs, and they often capitulate to these societal representations. A "good enough husband" must acknowledge the wear and tear on his wife's psyche caused by these constant incursions. In gatherings where references (either gross or subtle) are made to "woman's place," it is difficult for a woman to raise her voice yet one more time to nail subtle (or gross) sexism at its source. If she does, she is again perceived as deviant, aberrant, or—even today—"castrating." She wonders if it is worth continuing the battle. Attitudinal change is slow. A woman executive recently commented that male executives accept women as professionals, "but they're not ready to accept them as true peers" (8). Men must participate in the long and arduous task of changing attitudes; men in dual-career families are in a unique position to do so. They must raise *their* voices and take on the battle as their own. After all, it is.

REFERENCES

1. BERNARD, J. (1973). *The future of marriage*. New York: Bantam Books.
2. BURKE, R., & WEIR, T. (1976). Relationship of wives' employment status to husband, wife, and pair satisfaction and performance. *J. Marr. Family, 38*(2), 279–287.
3. FIDEL, L. S., & PRATHER, J. E. (1976). *The housewife syndrome: Fact or fiction*. Study report. Rockville, MD: Institute on Drug Abuse.
4. GADDY, C., GLASS, C., & ARNKOFF, D. (1983). Career involvement of women in dual-career families: The significance of sex role identity. *J. Counseling Psychol., 320*(3), 388–394.
5. HAYNES, S. G., & FEINLEIB, M. (1982). Women, work and coronary heart disease: Results from the Framingham 19-year follow-up study. In P. W. Berman and E. R. Ramey (Eds.), *Women: A developmental perspective* (pp. 79–101), Washington, D.C.: NIH Publications No. 82-2298. US Government Printing Office.
6. HILLER, D., & PHILLIBER, W. (1982). Predicting marital and career success among dual-worker couples. *J. Marr. Family*, Feb., 53–62.
7. JOHNSON, S. (1981). *Women today*, Nov. 1978 cited in Parker, M., Peltier, S., & Wolleat, P. Understanding dual career couples. *Personnel Guidance J.*, Sept., *60*, 14–18.
8. JONES, L. (President of Women in Management). Cited in Brophy, B., with Linnon, N. (Dec. 29, 1986/Jan. 5, 1987). Why women executives stop before the top. *U.S. News and World Report*, 72–73.
9. KILPATRICK, M. (1982). Job change in dual-career families: Danger or opportunity? *Family Relations*, July, 363–368.
10. LEWIS, R. A. (1985). Men's changing roles in marriage and the family. In R. A. Lewis (Ed.), *Marriage and family review*, Vol. 9, nos. 3/4 (pp. 1–10). New York: Haworth Press.

11. MEEKER, B. (1983). Equality and differentiation of time spent in paid work in two-income families. In P. A. Katz (Ed.), *Sex roles*, Vol. 9, no. 10 (pp. 1023–1033). New York: Plenum Press.
12. MOORE, K., SPAIN, D., & BIANCHI, S. (1987). Working wives and mothers. In B. B. Hess & M. B. Sussman (Eds.), *Marriage and family review*, Vol. 7, nos. 3/4, (pp. 77–98). New York: Haworth Press.
13. OSHERSON, S., & DILL, D. (1983). Varying work and family choices: The impact on men's work satisfaction. *J. Marr. Family, 45*(2), 339–346.
14. SEKARAN, U. (1983). How husbands and wives in dual-career families perceive their family and work world. *J. Vocational Behav., 22,* 288–302.
15. SHAW, G. B. *Man and superman.* Middlesex, England: Penguin Books (reprinted 1976).
16. TRYON, G., & TRYON, W. (1982). Issues in the lives of dual-career couples. *Clin. Psychol. Rev., 2,* 49–65.
17. VERBRUGGE, L. M. (1983). Women and men: Mortality and health of older people. Version I. In M. W. Riley, B. B. Hess, & E. K. Bond (Eds.), *Aging in society: Selected reviews of research* (pp. 139–174). Hillsdale, N.J.: Lawrence Erlbaum Associates.
18. WAITE, L. J. (1981). *U.S. women and work.* Population Bulletin 36(2), (43 pp.). Washington, D.C.: Population Reference Bureau.
19. WEITZMAN, L. J. (1985). *The divorce revolution, the unexpected social and economic consequences for women and children in America.* Stanford, CA: Stanford University Press.

15

UNEMPLOYMENT AND PSYCHOLOGICAL WELL-BEING

PHILIP ULLAH, PH.D.

Department of Psychology,
University of Western Australia,
Nedlands, Western Australia

Among the major life events, such as divorce or bereavement, which place the individual under considerable stress and strain, job loss is beginning to assume an increasing prominence. Since the beginning of the current economic recession in the 1970s, the number of people experiencing unemployment has grown steadily. National statistics on unemployment rates, which summarize the number of unemployed people at a given time, give little indication of the total number of people who may experience unemployment over a period of time. For example, in 1980, when the number of people unemployed in Britain during any one month never exceeded 2.15 million, it is estimated that over four million people appeared on the unemployment register at some point during that year. Since unemployment rates have risen sharply since then, the total number of people affected is also likely to have gone up.

Although the majority of people becoming unemployed still manage to obtain a new job within the next six months, gone are the days when unemployment was a voluntary reaction to unpleasant working conditions, to be followed quickly by a new job. The fact that job loss is today likely to be involuntary, and that the unemployed person is unlikely to know if and exactly when he might be re-employed, suggests that there are

I am grateful to the Health Promotion Research Trust for financial support during the writing of this chapter.

large numbers of people who are experiencing the stress that unemployment can often entail.

Mass unemployment is not a new phenomenon. During the 1930s national unemployment rates were even higher than they are today. There was a corresponding research effort into the psychological effects of unemployment on the individual, and a review of over 100 of such studies was presented by Eisenberg and Lazarsfeld (15). When viewed today, however, much of that early work appears conceptually and methodologically naïve. Current research is more rigorous and follows the standard procedures of scientific inquiry. In seeking to present what is now known about the psychological effects of unemployment, this chapter will therefore draw on the objective evidence produced by this recent research, rather than on the subjective appraisal of a relatively small number of case studies.

Clinical practice, if it is to be effective, requires more than simply a knowledge of the various ways in which a major life event, such as job loss, can affect an individual. The clinician also needs to know how the effects actually occur if he or she is to prevent or modify them. How are different groups within a population differentially affected by such processes? And how might the individual be counseled to deal with his problems by exerting his own influence? Issues such as these will be dealt with in the latter part of this chapter.

THE PSYCHOLOGICAL EFFECTS OF UNEMPLOYMENT

Research into the psychological effects of unemployment tends to take one of two forms. Cross-sectional studies seek to compare, on a range of psychological well-being measures, a sample of unemployed people with a carefully matched employed sample. In contrast, longitudinal studies obtain successive measurements, over a period of time, from one or more samples. In the latter type of study the effects of unemployment are gauged from comparisons between a person's psychological well-being at each measurement point. Although both types of studies indicate that unemployed people typically suffer lower psychological well-being than employed people, some caution is required in interpreting the results from the cross-sectional studies. In particular, these studies cannot differentiate those symptoms which may be an effect of unemployment from those which may be a cause of it. For example, is a person's depression an outcome of his or her unemployment, or did it in fact contribute to that person's job loss? Longitudinal studies, which permit the researcher to compare a person's level of well-being when he or she is unemployed with the level he/she exhibited before becoming unemployed, give greater confidence when asserting the direction of the causal influence. Such studies also allow comparisons between well-being during unemployment and that during a later state of re-employment, thereby allowing investigation of any improvements in well-being.

Psychological well-being is here being used as a general term to cover a variety of affective, cognitive, and behavioral states. Warr (61) has described low psychological well-being as that which is "illustrated in anxiety, depression, low morale, lack of confidence, low sense of personal autonomy, inability to cope with the problems of living, and dissatisfaction with oneself and the social and physical environment" (p. 417). Validated instruments now exist to measure these other aspects of well-being. Comparisons between groups of employed and unemployed people in terms of their scores on these instruments have produced the current knowledge of the psychological effects of unemployment. The variety of effects so far discovered will now be discussed (under the headings suggested by Fryer and Payne [26]).

Affective Symptoms

Bradburn (7) has produced measures of both positive and negative affect. The former taps the existence of positive feelings over and above simply the absence of such feelings, while the latter is concerned with the actual experience of states of boredom, depression, loneliness, and of feeling upset. The two scales tend not to be intercorrelated, supporting the view that they cover states that are independent of each other. From community surveys in the United States Bradburn (7) found significantly lower levels of positive affect among unemployed men than among those who were employed. No such difference was found in terms of negative affect. However, research in Britain by Warr (60) suggests that unemployment may entail more than simply the absence of positive feelings. Using much larger unemployed samples than those used by Bradburn (7), Warr found significantly lower positive affect and also significantly higher negative affect among steel workers who were unemployed six months after closure of their plant compared with those who had managed to find new jobs.

The study by Warr (60) is, of course, open to an alternative interpretation—namely, that the lower well-being of the unemployed men was a contributory factor in their failure to find a new job, rather than an outcome of this. However, longitudinal research focusing on other affective states fails to support such an interpretation. Studies that have obtained measures of present life satisfaction, satisfaction with self, experience of pleasure and of strain, and depressive affect both before and after the onset of unemployment have shown that poorer well-being follows from, rather than contributes toward, becoming unemployed (11, 21, 47, 53, 54).

Minor Psychiatric Morbidity

A number of instruments have been developed for use in community surveys to detect people likely to be suffering from psychiatric illness. These instruments typically take the form of self-report questionnaires, and their ease of administration makes them particularly suitable for use in unemployment studies. The General Health Questionnaire (GHQ), developed by Goldberg (28, 29) as a screening test for detecting minor psychiatric morbidity in the general population, has been used in the majority of such studies. There are different versions of the GHQ, which vary in length in order to differentiate between subsets of symptoms (e.g., depression, anxiety, psychosomatic symptoms). The shortest version, containing 12 items (GHQ-12), is most commonly used and has been described as a measure of general psychological distress (59).

There is now a growing body of evidence that unemployed people score significantly higher on the GHQ (indicating poorer well-being) than do similar employed people (14, 35, 52, 64). The size of the difference in scores is such to suggest that unemployed people are many times more likely to be diagnosed as a psychiatric case than are comparable employed people. Thus, following Goldberg's (28) suggestion of a threshold score of two on the GHQ-12 as an indication of psychiatric "caseness," Warr (62) points to five different samples of unemployed people where the proportion scoring above two varies from 54% to 62%. In contrast, the percentages from employed comparison groups vary from 15 to 25. Finlay-Jones and Eckhardt (23) describe a study of young Australians where unemployment raised the probability of psychiatric illness by a factor of six.

Once again, there is evidence from longitudinal investigations to strongly suggest that elevated GHQ scores occur as a result of unemployment (e.g., Ref. 2). Studies by Warr and Jackson (67) and Banks and Ullah (3) have also shown that people moving from unemployment to employment exhibit a marked reduction in GHQ scores, to a point that is comparable with other employed groups.

Depression and Anxiety

Studies using self-report measures of depression and/or anxiety typically show higher levels of these symptoms in unemployed people than in employed people (14, 19, 64). Zung's (73) self-rating depression and anxiety scales, the Beck Depression Inventory (6), and Rosenberg's (50) Depressive Affect Scale are among the instruments that have been used in such studies. Longitudinal surveys by Patton and Noller (46) and Feather and O'Brien (21) suggest that unemployment leads to an increase in depressive symptoms, rather than the converse. However, in a study of Australian school graduates, Tiggemann and Winefield (54) found that differences in depression between those who found jobs and those who became unemployed were largely due to an improvement in outlook on the part of the former rather than the unemployed becoming more depressed. Similarly, Banks and Ullah (3) found a significant fall in levels of depression and anxiety among young people moving from unemployment to employment. However, no measures were obtained prior to the onset of unemployment in order to indicate whether unemployment resulted in an increase in these levels.

Self-Esteem

Results from studies examining the association between unemployment and self-esteem have so far failed to produce a consistent pattern. Some cross-sectional studies (e.g., Ref. 17) have found lower levels of self-esteem among unemployed than among employed people, while others (e.g., Ref. 33) have not. In a longitudinal study of Australian school graduates, Patton and Noller (46) found that those people who became unemployed experienced a significant fall in their self-esteem, while there was some improvement among those who obtained jobs after leaving school. Gurney (31), however, found that the largest change in self-esteem among his sample of Australian school graduates occurred among those who obtained jobs. Those who were unemployed displayed no change from the level of self-esteem observed when they were still at school. Gurney suggests that the effect of unemployment among school graduates may be to prevent the development of psychosocial identity, which employment normally entails.

Although this interpretation is plausible, it is not supported by the findings from a more recent Australian study. Winefield and Tiggemann (71) found that those school graduates who became unemployed exhibited the largest improvement in self-esteem, compared with those who obtained jobs and those who returned to full-time education. This was mainly due to the particularly low scores the unemployed obtained while still at school; once they were in the labor market their level of self-esteem was not different from that of those who were employed. The authors suggest that low scholastic achievement may have contributed to this low level of self-esteem while at school and also to the subsequent unemployment of these people, whereas leaving school freed them from the unfavorable criticism by teachers, and thus contributed to an improvement in self-esteem.

Warr and Jackson (65) have suggested that one reason for the apparent disparity between research findings lies in the measures of self-esteem that have been used. Most of the studies cited above used adaptations of Rosenberg's (50) self-esteem scale. This measure contains both positively and negatively worded items which are typically summed to produce an overall score. Warr and Jackson argue that the two sets of items may be measuring different aspects (positive and negative) of self-esteem and that therefore they should not be combined. Keeping the two sets separate, they found greater negative self-esteem among unemployed British teenagers than among employed teenagers, but no difference in the levels of positive self-esteem. Moreover, longitudinal comparisons showed that a change in employment status was accompanied by a change in negative self-esteem, but no alteration in positive self-esteem. They concluded that positive feelings about oneself (e.g., "I feel I am as good a person as anyone else") were fundamental to the self-concept and resistant to changes in everyday circumstances. In contrast, negative feelings (e.g., "I feel I can't do anything right") may be less stable. Their argument is supported by further Australian research, which showed no difference between employed and unemployed graduates in terms of positive self-esteem, but greater negative self-esteem among the latter (19).

THE PROCESSES THROUGH WHICH UNEMPLOYMENT AFFECTS
PSYCHOLOGICAL WELL-BEING

Preventing or lessening the harmful psychological effects of unemployment is more likely to be achieved if the processes through which the effects occur are fully understood. There are currently two major explanatory frameworks. To a certain extent these explanations overlap, though they differ in some key respects.

Jahoda (38, 40, 41) presented the first real attempt at explaining why unemployment can prove so distressing. Obviously, the loss of income that unemployment entails is likely to be a major source of concern. Yet, as Jahoda has pointed out, if there is more to having a job than earning a living, there must be more to losing a job than a drop in income. Jahoda states that although increased income is the *manifest* benefit of having a job, there are also a number of nonintended, or *latent*, benefits. She lists five of these latent benefits of employment: the imposition of a time structure on the working day, regularly shared experiences and contacts with people, a link with transcending goals and purposes, a sense of identity and status, and the enforcement of activity.

Jahoda suggests that it is the loss of these five latent benefits of employment which causes the psychological harm inflicted by unemployment. All five, she says, are psychologically supportive and are essential to healthy psychological functioning. Thus, the primary causes of depression and distress during unemployment are the excessive amount of free time it usually entails, the isolation from friends and colleagues, the lack of purpose to each day, the sense of stigma and loss of an occupational identity, and the inactivity it can often induce.

Rather than focusing exclusively on what is lost when a person becomes unemployed, Warr (61–63) also considers the changes that occur during such a transition. Such a model incorporates the new burdens that an unemployed person takes on, as well as any possible improvements in his day-to-day life. Thus there are often new and potentially stressful activities for the unemployed to undertake, such as making job applications, looking for jobs, and claiming state benefits. These can account for some of the increased anxiety levels found in unemployed samples (e.g., Ref. 64), while failed job applications during unemployment have been shown to be linked with greater depression (20).

There is also a sense in which unemployment can be experienced as liberating, particularly when it follows a stressful job or one that is physically very demanding. Recognition of the potentially "good" features of unemployment is important if it is to be made easier to bear by the unemployed.

PSYCHOLOGICAL STAGES IN THE EXPERIENCE OF UNEMPLOYMENT

The notion that the unemployed individual passes through a number of distinct psychological stages during the course of unemployment is popular. Typically, it is claimed that the initial reaction to job loss is one of shock, followed by a period of optimism. This gradually changes to pessimism following unsuccessful attempts to regain employment. Following prolonged unemployment, it is claimed that there is a transition to a fourth and final stage, that of fatalism, where the unemployed individual resigns him/herself to a state of joblessness.

Stage accounts of the experience of unemployment initially emerged from the early psychological research into unemployment, conducted during the recession of the 1930s (1, 5). The theory resurfaced during the upsurge of psychological interest in unemployment that followed the rapid increase in unemployment levels during the 1970s. Assertions that there are distinct psychological stages in the experience of unemployment are to be found not only in academic books (e.g., Refs. 33a, 42), but also in journals and magazines intended for a much broader readership (e.g., Refs. 32, 39) and in popular books (45).

Despite the attractiveness and simplicity of the idea, stage accounts should not be uncritically accepted as valid descriptions of the psychological experience of unemployment. In a review of the literature on stage accounts, Fryer (24) suggests there are serious methodological and conceptual flaws in most of the expositions. In particular, he argues that they are "intuitive, poorly defined, and underspecified, and they appear to be theoretically groundless" (p. 263).

The evidence Fryer accumulates to support his claim is persuasive. For example, two of the key sources of the idea during the 1930s (5, 72) use as their evidence essays written by unemployed people. In the case of the Beales and Lambert (5) study, these were essays submitted to the *Listener* magazine, where the guidelines had been that the authors should state whether unemployment had left them optimistic or pessimistic and whether they expected to enter any new phases of life. Clearly, the writers of the essays had been primed to interpret their experiences of unemployment in terms of such phases. More recent studies are shown by Fryer to be similarly methodologically unsound.

Although there have been some acceptable studies that have found different levels of psychological distress (as measured by the GHQ) among people experiencing varying lengths of unemployment (66), others have produced results that fail to show an association between the length of time a person has been unemployed and some index of his mental health (3, 18, 68).

A true test of the stage account would involve a number of distinct psychological states being measured on different occasions over a considerable period of time. The logistics of conducting such a study have so far discouraged any attempts to do so. To this must be added the conceptual problems regarding the precise nature and number of stages there are thought to be (numbers range from two to seven), the possible differences in the pattern of change due to mediating factors such as age, gender, social class, and ethnicity, and the extent to which the psychological stages refer to global states or are merely confined to job prospects. Given these inherent difficulties in applying a stage account, Fryer's conclusion that such an account is not to be recommended seems entirely justifiable.

IS UNEMPLOYMENT LINKED WITH SUICIDE?

Although this issue has received considerable media coverage in recent years, it is unlikely that any firm conclusion can be reached. The reason for this lies in the methodological difficulties involved in identifying unemployment as an independent *causal* factor in suicide or attempted suicide (parasuicide). The relative rarity of its occurrence means that it cannot be investigated by longitudinal studies like those investigating changes in psychological well-being. Random population samples are unlikely to produce cases where suicide follows the onset of unemployment.

Research into possible links between unemployment and suicide have tended to adopt one of two procedures. Aggregate studies examine for possible statistical associations between national unemployment rates and suicide rates. Individual cross-sectional studies compare suicides with matched samples to see whether the former are more likely to be unemployed.

Generally, there appears to be some association between unemployment and suicide, though a more precise interpretation of this association cannot be made. Thus, although aggregate studies in the United States show that an increase in suicide rates tends to follow a period of economic decline, this can give no indication of how many suicides, if any, were the direct result of the person becoming unemployed. Similarly, cross-sectional studies have shown that the proportion of suicides who are unemployed can be as high as 46% (among men). Yet it is not possible to rule out the possibility that some additional factor, such as severe depression, may have been a major contributor to both job loss and suicide.

Interviews with parasuicides have rarely identified unemployment as the main reason why suicide was attempted. In most cases problems with interpersonal relationships are cited as the reason. Yet as Warr (63) has pointed out, unemployment may have been an initial cause of such problems, and so an indirect causal influence cannot be ruled out. Similarly, poverty has been linked with parasuicide, and unemployment remains one of the major causes of poverty.

Although firm conclusions cannot be reached regarding unemployment as a potential cause of suicide or parasuicide, the clinician needs to be aware that a link has been established. The fact that a patient is unemployed is itself likely to precipitate, or be an effect of, a number of other circumstances that in combination make suicide more likely to occur.

ARE DIFFERENT GROUPS IN SOCIETY DIFFERENTIALLY AFFECTED BY UNEMPLOYMENT?

Constant references to "the unemployed" may create the impression that they are a homogeneous group. Clearly, they are not. It is therefore pertinent to inquire how the psychological effects of unemployment differ according to the social and demographic characteristics of the person concerned. This has been the aim of much of the recent survey research into unemployment. Although survey research, particularly that which is longitudinal, is most suited to addressing such issues, one must be alerted to its limitations. Any statistical trend is likely to gloss over individual exceptions to that trend. There is, then, a sense in which each unemployed person is a unique individual. However, as long as this is borne in mind, it may also be extremely helpful for the clinician to know of the general patterns that have emerged regarding differences in the psychological reactions to unemployment. These will be discussed under the headings of age, sex, social class, and ethnicity.

Age

A number of studies (e.g., Refs. 13, 35, 37) have shown that age is curvilinearly related to psychological well-being among unemployed men. The relationship is such that men in the middle age groups tend to exhibit lower well-being than those at the two extremes. This may in part reflect the greater financial commitments and family responsibilities of those in middle life. It is also possible that more elderly unemployed men may view themselves as "early retired" and so may not feel the need to remain committed to finding another job. Young people without employment may similarly experience less need to find a job, since to a certain extent they have the options of further education or youth-training programs.

Sex

Any differences in well-being observed between unemployed men and women need to be interpreted within the light of wider contextual factors. Employment may have a different meaning for women who perceive their primary role to be carers of the home and family. Among women who are mothers, for example, there appears to be no benefit to psychological well-being from having a job (69). In addition to distinguishing between women who do or do not have children, it is also important to distinguish between those who are unemployed and those who are nonemployed (34). The latter may be defined as those women who, though not employed, do not view themselves as being in the labor market and do not want to obtain a job. Even in comparisons between men and women who are registered as unemployed and who desire employment, any observed differences in well-being need to be interpreted with caution. There is strong evidence to suggest that, generally, women have lower levels of psychological health than do men (10). Differences between the sexes among unemployed samples may therefore simply be reflecting this fact rather than pointing to a greater inability to cope with unemployment. Thus in a study of unemployed British teenagers, Warr, Banks, and Ullah (64) found that females had significantly higher levels of psychological distress, depression, and anxiety. However, it was not possible to determine how far this reflected differences found in commitment to finding employment and in activity levels, and how far it reflected the general pattern of sex differences normally present in community-based samples.

Social Class

Because of the greater insecurity of jobs at the lower occupational level, unemployment is typically more common among blue-collar workers than among white-collar workers. However, middle-class unemployment is becoming increasingly more common, and so the clinician should be alert to the specific problems experienced by both working and middle-class unemployed people.

In some respects unemployment may be less of a problem among professional workers, since they may be able to call on greater financial, educational, and personal resources than can blue-collar workers (22). However, there is also a sense in which the middle-class professional has more to lose, with respect to income and status, than the blue-collar worker (e.g., Ref. 42).

The results from one British study (48) suggest that white- and blue-collar workers suffer the same degree of psychological harm caused by job loss. The study is a particularly impressive one, since the investigators controlled for age, marital status, and length of time unemployed, while still managing to obtain relatively large sample numbers. A total of 399 unemployed men were interviewed. All were aged between 25 and 39, all were married, and they had all been unemployed for between 6 and 12 months. Half of the sample had been previously employed in unskilled and semiskilled occupations, and the other half had been unemployed in managerial or professional occupations. The two groups were found to have very similar low levels of psychological well-being, as measured by the GHQ-12. They were, however, different in other important respects. Working-class respondents reported significantly greater financial problems and more difficulties in filling the time than did middle-class respondents. Although both these features tend to be associated with poorer psychological well-being during unemployment, it appears that the overall psychological effect of unemployment is a homogenizing one for middle- and working-class men.

Ethnicity

There is much evidence from sociological studies that members of nonwhite ethnic minorities face considerable discrimination in the labor market. They are more likely to lose their jobs than are whites in similar occupations; once unemployed it tends to take longer for nonwhites to find new jobs than it does whites; nonwhites who obtain jobs have usually had to make many times more job applications than have whites who obtain new jobs; and educational qualifications do not appear to increase job prospects among nonwhites, though they quite considerably improve the chances of whites obtaining jobs (12, 51).

Given the extent of disadvantage among ethnic minorities, it might be expected that they experience poorer psychological well-being during unemployment than do whites. It is also often assumed that young Afro-Caribbeans are particularly prone to becoming alienated. Yet the small amount of British research available shows that both these assumptions are unsupported. One study of unemployed British teenagers found that Afro-Caribbeans had higher levels of psychological well-being (as measured by the GHQ-12 and Zung depression scale) than similar whites one year after leaving school (64). This appears to have been partly due to the lower commitment to seeking paid employment that was found among blacks in the sample, since less commitment was strongly associated with better well-being. It is possible that the lower commitment among blacks may reflect a realistic adaptation to poor job prospects. The authors argue: "Continuing to seek jobs is particularly stressful in a labour market where rejection is almost certain, and temporary withdrawal from job search provides some defense against that threat" (p. 85). Interestingly, these results were from the first stage of a two-stage longitudinal study. When these young people were interviewed one year later, those whites who were still unemployed had reduced their job-seeking efforts to that of the level of blacks and no longer exhibited poorer psychological well-being (3). It appears that with more unemployment young whites adopted some of the coping strategies adopted at an earlier stage by young blacks.

Support for the "alienation hypothesis" also appears to be lacking. One British study found no difference between unemployed blacks and unemployed whites in terms of their rejection of the norms and institutions of British society (27). In fact, both groups expressed positive attitudes toward these institutions. Similarly, Ullah (55) found that unemployed blacks were no more disaffected with the youth labor market and the agencies operating within it than were unemployed whites.

Although this research has provided vital information regarding ethnic differences, many areas are still largely unresearched. Little is known about the effects of unemployment on older age groups of ethnic minorities. There is also a need for comparisons between Asians and both whites and Afro-Caribbeans. And, of course, similarities in terms of ethnicity must not be allowed to obscure important differences within ethnic groups. Generally, comparisons between groups in terms of mean scores fail to capture intragroup differences (49). Qualitative research by Ullah (56) has highlighted important differences in the psychological experience of unemployment among young Afro-Caribbeans.

PSYCHOLOGICAL AND BEHAVIORAL MODERATORS
OF THE EXPERIENCE OF UNEMPLOYMENT

Variables such as age, gender, ethnicity, and social class do not *in themselves* explain differences in the psychological reactions to unemployment. It is more appropriate to regard them as proxies for other variables, which in turn are the true causes of the differences observed. Thus the lower levels of well-being found among unemployed men from the middle age groups, when compared with younger and older men, are likely to be reflecting the effects of financial strain. It is important, therefore, to consider the psychological and behavioral variables that are associated with differences in psychological well-being among the unemployed. Research has so far identified the following variables.

Employment Commitment

This refers to a person's commitment to obtaining paid employment and is measured by multiitem scales. Contrary to popular stereotypes, unemployed people have been found to be highly committed to obtaining a job. However, a number of studies have shown that this can have a detrimental effect on the person concerned, since greater commitment tends to be associated with lower psychological well-being during unemployment. Not surprisingly, those people who most strongly desire a job tend to suffer more psychological harm from being unemployed.

Higher employment commitment tends also to be associated with greater effort being made to find a job (57). Several studies have shown that the number of unsuccessful job applications made during unemployment is positively associated with the amount of depression reported.

Financial Strain

Unemployment may be associated with varying degrees of financial strain, according to differences in age, previous occupation, total family income, and benefit entitlements. Several studies have confirmed that greater financial strain during unemployment is associated with lower psychological well-being. Although financial strain has been found not to increase with the length of time spent unemployed (66), it nevertheless tends to be associated with a deterioration in well-being during that time (4).

Level of Activity

Unemployment is typically associated with problems with filling the time, boredom, and inactivity. For those who suffer least from these problems, unemployment tends to be less stressful. In studies of unemployed people, higher levels of activity tend to be associated with higher levels of psychological well-being. Thus Warr, Banks and Ullah (64) found that unemployed young people reporting the most ease in filling their time, the most time spent out of the house, the most day-to-day variety, and the most time spent with friends, tended to have lower levels of distress, depression, and anxiety.

One study used time diaries to discover how the unemployed tended to spend their time (43). Four distinct types of life-style were identified, described by the authors as active, social, domestic, and passive. Comparisons between these clusters in terms of GHQ scores showed that the lowest scores were obtained by the active group, followed by the social, domestic, and passive groups, in that order. Particularly high scores were found for the latter two groups.

Fryer and Payne (25) report a study in which they set out to investigate those people who were actively using their time while unemployed to pursue interests and hobbies they would otherwise not have time for if they were employed. They studied 11 such people in one northern city. Although these people differed in their goals and interests, each was characterized by a degree of commitment and level of activity which was extremely high and which entailed more than the usual eight hours of work demanded by a job. Psychological well-being in this sample was high and quite untypical of that found in more representative unemployed samples.

Social Support

There is much evidence from clinical studies that support from other people tends to lessen the psychological harm caused by stressful life events, such as bereavement (8, 9). Only a small number of studies have investigated whether this is true of unemployment, and the results need to be interpreted with some caution.

In one American study, greater social support tended to be associated with fewer psychological symptoms during unemployment (30). However, Warr (61) has since questioned how far the results actually illustrate this. Ullah, Banks, and Warr (59) measured the availability of five different forms of social support among a sample of unemployed British teenagers and found only two to be significantly associated with better well-being: having someone to turn to for help with money and having someone to suggest interesting things to do. Warr and Jackson (67) distinguished between instrumental and emotional forms of support. The former was measured by the presence or absence of someone to turn to for help with money; emotional support was measured by asking the respondent if he had someone "who can cheer you up when you're feeling low," "who can help you find interesting things to do," and "with whom you can talk about your everyday problems." Only instrumental support was found to be associated with better psychological well-being among their sample of unemployed men.

Clearly, some forms of social support do appear to lessen the harmful psychological effects of unemployment. These appear to be those forms of support which replace the things that are lost when a person becomes unemployed — money and, to a lesser extent, activity.

THE EFFECTS OF UNEMPLOYMENT
ON OTHER FAMILY MEMBERS

Although the unemployed man has been the focus of most of the psychological research, it is important not to overlook the effects on other family members. Studies by Fagin and Little (16) and Jackson and Walsh (36) have shown that the wives of unemployed men can experience a similar degree of psychological ill-health.

Madge (44) has reviewed the literature on the effects on the children of the unemployed and has concluded that the economic deprivation entailed by unemployment can ultimately cause a deterioration in their emotional well-being. There is also evidence that children tend to hold negatively stereotypical views of the unemployed, explaining their joblessness in terms of simple individualistic causes (70). It is possible, therefore, that those who have fathers who are unemployed are fully aware of the stigma this entails.

COUNSELING THE UNEMPLOYED

Finally, it is important to consider the counseling implications of the research described above. In particular, what facts should the clinician bear in mind when treating a patient who is experiencing distress due to unemployment, and what practical advice can be given to lessen that distress?

Although it is hardly surprising that most people feel depressed about being unemployed, this needs to be seen as part of a more general reaction to unemployment. Unemployment can and does cause an increase in psychological symptoms to the point where the individual is significantly more likely than an employed person to be diagnosed as suffering from nonpsychotic minor psychiatric disorder. It is important, therefore, not to underestimate the psychological impact of unemployment.

Having stated this, it is also true that different groups within society tend to be affected to varying degrees. Among men, those in the middle age groups tend to suffer the most. This is likely to be due to a combination of factors reflecting the greater financial commitments and family responsibilities that come with age. Among young people, there is some evidence that whites in Britain are initially worse affected than blacks, although this difference disappears after more than one year in the labor market. Other research findings are important because they show that certain groups do not differ in their psychological well-being during unemployment. In particular, there appear to be no differences in the degree of psychological distress found among middle- and working-class men. Similarly, the effects of unemployment are just as great among women who view themselves to be in the labor market as they are among men. It is also important to point out that although some groups of unemployed people experience better psychological well-being than do others, the majority of research shows that they are still much less psychologically healthy than people who are unemployed.

Stage models of the psychological experience of unemployment, suggesting that pessimism follows initial optimism and that this soon changes to resignation, are not well supported by research findings. The clinician should therefore keep an open mind when considering the possible development of psychological well-being during a patient's period of unemployment. The clinician should also be aware of the probable spinoff effects of unemployment on other members of the family. In particular, the spouse of the unemployed person, and perhaps their children, may be undergoing similar psychological reactions to the event of unemployment. Conversely, when the patient is the wife or child of an unemployed man, the possible role of the husband's/parent's unemployment in the genesis of the patient's psychological symptoms needs to be considered.

Improvements in the psychological well-being of the unemployed may be achieved through practical advice based on the research findings. If some of the psychological harm of unemployment is caused by loss of the latent benefits of employment, then replacing these might lessen that harm. A time-consuming and intrinsically motivating pursuit may provide the unemployed person with some of the time structure, goals, and activity that are normally provided by having a job. At the very least, some form of activity, preferably that which takes the unemployed person out of the house and brings him into contact with other people, should be encouraged.

One piece of advice often given to the unemployed is that they should keep trying to get a job, and not lose hope in the future. However, findings from several studies suggest that under certain circumstances this may make matters worse, since greater commitment to finding a job tends to be associated with lower psychological well-being. However, research has also shown that greater efforts to find employment do predict future success in obtaining it (58). One possible solution to this dilemma might be to limit job hunting to those methods which are most likely to be productive, rather than making an all-out "attack" on the labor market. In the meantime the unemployed person should be encouraged to participate in other activities, thereby reducing the salience of employment in that person's life.

Changes such as these, which must originate from the unemployed themselves, reflect only part of what can be done to lessen the psychological harm caused by unemployment. In recommending them the clinician should also be aware of the considerable changes required in society as a whole.

REFERENCES

1. BAKKE, E. W. (1940). *Citizens without work*. New Haven: Yale University Press.
2. BANKS, M. H., & JACKSON, P. R. (1982). Unemployment and risk of minor psychiatric disorder in young people: Cross-sectional and longitudinal evidence. *Psychol. Med.*, *12*, 789–798.
3. BANKS, M. H., & ULLAH, P. (1986). Unemployment in less-qualified urban youth: A longitudinal study. *Employment Gazette*, *92*, 343–346.
4. BANKS, M. H., & ULLAH, P. (1987). *Youth unemployment: Social and psychological perspectives*. Department of Employment Research Paper. London: HMSO.
5. BEALES, H. L., & LAMBERT, R. S. (1934). *Memoirs of the unemployed*. Wakefield, UK: E. P. Publishing.
6. BECK, A. T., & BECK, R. W. (1972). Screening depressed patients in family practice: A rapid technique. *Postgrad. Med.*, *52*, 81–85.
7. BRADBURN, N. M. (1969). *The structure of psychological well-being*. Chicago: Aldine.
8. BROWN, G. W., & HARRIS, T. (1978). *Social origins of depression: A study of psychiatric disorder in women*. London: Tavistock.
9. CAPLAN, G. (1974). *Support systems in community mental health*. New York: Behavioral Publications.
10. COCHRANE, R. (1983). *The social creation of mental illness*. London: Longman.
11. COHN, R. M. (1978). The effect of employment status change on self-attitudes. *Social Psychology*, *41*, 81–93.
12. Commission for Racial Equality (1978). *Looking for work*. London: Commission for Racial Equality.
13. DANIEL, W. W. (1974). *A national survey of the unemployed*. London: Political and Economic Planning.
14. DONOVAN, A., & ODDY, M. (1982). Psychological aspects of unemployment: An investigation into the emotional and social adjustment of school leavers. *J. Adolescence*, *5*, 15–30.

15. EISENBERG, P., & LAZARSFELD, P. F. (1938). The psychological effects of unemployment. *Psychol. Bull.*, *35*, 358–390.
16. FAGIN, L., & LITTLE, M. (1984). *The forsaken families.* Harmondsworth: Penguin.
17. FEATHER, N. T. (1982). Unemployment and its psychological correlates: A study of depressive symptoms, self-esteem, Protestant ethic values, attributional style, and apathy. *Aust. J. Psychol.*, *34*, 309–323.
18. FEATHER, N. T., & BARBER, J. G. (1983). Depressive reactions and unemployment. *J. Abnorm. Psychol.*, *92*, 185–195.
19. FEATHER, N. T., & BOND, M. J. (1983). Time structure and purposeful activity among employed and unemployed university graduates. *J. Occup. Psychol.*, *56*, 241–254.
20. FEATHER, N. T., & DAVENPORT, P. R. (1981). Unemployment and depressive affect: A motivational and attributional analysis. *J. Personality Social Psychol.*, *41*, 422–436.
21. FEATHER, N. T., & O'BRIEN, G. (1986). A longitudinal study of the effects of employment and unemployment on school-leavers. *J. Occup. Psychol.*, *59*, 121–144.
22. FINEMAN, S. (1979). A psychological model of stress and its application to managerial unemployment. *Hum. Relations*, *32*, 323–345.
23. FINLAY-JONES, R., & ECKHARDT, B. (1984). A social and psychiatric survey of unemployment among young people. *Aust. J. Psychiatry*, *18*, 135–143.
24. FRYER, D. M. (1985). Stages in the psychological response to unemployment: A (dis)integrative review. *Current Psychol. Res. Rev.*, *4*, 257–273.
25. FRYER, D. M., & PAYNE, R. (1984). Proactive behaviour in unemployment: Findings and implications. *Leisure Stud.*, *3*, 273–295.
26. FRYER, D. M., & PAYNE, R. (1986). Being unemployed: A review of the literature on the psychological experience of unemployment. In C. L. Cooper & I. Robertson (Eds.), *Review of industrial and organisational psychology.* Chichester: Wiley.
27. GASKELL, G., & SMITH, P. (1981). "Alienated" black youth: An investigation of "conventional wisdom" explanations. *New Community*, *9*, 182–193.
28. GOLDBERG, D. (1972). *The detection of psychiatric illness by questionnaire.* London: Oxford University Press.
29. GOLDBERG, D. (1978). *Manual for the general health questionnaire.* Windsor: National Foundation for Educational Research.
30. GORE, S. (1978). The effect of social support in moderating the health consequences of unemployment. *J. Health Social Behav.*, *19*, 157–165.
31. GURNEY, R. M. (1980). Does unemployment affect the self-esteem of school-leavers? *Aust. J. Psychol.*, *32*, 175–182.
32. HARRISON, R. (1976). The demoralizing experience of prolonged unemployment. *Dept. Employment Gazette*, *84*, 339–348.
33. HARTLEY, J. (1980). The impact of unemployment upon the self-esteem of managers. *J. Occup. Psychol.*, *53*, 139–145.
33a. HAYES, J., & NUTMAN, P. (1981). *Understanding the unemployed: The psychological effects of unemployment.* London: Tavistock.
34. HENWOOD, F., & MILES, I. (1987). The experience of unemployment and the sexual division of labour. In D. M. Fryer & P. Ullah (Eds.), *Unemployed people: Social and psychological perspectives.* Milton Keynes: Open University Press.
35. HEPWORTH, S. J. (1980). Moderating factors of the psychological impact of unemployment. *J. Occup. Psychol.*, *53*, 139–145.
36. JACKSON, P. R., & WALSH, S. (1987). Unemployment and the family. In D. M. Fryer & P. Ullah (Eds.), *Unemployed people: Social and psychological perspectives.* Milton Keynes: Open University Press.
37. JACKSON, P. R., & WARR, P. B. (1984). Unemployment and psychological ill-health: The moderating role of duration and age. *Psychol. Med.*, *14*, 605–614.
38. JAHODA, M. (1979a). The impact of unemployment in the 1930s and 1970s. *Bull. Br. Psychol. Soc.*, *32*, 309–314.

39. JAHODA, M. (1979b). The psychological meanings of unemployment. *New Soc.*, Sept. 6, *49*, 492–495.
40. JAHODA, M. (1981). Work, employment, and unemployment: Values, theories, and approaches in social research. *Am. Psychologist, 36*, 184–191.
41. JAHODA, M. (1982). *Employment and unemployment*. Cambridge: Cambridge University Press.
42. KAUFMAN, H. G. (1982). *Professionals in search of work: Coping with the stress of job loss and underemployment*. New York: Wiley.
43. KILPATRICK, R., & TREW, K. (1985). Life-styles and psychological well-being among unemployed men in Northern Ireland. *J. Occup. Psychol., 58*, 207–216.
44. MADGE, N. (1983). Unemployment and its effects on children. *J. Child Psychol. Psychiatry, 24*, 311–319.
45. MELVILLE, J. (1981). *The survivor's guide to unemployment and redundancy*. London: Corgi Books.
46. PATTON, W., & NOLLER, P. (1984). Unemployment and youth: A longitudinal study. *Aust. J. Psychol., 36*, 399–413.
47. PAYNE, R. L. (1985). *Predictors of affective reactions to long-term unemployment: A longitudinal study*. MRC/ESRC Social and Applied Psychology Unit Memo No. 727. Sheffield: University of Sheffield.
48. PAYNE, R., WARR, P. B., & HARTLEY, J. (1984). Social class and psychological ill-health during unemployment. *Sociol. Health Illness, 6*, 152–174.
49. POTTER, J., & LITTON, I. (1985). Some problems underlying the theory of social representations. *Br. J. Social Psychol., 24*, 81–90.
50. ROSENBERG, M. (1965). *Society and the adolescent self-image*. Princeton, NJ: Princeton University Press.
51. SMITH, D. J. (1981). *Unemployment and racial minorities*. London: Policy Studies Institute.
52. STAFFORD, E. M., JACKSON, P. R., & BANKS, M. H. (1980). Employment, work involvement and mental health in less qualified young people. *J. Occup. Psychol., 53*, 291–304.
53. TIGGEMANN, M., & WINEFIELD, A. H. (1980). Some psychological effects of unemployment in school leavers. *Aust. J. Social Issues, 15*, 269–276.
54. TIGGEMANN, M., & WINEFIELD, A. H. (1984). The effects of unemployment on the mood, self-esteem, locus of control, and depressive affect of school leavers. *J. Occup. Psychol., 57*, 33–42.
55. ULLAH, P. (1985). Disaffected black and white youth: The role of unemployment duration and perceived job discrimination. *Ethnic Racial Stud., 8*, 181–193.
56. ULLAH, P. (1987). Unemployed black youths in a northern city. In D. M. Fryer & P. Ullah (Eds.), *Unemployed people: Social and psychological perspectives*. Milton Keynes: Open University Press.
57. ULLAH, P., & BANKS, M. H. (1985a). Youth unemployment and labour market withdrawal. *J. Econ. Psychol., 6*, 51–64.
58. ULLAH, P., & BANKS, M. H. (1985b). How to get a job if you're young and unemployed. Paper presented at the Annual Conference of the BPS (Occupational Psychology Section), Sheffield.
59. ULLAH, P., BANKS, M. H., & WARR, P. B. (1985). Social support, social pressures, and psychological distress during unemployment. *Psychol. Med., 15*, 283–295.
60. WARR, P. B. (1978). A study of psychological well-being. *Br. J. Psychol., 69*, 111–121.
61. WARR, P. B. (1984a). Work and unemployment. In P. J. D. Drenth, H. Thierry, P. J. Willems, & C. J. de Wolff (Eds.), *Handbook of work and organizational psychology*. London: Wiley.
62. WARR, P. B. (1984b). Job loss, unemployment and psychological well-being. In V. L. Allen & E. van de Vliert (Eds.), *Role transitions*. New York: Plenum Press.

63. WARR, P. B. (1985). Twelve questions about unemployment. In B. Roberts, R. Finnegan, & D. Gallie (Eds.), *New approaches to economic life*. Manchester: Manchester University Press.
64. WARR, P. B., BANKS, M. H., & ULLAH, P. (1985). The experience of unemployment among black and white urban teenagers. *Br. J. Psychol.*, 76, 75–87.
65. WARR, P. B., & JACKSON, P. R. (1983). Self-esteem and unemployment among young workers. *Travail Humain, 46*, 355–366.
66. WARR, P. B., & JACKSON, P. R. (1984). Men without jobs: Some correlates of age and length of unemployment. *J. Occup. Psychol, 57*, 77–85.
67. WARR, P. B., & JACKSON, P. R. (1985). Factors influencing the psychological impact of prolonged unemployment and of re-employment. *Psychol. Med., 15*, 795–807.
68. WARR, P. B., JACKSON, P. R., & BANKS, M. H. (1982). Duration of unemployment and psychological well-being in young men and women. *Current Psychol. Res., 2*, 207–214.
69. WARR, P. B., & PARRY, G. (1982). Depressed mood in working-class mothers with and without paid employment. *Social Psychiatry, 17*, 161–165.
70. WEBLEY, P., & WRIGLEY, V. (1983). The development of conceptions of unemployment among adolescents. *J. Adolescence, 6*, 317–328.
71. WINEFIELD, A. H., & TIGGEMANN, M. (1985). Psychological correlates of employment and unemployment: Effects, predisposing factors, and sex differences. *J. Occup. Psychol., 58*, 229–242.
72. ZAWADSKI, B., & LAZARSFELD, P. F. (1935). The psychological consequences of unemployment. *J. Social Psychol, 6*, 224–251.
73. ZUNG, W. W. K. (1965). A self-rating depression scale. *Arch. Gen. Psychiatry, 12*, 63–70.

16

WORK DYSFUNCTION

Irving Bieber, M.D., P.C.

Clinical Professor of Psychiatry,
New York Medical College,
New York, New York

The views stated in this article are based on long-term clinical investigation and address the psychodynamics of work maladaptiveness. Optimal work functioning may be characterized as a continuing ability to develop one's potentialities, participate in a chosen field of interest, and use one's resources consistently and effectively. It also includes the capacity to reveal publicly one's abilities and accomplishments and to sustain a creative interest and pleasure in chosen work. Work can be conflict-free, it may flow without undue strain, and under normal conditions it is pleasurable despite occasional disappointments, pitfalls, and obstacles. The pleasure in work tends to increase as larger and larger reservoirs of personal resources are tapped. The absence of conscious pleasure in effective work and achievement is a symptom of work-connected anxiety and inhibition.

Inhibition is a biological defense against threat. It is a defense characterized by an involuntary termination of an impulse or activity perceived as a threat to one's self. The threat, real or imagined, conscious or unconscious, may involve physical danger, rejection, humiliation, or loss of something valued. Work inhibitions vary in severity and are not uncommon; in fact, few individuals escape them entirely. Work-connected difficulties often appear at adolescence in association with sexual development. The adolescent surge of sexuality at this stage may reactivate oedipal problems so that a boy may fear that achievement will evoke affection from his mother and trigger competitiveness and hostility from his father. A girl may run into the same problem but with the opposite parents.

Symptoms associated with work may emerge as recurrent episodes or as chronic anxiety and tension, with or without psychosomatic symptoms.

Symptoms may also be manifested in the inability to develop one's resources in work of interest, or in the inability to consistently tap personal resources that *have* been developed. Not infrequently, there is a failure to know clearly what sort of work one is interested in pursuing, or there may be difficulty in beginning a project of interest which, once begun, cannot be completed.

The Initial Interview

In initial interviews, my goal is to obtain the data necessary for making a diagnosis and a prognosis and to formulate a treatment plan suitable to the patient. Physicians in other branches of medicine arrive at an evaluation of an organ only after finding out how it functions. Similarly, I evaluate patients only after eliciting cogent information related to their biosocial adaptation. This evaluation encompasses their work, sexual history and current status, interpersonal and romantic relationships, pleasure activities, and general life-style.

Work begins when school begins. The work history includes, when obtainable, information covering the first grade, through graduate school, and on to jobs and career. Clear-cut disparities between intelligence and performance identify the underachievers, adult or child. When a child has been doing well at school, a drop in school performance is cause for concern and investigation. The problem may be the result of difficulties with a specific teacher or with peers. More usually, it is the problems being experienced within the family that have inhibiting effects on performance. If school work continues to be defective over a significant period of time, a psychiatric consultation is indicated. The two most telling indications of childhood psychopathology are significant work problems, on the one hand, and an inability to integrate into a same-sex peer group, on the other.

A probe of intellectual curiosity reveals specific interests. Does the patient read? Is there interest in sports, music, and so forth? I invariably ask what he or she aspired to as a child or adolescent. If a late adolescent has not cultivated an area of special interest or if the type of work to be undertaken has not as yet been contemplated, this is taken as evidence of a work problem.

In the first interview I inquire whether the patient ever had difficulties in reading, spelling, and arithmetic. Consequently, I have been able to identify dyslexia and dyscalculia in a surprising number. Not infrequently, such problems seem to have been missed in the classroom, even when the patient attended a highly rated school. In a recent television interview, the British actress Susan Hampshire related that she first discovered she was dyslexic when she was in her twenties. In describing the deleterious influence this condition had on her self-esteem during her school years, she commented, "I thought I was stupid." Dyslexia is related to handedness. It is frequently associated with left-handedness, yet dyslexics who are right-handed may have a left-handed member of the nuclear family who is not dyslexic. Dyslexics may also have some confusion with left-right discrimination. Children who have learning disabilities tend to become discouraged and more often than not lose interest in school. Some develop behavior disorders and eventually drop out. With rare exceptions, school dropouts, whether from high school or graduate school, do so because of work-related difficulties of one sort or another.

The school history having been completed, I then probe for disparities between intellectual and academic development and the kind of work the patient is currently engaged in. Taking into account the economic, occupational, social, and ethnic realities, I inquire about work goals, whether the work represents the patient's area of interest, and whether it is pursued with resolve. I inquire about salary, frequency of job change, reasons for terminating, creativity in work, and I inquire about symptoms accompanying work, such as anxiety, tension, concentration difficulties, and psychosomatic complaints. Work disorders may give rise to these symptoms and also to its apparent opposite, compulsiveness, seen in the so-called workaholic. The two syndromes are not mutually exclusive. Workaholics may also be work inhibited, particularly in creative aspects which will be discussed later.

PSYCHODYNAMICS OF WORK DISORDERS

Subsumed under symptoms related to work disorders are two salient dynamics: the fear of success and the fear of failure, which may operate in tandem (1).

Fear of Failure

Normal newborns have a developmental potential for organizing an extensive and complex intellectual repertoire. Depending on the quality of parenting and the cultural setting, potentialities may be stimulated, even overstimulated, or natural interest and curiosity may be neglected and inhibited to the point where exploratory behavior, creativity, and interest in the environment are almost extinguished. For the underprivileged, black and white, the culture of poverty has constricting effects on aspirations, intellectual curiosity, and personality development. A substantial number of deprived children arrive at the first grade suffering from the effects of understimulation, and they may have such marked disturbances in the ability to communicate and may already be so intellectually impaired that they are unable to learn to read or comprehend with even passable competency. Since such children are programmed for failure, they have ample reason to fear it.

Much of a child's self-esteem and confidence derives from parental attitudes and reactions. Normally, a parent responds with enthusiasm to a child's development and accomplishments from the time it begins to react with smiling and laughter, on to walking, talking, playing, exploring, and so forth. Parental failure to respond appropriately to these stages, and later to achievements, leaves the child with a sense of inadequacy because he or she feels unable to evoke parental approval. Parents also provoke feelings of inadequacy when they do not stimulate and encourage their child's activities or when they do not respond positively to the interests that differ from theirs or that they do not value.

Parents who themselves fear failure may react with anxiety and anger toward a child who is having difficulty with schoolwork and is not performing at the levels of achievement they demand. Highly competitive parents who require that their children be superior to others and who regard average performance as less than adequate engender fears of failure and neurotic competitiveness toward others, a situation that seriously interferes with good peer relationships.

When either parent prefers another sibling, this, too, stimulates feelings of inferiority in the nonpreferred child, particularly in the areas for which the other sibling is preferred (2). Competitiveness with others who are perceived as preferred, hence superior, is accompanied not only by fears of failure but by fears of success. Displacing a higher-status, preferred rival is felt to be a very aggressive act. Feelings of guilt and especially fears of retaliation have constricting effects on performance and may inhibit it entirely. Parents who block a child's opportunity to solve problems that may be difficult but within his grasp engender feelings of incompetency and fears of failure by habitually taking the problem out of the child's hands. Parents may do so because they are impatient or overdirective, overprotective, or covertly competitive with the youngster.

Teachers and other adults important to children may induce inferiority feelings and fear of failure by shaming and humiliating them for making mistakes or for having difficulties in comprehension and problem solving. Teachers who prefer certain students over others and favor their "pets" encourage the same psychopathology as do parents who prefer another sibling. Children may relate to peers in similar ways and with similarly destructive effects. In one case, the patient was intensely fearful of making mistakes. Whenever she was faced with having to choose between two difficult judgments, she froze and was totally unable to proceed toward a resolution. She ascribed the origin of these difficulties to a preadolescent relationship with a girl to whom the patient was deeply attached but subservient. Cassandra-like, the girl would constantly warn her of the terrible things that would happen if she did anything wrong. There were, to be sure, other determinants, but the warnings of her friend remained salient in the patient's view of her problem.

Fear of failure may also result from past experiences of inhibition. An actor who forgot his lines during a performance had fears of a recurrence. In another case, a surgeon became so blocked during operations that he contemplated leaving medicine. Masochistic defenses that sabotage resources necessary for a task are common in work inhibitions (3). Such defenses always result in fears of failure, which, in turn, exert a constricting effect on development and performance. The fear of failure keeps many potentially creative individuals in occupations that neither challenge their abilities nor require spontaneity; these persons avoid new experiences and activities that involve a learning period lest their ineptness be discovered.

Fear of Success

Most patients have little difficulty recognizing their fears of failure and they tend readily to understand the corollary fears of rejection, loss of self-esteem, fear of humiliation, and so forth, but many, especially among the less sophisticated, have difficulty understanding their fear of success. The idea eludes them. It does not seem logical. Success, they protest, is exactly what they are after. Yet, the fear of success is more often the stronger determinant of work inhibition, particularly among the talented and educated.

By itself, fear of success is simply the headline that can direct the patient to the source of the difficulty. The specific irrational beliefs underlying such a fear require detailed analysis. A belief that achievement will antagonize and evoke jealousy in rivals, particularly power figures who will retaliate by attack, needs to be delineated and traced to its origins. Pathologically dependent individuals may harbor the fear that their success will jeopardize the prerogatives of protection by an omnipotent figure, and that success will antagonize those depended on and support will therefore be withdrawn—a very frightening idea. Others may fear that success will isolate them, and that they will lose friends and the affection of loved ones, especially family members and especially if success is associated with upward mobility and entry into a higher social stratum. Such fears need not be irrational. In order to maintain the cohesion of the family and community, initiative and success may be discouraged. Conforming to tradition is a way of defending against the threat of group disruption, and if group standards are not those of excellence, creativity, and achievement, the guilt and fear of antagonizing one's fellows by superseding them become powerful deterrents. Not infrequently, good students will hold back their abilities as a way of conforming to the lower standards of a particular peer group. Such children are afraid that if they reveal their intellectual talent they will be isolated or, worse, become targets of humiliating epithets.

In families where there are child preference patterns, it is not only the nonpreferred one who suffers; the preferred child usually develops deep-seated guilt feelings. The guilt is based on the idea that the unfavored sibling has been deprived of a rightful share of affection and privilege. The favored child masochistically renounces attributes and skills. This type of inhibition is, in part, an altruistic attempt to neutralize competition; in part, it is a defense against hostility and retaliation from the less favored one.

Oedipal dynamics are almost always salient in work inhibition and are based on fears about superseding a parent, especially when that parent has been competitive with the child or when the child has been favored by the cross-sex parent. Sibling rivalry and peer group rivalry reinforce the oedipal fear of retaliation.

Work disorders may be linked to antisocial motives. The wish to exploit or dominate others will exact a price in guilt, anxiety, and inhibition. Fear of the limelight may account for the avoidance of achievement when exposure to public attention is anticipated as a threat. The analyst must work out with each patient the specific fears that short-circuit consistent use of one's effective resources.

The Masochistic Defense

From its original meaning as a sexual aberration, the term "masochism" has evolved as a description of self-defeating behavior. I have defined masochism as a defensive adaptation involving self-injury through a wide range of behaviors oriented to preventing attack by power figures. Masochism may also be an attempt to elicit positive affects from power figures. Children who are given affection and solace only when ill or defeated tend to establish a masochistic adaptation. Masochism and inhibition may play a role at all levels of endeavor. From the initial stages of interest and motivation to its conclusion, objectives may be blocked in one way or another, the work itself sabotaged, and monetary or prestige rewards minimized or destroyed. The term *loser* has come to be used to describe the individual who undermines personal attributes and opportunities. Many failures in educational and occupational endeavors may be traced to masochistic defenses against the fear of success.

In clinical practice, I have found that masochistic behavior occurs much more often in work than in sexuality. The work-related masochism of everyday life may be acted out in lateness, procrastination of tasks, forgetting appointments, making foolish, inappropriate errors, minimizing accomplishments, getting into accidents, getting sick at inopportune times, and so forth. Lost-and-found departments are repositories of masochistic acting out. In one case, the patient finally succeeded in effecting a pregnancy after years of failure. He and his wife very much wanted the pregnancy but they also had fears of having a child. During the week that they learned of the pregnancy, the wife left her purse in a taxi and the patient left his wallet behind in a restaurant.

Work Inhibition in Women

Before women entered the workforce in substantial numbers, most were chiefly occupied in homemaking and child rearing. Work inhibition and its symptoms were recognized mainly in men. Women were relatively protected from the vicissitudes often associated with making a living and from the responsibility of supporting a family. Work dysfunction was not obvious unless it interfered with domestic demands. Work inhibition became apparent only if a woman had to function in an area where she was inhibited, say, having to support her family financially or finding an interest outside of her family when the children had grown up and left home. I have rarely seen a menopausal depression in women who were not significantly work inhibited. Women who cannot become meaningfully involved in activities not immediately related to their family are at risk for depression when the nest has emptied. With little left to do, they may make new, unfamiliar demands for attention from their husband that strain the marriage and add even more weight to feelings of abandonment, loss, and depression.

With the entry of masses of women into the labor force and into professions and managerial jobs that were previously held almost exclusively by men, the work inhibitions seen in men are now as common among women. The psychodynamics of work dysfunction do not essentially differ between men and women. Rationalizations may differ based on gender roles, but the underlying fears that result in inhibition do not vary significantly. Uninhibited women are not sidetracked by conflicts such as having to choose between love and having children or opting for a career, nor do they fear that competing with men will result in a loss of femininity, thus sacrificing love and sex.

In the following case, the psychodynamics of the patient's work inhibition could have been as relevant for a man as for a woman. The patient and a twin brother were the younger of four children. The boy was openly preferred by the mother, a preference so pronounced that when the mother became senile, he was the only one of her children she recognized and she referred to him as her husband. In early childhood, the patient was the more aggressive and precocious of the two. She walked and talked earlier and was more verbal. Her brother repeatedly complained, "She takes my words." As a child the patient had thought there was a fixed quantity of words; if she used more, her brother had less. The mother actively interfered with her daughter's intellectual progress, provoking guilt in oblique and direct ways. She would complain that the patient was too precocious, too energetic, her talents were inappropriate for a girl, and so on. The mother was afraid that her daughter's abilities would somehow interfere with the son's development. Actually, the boy was very bright and soon caught up with his sister. He was an outstanding student, earned a doctorate, and entered upon an interesting career. The patient, however, developed a severe work block in adult life. It was determined, in part, by her mother's destructive behavior and, in part, by the patient's strongly competitive feelings toward her twin. In a dream she had when she was about eight years old, she threw the book of knowledge at her brother. It hit him in the head and killed him.

Despite her fine intellectual endowment and artistic talent, the patient was unable to complete college. She denied her abilities, denied that success had meaning to her, and shut out awareness of her normal ambitions. Her work inhibition was based on the irrational belief that her effectiveness would destroy her brother. In her psychoanalysis she began to work through these problems. Her job required her to write reports. Initially, this was difficult. She procrastinated and often failed to hand in requested reports, but as a patient she was conscientious and not resistive. One day, as a consequence of insight into her irrational beliefs about the dangers of successful work, she was able to write an unusually good report. That night, she dreamed that her twin brother had suffered an epileptic seizure. In her dream she had the thought that it would take at least a year before it would be safe to expose him again to her productivity. Several weeks later, she again submitted a good report. That night she had a dream that her brother and daughter had died. She awakened feeling depressed. Several months later, her brother, who was then living in another country, became seriously ill with an infectious disease. She realized fully that her work could not possibly have affected him, yet she could not completely escape the idea that in some undefined way, her creativity had finally injured him. There was no indication during her analysis that she thought her brother's success hurt her, but she had great difficulty ridding herself of the belief that the expression of her abilities would injure him.

Even when a patient recognizes its irrationality, the resolution of irrational beliefs associated with an expectation of injury are not easily or rapidly accomplished. This patient had to accumulate a great deal of evidence that her work inhibitions were determined by her belief that her success would damage her brother. As she developed increasing conviction that her beliefs were not based on reality, her work problems began to dissipate. She completed her graduate work and, finally, went on to enjoy a productive career. Had the patient been the preferred child and psychologically free to pursue her work goals, her twin would probably have been beset by work problems. The psychodynamic underpinning would have been similar to that observed in the patient.

Compulsive Workers: The Workaholic

Like other neurotic individuals who are driven by their compulsions, the workaholic develops a medley of defensive, affective reactions should their compulsive patterns be interfered with or interrupted; anxiety, rage, boredom, depression, and restlessness are typical. As contrasted to workaholics, dedicated workers who spend much time and energy at their occupation are motivated by intense interest, curiosity, and a creative capacity for self-expression, yet retain the ability to relax and enjoy free time. Workaholics when faced with free time are uneasy and they tend to be creatively constricted. Apart from structured periods of leisure during usually short vacations, they remain immersed in their work, thus avoiding the anxiety associated with having time for themselves. An example is the case of a woman who, for several years, was indecisive about retiring and then one day impulsively resigned. She was a competent professional who had been a compulsive worker all her life. When the realization sank in that she no longer had a defined work life and now had unlimited free time, she became anxious and severely depressed. Her work had given her a sense of value, identity, and self-esteem, and it provided her with easily accessible social opportunities. The feeling that she was no longer productive flooded her with a sense of worthlessness; the ample time she now had left her with a sense of emptiness and apprehension.

Among the many idiosyncratic determinants of compulsive work behavior is the fear of being overtaken by a rival should one relax, as did the hare in its race with the tortoise. Highly competitive individuals, particularly those with a need to be best, drive themselves lest they be surpassed. Carrying an unremittingly heavy workload is also a way of avoiding pleasure or intimacy with people, even with spouse and children. Talented people who are inhibited in the creative aspects of their work or fear exhibiting their originality may overload themselves with humdrum tasks and then have the rationalization that they lack the time to attend to their genuine interests.

A compulsive preoccupation with work is a hazard of certain professions, especially in the performing arts as seen among ballet dancers, musicians, and singers, and also among athletes, such as tennis players, golfers, and gymnasts. Constant practice and strict discipline often preclude the pursuit of other interests.

Resolving the problems of compulsive working requires delineation of the primary psychopathology and the defenses that have been described. If a patient needs to work compulsively to preserve a sense of self-esteem, the therapeutic effort must be directed toward resolving the psychopathology that feeds the impaired self-esteem.

Disorders of the Work Function and Depression

It is well known that work, interpersonal relationships, romance, and pleasure can be inhibited in a major depression. In current thinking, such inhibitions are deemed to be the consequence of depression, and the depression itself is viewed as primarily biological in etiology. I view depression as a basic inhibitory reaction, as contrasted with anxiety, which is an excitatory reaction. The depressive, inhibitory state is precipitated by inhibition in one or more of the major functional areas, as referred to earlier.

Work inhibition is a commonly occurring determinant of depression (4). The following case illustrates the psychological relationship between fear of success, work inhibition, and a depression that currently would be regarded as endogenous.

The patient is a man now in his late 60s whom I have seen periodically over many years. His presenting symptoms were work related. Until his retirement, he worked as a commercial artist with abilities as a graphic artist and photographer at a professional level. His talent was recognized by employers, and he was periodically offered the directorship of the art department of several prestigious department stores, offers he refused for years. Following long-term psychotherapy, he finally accepted an offer. A synopsis of his fear of success and his inhibition appeared in a dream about his car. The accelerator and footbrake were on the same pedal, an arrangement that would make it difficult to be arrested for speeding. His ambition on retirement was to set up a professionally equipped laboratory in his home so that he could continue with his photography. When he did retire, he proceeded to implement this plan but he became phobically concerned about the toxicity of some of the chemicals he had to use. Nevertheless, he completed his laboratory including the installation of all necessary safety equipment. When he was ready to proceed with the project he had in mind, he became totally inhibited and was unable to go ahead with any photographic work. He became increasingly depressed. The clinical picture was that of an endogenous depression with the somatic symptoms that typically accompany this condition.

In every depression I have seen that was diagnosed as endogenous, I found that preceding the depression there were profound disorders in one or more of the major functions, disorders that ultimately precipitated the depression. As has been emphasized, work disorders are most frequently involved. People who work below their abilities are usually aware of it. Consciously or not, they do not put forth the effort needed to achieve their goals. They recognize that others with no greater talent are more successful. The awareness of constricted work performance generates feelings of depression. It is my view that depression is a reaction to loss or the threat of loss of something or someone highly valued—a loved one, body part, an ability, self-esteem, money, an artifact, or a function such as work. The high value placed on the loss, the belief that the loss is irreplaceable and irretrievable, and the general sense of hopelessness accompanying these beliefs are the common denominators of depression.

In most cases of depressive reaction seen in clinical practice the patient has a guilt-ridden belief that he or she played some part in the loss. A major depression stemming from a source other than work may inhibit the work function; however, I have noted that in many patients, the depressions they experience most frequently are those induced by the sense of loss associated with work inhibition. The greater the discrepancy between talent and the capacity to use it, the greater the depressive reaction. Paranoid characters may project psychologically rooted failure onto an external situation, such as discrimination, bad luck, and so on. As individuals with work inhibitions move into their middle years, the growing awareness of the intractability of their work problems and the unlikelihood that they will achieve their career aims puts such people at risk for a significant clinical depression.

Disorders of the Work Function and Addiction

Addiction is linked to work disorders in much the same way as depressions are linked to them. Addiction of all types is primarily the outcome of serious disorders in one or more of the major functions I have referred to. Among the most profoundly work-inhibited people I have ever examined are heroin addicts. In an unpublished study, S. Foster and I interviewed 50 consecutive cases of heroin addicts who were admitted for detoxification to Metropolitan Hospital in New York City. Careful school and work histories were obtained, and in each case a sharp drop in performance occurred between a year and a half to two years before the addiction began. Symptoms noted were loss of interest in schoolwork or job, an inability to concentrate, and feelings of boredom and restlessness. If the patients had been attending school, they began to cut classes and ultimately dropped out. As a group, the sample of addicts was above average in intelligence. To support their habit, the addicts stole or otherwise illegally obtained between $50,000 and $100,000 a year without getting caught, a way of life that requires resourcefulness and intelligence. After detoxification, many of the addicts renewed an attempt to work. Their abilities were often soon recognized, leading to promotion and an increase in salary. Predictably, there was a return to the use of heroin within a matter of weeks.

Addiction masks an underlying depression. Almost all addicts suffer from depressions. The attempt to replace the gratification lost through inhibition of function by the use of drugs and the need to narcotize the pain of failure do not stave off depressions.

Alcohol, like other agents used in substance abuse, serves as an anxiolytic to lessen or extinguish function-related anxiety or as a masochistic mechanism to subvert one's abilities or to damage one's social and economic situation, self-esteem, health, and so on. An example of the use of alcohol as an anxiolytic may be seen in an anecdote about Jackie Gleason that appeared in a recent biography (5):

> "We had a very happy thirteen years together, longer than many marriages. Much of that time—and people don't know this—Jackie was dry, never touched a drop. . . . He would go months at a time without taking one drink. The reason people never knew about it is that Jackie always liked to keep up his image of a heavy drinker. . . . I noticed that whenever he did return to drinking during those thirteen years, it always coincided with a return to work. Don't ask me why. (p. 146)

The psychodynamics of masochism are prominent in the alcoholic as differentiated from the more usual anxiolytic use by the social drinker. Although the choice of substance in addiction may have cultural and even genetic determinants, the addiction itself is primarily the consequence of psychopathology.

CONCLUSION

In sum, work dysfunction is a salient variable in the diagnosis of many psychiatric conditions, especially depression and addiction. It is a central component of psychopathology, yet much less attention has been paid to work inhibition than to sexual inhibition. In recent years, however, work topics have begun to appear in the literature with more frequency than in the past, as attested to by this volume.

REFERENCES

1. Bieber, I. (1980). Disorders of the work function. In: Cognitive Psychoanalysis. New York: Jason Aronson.
2. Bieber, I. (1980). Pathogenicity of parental preference. In: Cognitive Psychoanalysis. New York: Jason Aronson.
3. Bieber, I. (1980). The meaning of masochism. Sadism and masochism. In: Cognitive Psychoanalysis. New York: Jason Aronson.
4. Bieber, I. (1985). Linking biological and psychological psychiatry. J. Am. Acad. Psychoanal., 13, 413–421.
5. Bacon, J. (1985). How sweet it is — The Jackie Gleason story. New York: St. Martins Press.

17

PERSONAL DISASTER

BEVERLEY RAPHAEL, F.R.A.N.Z.C.P.,
M.B.B.S., M.D., F.R.C.PSYCH.

*Head, Department of Psychiatry,
University of Queensland, Royal Brisbane Hospital,
Herston, Queensland, Australia*

and

WARWICK MIDDLETON, M.B.B.S.,
F.R.A.N.Z.C.P.

*Staff Psychiatrist,
Royal Brisbane Hospital,
Herston, Queensland, Australia*

The concept of personal disaster encompasses shocking, overwhelming personal experiences that test the individual beyond his adaptive capacity and bring major stresses and sometimes changes to his life. This concept reflects, at an individual level, many variables similar to those affecting communities in major catastrophes, such as tornadoes, fires, volcanic eruptions, and earthquakes, or those resulting from "man-made" forces such as bombing, air crashes, hotel fires, and so forth.

Life event research has highlighted the levels of stressfulness of unanticipated, uncontrollable, and unpreventable events for those individuals who experience them (61). Such personal-disaster events include sudden, unexpected bereavements, particularly when the young die; separations or other serious and unanticipated losses; severe and serious accidents, injuries, and illnesses; assault, rape, and other life threat or death encounter situations; and dislocation from home and place.

In the total picture of catastrophic personal experience however, one must also include and even emphasize the individual's experience of war;

of famine, such as that presently affecting the African continent; and of cyclones, earthquakes, floods, and so forth in underdeveloped countries.

Even if they do not experience these communal events, most people face, at some time in their lives, a level of loss or personally traumatic experience that intrudes on even the most protected and affluent life situation. Suffering is an intrapsychic and highly personal experience (35). Under favorable social circumstances, individual and community resources may provide a buffering and supportive background that is so often absent for those who experience ongoing catastrophe and deprivation in many underdeveloped countries.

The key elements or components of personal disaster are several. There is suffering. There may be threat to life of the self or significant other. There may be encounter with death, perhaps personally or through the massive, mutilating, or "gruesome" deaths and injuries of others. Often there are shock and helplessness and a sense of being powerless and overwhelmed. There is frequently destruction, loss or threat of loss, of those one loves, or of home or community or dearly treasured aspects of life or possessions.

The nature of stressful effects may lie in any or all of these, proving overwhelming for the ego and breaking the "stimulus barrier," as it may be considered in psychodynamic terms. There are likely to be immediate effects such as the sensations and reactions during the time of the stressor experience and the intense response in its immediate aftermath. Fear and anxiety levels may be high; arousal and vigilance increased. There may be a control or shutting out of some aspects of emotional reaction. There may be regression, adaptive or nonadaptive. There may be panic or despair. Both during the impact of such dreadful experience and for some time afterward there may be an element of denial, shutting out, or numbing, so that the experience seems unreal, and the person feels as if in a dream, a nightmare from which he will awake. Later in the immediate aftermath these feelings may give way to a return of anxiety as well as anger, sadness, depression, despair, guilt, and a range of other affects, depending on the nature and extent of the stressor components. In many instances there will be intense preoccupation with what has happened, intrusive images breaking in with a return of anxiety, helplessness, and terror, and intermittent or prolonged inhibitory processes attempting to shut out control and mitigate the emotional shock, as Horowitz described (27). Gradually such responses settle.

It is probably true to say that from the study of individual traumatic events such as bereavement (62), accidents (50), assault (76), rape (53), and so forth, there is much to suggest that the severity of the initial reaction relates to at least some degree to the severity (including intensity, proximity, duration, propinquity), expectability, controllability, and preventability of the stressful event. Similarly, research in the field of the individual's response to communal disaster has also highlighted the influence of exposure to threat and loss stressors to the extent of post-traumatic reactive phenomena that are likely to occur (65).

There is also much to suggest from studies in both these fields not only that there may be suffering and intense initial reactions, but also that such events may also lead to the development of post-traumatic psychiatric morbidity, especially post-traumatic stress disorder, generalized anxiety and depressive illnesses, and a range of other phenomena. It behooves us then to study such experiences in depth, not only from the point of view of lessening human suffering, but also from the need to develop our understanding of stress effects, their management, and the prevention of undue psychiatric morbidity in association with them.

There are several common themes in the nature of personal disaster: response to particular stressful components of catastrophic life experience; a range of adaptive processes; and a particular spectrum of morbid psychopathology that may be the outcome.

While the most prominent *elements of stress* are likely to be the encounter with death and loss, a more comprehensive list includes variables such as those delineated by Wilson et al. (79) in their comparative study of post-traumatic stress disorder in a range of persons who had experienced major life stress ranging from Vietnam combat to rape, from disasters to divorce. This list follows (p. 149).

1. Degree of life threat
2. Degree of bereavement
3. Speed of onset
4. Duration of trauma
5. Degree of displacement in home community
6. Potential for recurrence
7. Degree of exposure to death, dying, and destruction
8. Degree of moral conflict inherent in the situation
9. Role of the person in the trauma
10. Proportion of community affected by the trauma

Thus each personal-disaster experience, be it a war, famine, family bereavement, or assault, may be viewed for its stressfulness along such potential parameters.

Another conceptual aspect of personal-disaster experience is the way in which the individual *attempts to adapt or cope*. In similarity with the crisis model, usual coping styles are inadequate, at least initially, and the individual is vulnerable. Of course, if life or existence is, or seems, threatened by the event, then survival is critical. Adaptations that help survival include the powerful primary-attachment bonds, hope, prayer, and in a group situation aspects of leadership. The bereaved widow will say, "I had to keep going even though I felt I'd never survive—the children were all that made me survive." And, as Henderson and Bostock (24) showed with survival following shipwreck and Dimsdale with survival in the concentration camp (12), the images of loved ones proved powerful survival forces. Having survived and ensured the safety of those he loves, or having realized their loss, the individual turns to others for support. A variety of intrapsychic and interpersonal processes occur whereby he deals with the event and eventually integrates it into his view of himself and the world. These processes include "making meaning" of what is extraordinary and outside the day-to-day range of experience; comprehending and coming to terms with the reactions it evoked in the self and perhaps also significant others; dealing with the feelings the experience has produced and which may continue; and adjusting to the changed circumstances that the event has produced, either in the self, the personal, or the relevant world.

Almost all such stressful experiences *must* lead to some *reactions* in the immediate aftermath, including shock, fear, denial, anxiety, depression, numbing, perhaps guilt, and cognitive processes of review and remembering. Whether or not such reactions become extreme or prolonged or develop into a focus of disabling pathology varies enormously, and assessing impact is difficult methodologically (20). Particularly important in this outcome is the severity of the original stressor experience, with death encounter plus traumatic loss contributing most, and dislocation from home and community also potentially pathogenic. While preexisting vulnerability in terms of past psychiatric problems (7, 77) and neuroticism may also contribute in some instances (48), it is also clear that a variety of factors may assist, including support and opportunities for active mastery and resolution, which it seems may facilitate the intrapsychic and interpersonal adjustment processes. And, as is true in so many situations of both acute and chronic stress, factors such as higher education, occupation, affluence, and social status may all contribute to a degree to buffering the adversity. While Hocking asks (26), "Does every man have a breaking point? Or can a normal human being adjust to any amount of biological stress without developing neurotic symptoms?" (p. 542), many would say that every man does have a breaking point — e.g., Rappaport's (68) view that the regenerative powers of the ego are not limitless, and that the human spirit can be broken beyond repair.

It is clear that while not all persons respond to catastrophic events in a similar way, no one is immune from them. Whereas many victims will show regressive tendencies (e.g., a need to be nurtured/protected), in some the stress may lead to acceleration of ego development (60).

Apart from a generally increased vulnerability psychologically and physically, personal experience of disaster may lead to risks not only of psychiatric disturbance, but also of physical ill health: for instance, increased incidence of leukemia, spontaneous abortion (28), diabetes, hypertension (8), and fatal heart attack (59) have been found in association with postdisaster stress.

The most common morbid patterns psychiatrically (65) are: post-traumatic stress disorder, which may follow directly or after a latent period of delay; survivor syndromes; generalized anxiety disorder and some other anxiety manifestations, including sometimes phobic responses in association with the event or its circumstances; depression in its many diagnostic forms; and various patterns of pathological bereavement, which are classified by some workers within the framework of post-traumatic stress disorder or adjustment reaction but, nevertheless, clearly represent either chronic grief or other distortions of the grieving process.

It is now useful to consider some of the many personal disaster circumstances. These will be divided into three main categories: personal disasters of everyday life; personal experience of catastrophe and disaster affecting the wider community; personal disaster of war.

PERSONAL DISASTERS OF EVERYDAY LIFE

The *loss of a dearly loved person*, particularly when sudden, unexpected, untimely, and/or violent, is likely to lead to a particularly traumatic bereavement experience and often constitutes a personal disaster for those involved. When the person dies through suicide, murder, or accident, the mutilation of the body may add gruesomeness and a more painful encounter with death. Certainly it has been shown that such bereavements are more likely to be associated with ongoing problems and morbidity (62). The death of a child, too, often evokes the overwhelming sense of personal disaster and rage at the world for the loss of the innocent and blameless and guilt for the inability to totally protect and nurture (70).

Initially the bereaved shows shock, numbness, and disbelief. This phase of denial may be prolonged, particularly if there has been no opportunity to see and say goodbye to the person after death. They are last remembered as alive and the mind fantasizes that they are elsewhere and could return.

When the bereaved person has been involved in the circumstances of the death, he may be shocked and traumatized by these — for instance, witnessing it and being helpless to respond, or personally threatened, or, in some sense, responsible. Then there may be great preoccupation with these circumstances, and they may constitute a focus for a traumatic neurosis and post-traumatic stress phenomenology throughout the bereavement period. With this there may be intrusive images and memories of the scene of the death; inhibitory processes of cutting out; anxiety and depression; a psychic numbing; and, as well, much irritability and sometimes guilt. The natural processes of mourning and relinquishment of the lost person may be unable to proceed because the bereaved is locked to the need to resolve this traumatic component. Such blocks to grief and resolution have been noted by many workers in the field (42, 65).

Even when such trauma does not complicate bereavement, it is, of course, still immensely painful, and when the relationship to the dead person has been close and intense, there is still likely to be a sense of personal catastrophe. The more dependent the relationship with the deceased, the more the bereaved may feel his or her whole existence to be threatened, and thus he is overwhelmed. Intensely ambivalent relationships also bring their problems, for they may confront the grieving person with the seemingly "murderous" nature of his negative feelings, and sometimes with unresolvable guilt.

The more common losses of separation and divorce may in some circumstances be personally catastrophic as well — particularly, it seems, if there are features such as shock, severely rejecting circumstances, and extremely dependent relationships. It is difficult in all these situations to draw the line between what can be defined as a normal loss situation and what is catastrophic or personally disastrous for the individual. Certainly individual perceptions are highly significant, but also the variables outlined previously, viz., degree of life threat, degree of bereavement, speed of onset, duration of trauma, displacement, potential for recurrence, degree of exposure to death, dying, and destruction, plus degree of moral conflict inherent in the situation, must all come into account. In addition, it must be remembered that multiple traumatic circumstances occurring together, increased life stresses in the immediate period, and concurrent crises have all been demonstrated to increase the risk of intense or distorted reaction and morbid outcome.

Other sources of personal disaster in everyday life may be situations such as *assault, rape, robbery,* and so forth. Such episodes are becoming increasingly frequent in society and have clearly demonstrated traumatic phenomena associated with them (53, 76), which often become entrenched and chronic. Similarly, the violence of family life in the form of abuse of children, sexual abuse, and violence to women have all been demonstrated to have major traumatic effects. Obviously, violence such as child abuse brings not only morbidity such as post-traumatic stress disorder (18), but also impairments of development and personality which may carry vulnerability and abuse into the next generation.

The patterns of personal-disaster morbidity found in association with trauma such as motor vehicle *accidents* are only just being realized, and some papers such as those of Shanfield (72) delineate the severe morbidity that may follow for many of those bereaved in this way. The levels of post-traumatic stress disorder and other disturbances associated with injury or survival have yet to be adequately documented, yet appear in significant costs to the community as attested by court actions for compensation.

Similarly, the personal-disaster experience of being involved, in terrorist or other forms of *civilian violence*, is likely to be substantial (55), but again, this requires ongoing systematic study.

Loss of home, as through house fires and dislocation through ejection, may constitute powerful personal disasters for those experiencing them. Krim (33) discussed the decompensation and morbidity that may follow the former. Similarly, *loss of job* may become a personal disaster in times of high unemployment, and with the need to provide for the self and family and few material resources. High levels of morbidity are associated with unemployment, which often moves from personal disaster to chronic and maladaptive life stress.

In all these personal disasters coping processes as described earlier are relevant. For instance, it has been clearly shown with the crisis of bereavement that support which facilitates the expression of feelings of grief and the review of the real relationship in the mourning process is likely to assist resolution (64). The lack or perceived inadequacy of such support may make the development of depression or other pathology more likely for the bereaved. Similarly, very dependent and ambivalent relationships are more frequently associated with problems of grief, and the presence of multiple crises may add a further loading of risk unless support is available to deal with these specific issues (63). Parkes has also shown that a stress such as amputation (57) may lead to grief, and support may be important for the outcome too.

Here, as in other disastrous experiences, those affected often have an intense need to talk through, share, and make meaning of their experience, and with this there is often cathartic release of feelings which may also assist adaptation. The bereaved, like other disaster victims, are often helped by sharing experiences with others who have been through the same thing—thus the growth of self-help associations which not only offer emotional and practical support, but also facilitate role transition. Studies, too, have shown that counseling of the bereaved (58, 67) can lessen the risk of pathological outcome, particularly when it facilitates the processes of grief and mourning. Similarly, those experiencing severe and often life-threatening illnesses, injuries, or accidents may be helped by counseling support (6, 75), so that they are less likely to develop psychiatric morbidity in association with such personal disasters.

PERSONAL EXPERIENCE OF CATASTROPHE
AND DISASTERS THAT AFFECT A SIGNIFICANT
PROPORTION OF THE COMMUNITY

As noted earlier, vast numbers of people may be involved in the many disasters that affect human communities.

Most of the studies of the psychological sequelae of disasters have looked at events which, when viewed in the historical context, have been relatively small disasters. We tend to ignore the magnitude of even recent disasters occurring in non-English-speaking or Third-World countries.

As recently as 1969–1971 some 20,000,000 persons died in a famine in Northern China (49). In 1976 an earthquake in Tangshan in China killed 750,000 (49). In 1977 15,000 were killed in a cyclone and tidal wave in India (49), and in late 1984 2,500 died and over 200,000 were injured in a chemical leak in Bhopal, India (3).

The year 1985 typified the range of disasters that stalk the world community. Over 7,000 people were crushed to death in a series of earthquakes that struck Mexico City (4), and between 25,000 and 40,000 people perished when the 5,400 meter Nevada del Ruiz volcano in central Colombia erupted. In addition, 150,000 were left homeless.

There were many major air crashes including that of the Japan Air

Lines 747 that smashed into Mt. Mikuni, killing 520 of the 524 people on board (1a).

Major train collisions killed 49 people in Portugal and another 47 in a French disaster (3). "Grave negligence" was given as the cause of a dam burst at Tesero, Italy, in which more than 300 people perished (4).

A fire at the U.K.'s Bradford football ground killed 58 and injured 252 more (45). Worse was to follow: prior to the European Cup soccer final held in June in Brussels, British soccer fans attacked Italian fans in a neighboring section of a grandstand. Thirty-eight people, mostly Italians, died and almost 400 were injured.

In Spain's Bay of Algeciras the tanker Petragen One blew up, killing 33 and injuring 36 (36), while in Philadelphia 11 died and 250 were left homeless following the Police Department's bombing of the headquarters of the radical cult Move (37).

While the death count of the AIDS epidemic climbed beyond 8,000 (54), the most significant disaster of the year was the continued slow death through starvation of hundreds of thousands of people in Sub-Saharan, Africa (4).

Disasters may be man-made (e.g., Chernobyl nuclear accident), natural (e.g., Cyclone Tracey), or a combination of both (e.g., Ash Wednesday bushfires). Disasters may be localized (e.g., tornado) or generalized (e.g., famine); victims' houses may or may not be destroyed; disasters may strike without warning (e.g., transportation accident), with some warning (e.g., bushfires), or with considerable warning (e.g., slowly rising flood waters).

Disasters vary in their duration of impact; e.g., famines and epidemics may take years to demonstrate their worst effects, while in other cases the impact phase may last only seconds, e.g., collapse of Hyatt Hotel skywalk.

Primary victims directly experience the physical, personal, and material losses associated with the disaster, while secondary victims witness the aftermath without experiencing the actual impact or may be those bereaved by disaster deaths. Indeed, disaster workers themselves, both those involved in rescue and recovery and those in support and welfare, may also become indirect victims of the disaster and suffer its psychologically traumatic effects.

With disasters, populations frequently show a predictable progression of response. Initial reactions to disaster warning (if there is warning) are frequently delayed or absent, as denial and the sense of personal invulnerability make those likely to be affected feel that it could not happen to them. As threat becomes increasingly near, denial usually is replaced by activities designed to protect the self and significant others. During the impact phase there is confrontation with the threat or likelihood of death and injury, and with helplessness in the face of overwhelming forces.

Immediately after impact, there may be a sense of euphoria at having survived, although many are shocked and numb; a few are affected to the degree that they present a disaster syndrome. For most, however, there is a rapid mobilization into activities of rescue and attempts to deal with the consequences of the disaster. These activities and the initial denial of loss may interfere with the capacity of the individual to grieve for the losses he has experienced, although the reality of these will increasingly impinge on him (65).

The grief of disaster victims relates to both the personal losses of loved ones and the losses of personal and material possessions, home, place, and neighborhood. The grief and problems of grieving have been studied following major rail disasters (73), hotel fires (19, 41, 43), and bushfires. Many problems arise for those bereaved in disaster, such as the difficulties of seeing the bodies of loved ones, the concurrent crises and traumas of the disaster, and the breakdown of social networks and systems of support that would at normal times facilitate recovery.

In the longer term, recovery-phase restitutional processes in the individual and in the community come into play. Chronic stresses and difficulties are frequent in this phase, as the realities of loss, the long time for recovery, and the difficulties of bureaucracies become more apparent. The problems of replacing what has gone, issues of compensation, questions of who is responsible and who will pay may become pronounced.

As with other personal experience of disaster, many of the same variables come into effect in determining stressfulness of the event, coping, and ultimate psychiatric morbidity. Many studies, reviewed elsewhere (65), have shown the relationship between life threat (16, 56, 77), bereavement (19, 43), displacement or dislocation (5, 78), exposure to death, dying and destruction, including gruesomeness (16), degree of moral conflict, and multiple such factors, and perceived stress and outcome. Studies have also explored those effects with indirect victims; such helpers for instance as those exposed to gruesome body recovery have been shown to be vulnerable. Repeatedly, in personal experience of disasters as disparate as Buffalo Creek Dam burst, Mt. St. Helens volcanic eruption, Ash Wednesday bushfires, a major rail disaster, and hotel and night club fires, those same variables have appeared, and again, intensity and extent of exposure and severity of stress have been significant factors in leading toward more pathological outcomes.

Many studies of the consequences of disasters are hampered by methodological difficulties. Frequently there is difficulty in establishing and maintaining contact with disaster victims, particularly if they have been evacuated. As disasters generally occur with little notice, research protocols have to be developed in haste. Predisaster data for populations, other than for general information about utilization of community services, crime statistics, etc., are not available, and frequently studies rely on questionnaire or structured-interview information which is provided by a relatively small sample of the target population approached. Compensation issues and the frequent unintegrated approach of researchers representing different interests introduce additional uncontrolled variables.

Of many disasters studied, the Buffalo Creek disaster has frequently been cited as one associated with particular psychiatric morbidity. In February 1972 a slag dam created by the Buffalo Mining Company gave way after several days of heavy rain, and a wall of "black water" raced down the narrow creek hollow, devastating mining hamlets along the 17-mile valley. A total of 125 people were killed and nearly 5,000 made homeless. Survivors were resettled in scattered localities, and a lawsuit on behalf of 600 of them was settled out of court for 13.5 million dollars.

Lifton and Olson (39) reported that the "psychological impact of the disaster had been so extensive that no-one in Buffalo Creek had been unaffected" (p. 1) and they went on to document their observations of the manifestations of that impact, which included survivors retaining indelible images of the disaster which were associated with death anxiety and which were revived by environment triggers such as rain, muddy water etc. Survivor guilt and psychic numbing—a diminished capacity for feeling—were described. Previously stable relationships became unstable while survivors struggled to give the disaster meaning. Gleser et al. (16), in noting that victims were not uniformly affected, concluded that a major discriminating factor was the nature and extent of traumatic loss and bereavement. The extent of death and destruction and the impact of such losses on their immediate life circumstances were cited as being crucial variables in producing stress following a disaster; in addition, there was a "gruesomeness factor" such that the aftereffect of disaster for survivors related to the manner in which victims died, the number and condition of bodies witnessed by survivors, and the duration of contact with these horrifying details.

The loss of a home (5) may represent an additional stress, above and beyond the general distress of the disaster experience, while the degree of dislocation and number of moves contribute to problems of adjustment in the postdisaster period.

While Cohen and Ahearn (9) suggested that the elderly and children were especially vulnerable to extreme stress, no studies give clear evidence that the aged are more at risk. McFarlane's recent studies (47) of school-children exposed to the Ash Wednesday fires revealed that while children appear very "good" in their immediate response to disaster, substantial morbidity may appear later and continue well into the second year, and this morbidity is correlated to some degree with parents' ongoing preoccupation with their own disaster experience and post-traumatic stress disorder.

Clearly, stress-related disorders in the immediate postdisaster period can be widespread; e.g., Weisaeth (77) was able to show that after a factory fire more than 90% of the total population sample experienced an anxiety reaction in the first five hours, and at one week after the fire 43% of those most directly exposed had symptoms equivalent to those of post-traumatic stress disorder.

Overenthusiastic evacuation of survivors to scattered and suboptimal living conditions has been cited as contributing to the disaster impact rather than ameliorating it. In describing the effects of the evacuation of 20,000 people following the Wilkes-Barre flood, Quarantelli (60) cites the Disaster Research Center (1976) finding that for many greater social and psychological damage resulted from the "helpful" response of putting evacuees in unsuitable trailers in undesirable areas than was done by the actual disaster agent, the flood water.

In Milne's (52) longer-term follow-up of survivors of Cyclone Tracey it was found that victims who had never left the devastated city showed a better adjustment than returning evacuees, while evacuees who had not yet returned to Darwin exhibited the most psychological problems.

In looking at the massive relief effort that followed the Buffalo Creek disaster, Harshbarger (23) suggests that "the end result insofar as rehousing was concerned was rather like that which would be expected if a brilliant madman set about in the most ingenious ways to maximize personal and social pathologies" (p. 165).

Long-term morbidity following disaster is still debated; e.g., while Titchener and Kapp (74) described large-scale psychological impairment and character change in both individuals and families two years after the Buffalo Creek disaster, it is interesting that in the wake of the Xenia, Ohio tornado, research of victims 18 months afterward (60) revealed "an extremely low rate of severe mental illness, if any at all, as a consequence of the tornado" (p. 192), while a large percentage of the population studied reported extremely positive reactions to the disaster in that they had gained personal confidence.

This latter finding highlights the fact that disasters vary enormously in their personal impact. It may be, as Luchterhand (44) suggests, that "man-made" hazards are more likely to be associated with negative morbid outcomes, perhaps because of issues of the personal human meaning of neglect, negligence, and violence that are so often part of them, or the sudden, devastating, and unexpected nature of their impact in situations of security and trust.

Be that as it may, there is obviously a need for comparable methodologies that examine the various stressful components of many different disasters, taking inventory of the individual's experience. These should encompass loss, death, destruction, and so forth — their intensity, severity, and duration. Such assessments should be followed by short- and longer-term evaluations of outcome on widely accepted and valid criteria, exploring as well positive and negative adaptations and the factors that contribute to them. Some recent studies (66) are attempting to do this, and review of previous work highlights the influence of these stressors in contributing to postdisaster morbidity for the individual (65).

It is important to realize that in this personal experience of community disaster once again the evidence seems to indicate that coping processes for the individual follow paths similar to those for the personal disasters of everyday life. First, there is a need for victims to ensure their own survival. Powerful attachments and hope may contribute strongly here. Shock and denial may delay affective response to the experience of life threat or loss so that the individual only gradually faces the reality of what has happened. His usual coping styles may prove inadequate to the degree that he stays numb and stunned, continuing to be cut off from the devastation as is found in the "disaster syndrome." Or these may give way in the first day or shortly after to reexperiencing of intense distress and anxiety. There is a need to review what has happened. Cognitions of intrusive thoughts may disrupt daytime experiences and bring back all the intensity of the disaster impact. Triggers that are reminders may reawaken such thoughts and feelings of fear or even panic. Sleep may be disrupted by nightmares which also reflect a vivid reexperiencing of the trauma. Gradually for many or most, these phenomena fade over the early weeks.

There may also be an intense need to talk through what has happened, and this may be facilitated by the euphoria and spontaneous group processes that affect many in the immediate aftermath. This has often been called the "therapeutic community" of the postdisaster phase and may be one of the factors leading to the positive resolution of the experience in some cases, as noted previously. This facilitating social support usually assists review and integration and is a much more universal phenomenon than the individual is likely to experience after the personal disasters of everyday life.

In his efforts to make meaning of his experience the person may also find more support than in the personal disasters of everyday life, for others are having the same struggle, and while there are many individualistic perceptions, there is also much in common. The shared meaning may reinforce mastery as it becomes integrated into the psyche and the community as *the* interpretation of what has happened. Of course, if the individual's experience and belief is very dissonant from this, then he may be stressed additionally.

It has also been noted that previous disaster experience and training may facilitate adaptation and lessen the likelihood of morbidity. Perhaps these strengthen the ego or assist cognitive progress by lessening the helplessness, fear, and sense of being overwhelmed, as well as leading to more positive capacity for meaningful activity in the postdisaster period. Active involvement in rescue and recovery processes seems particularly valuable to many and may undo the feeling of helplessness so often associated with impact — such feelings may be instrumental in imprinting the experience and leading to more difficulties in recovery.

The bereaved of disasters, as noted earlier, also confront many problems for the sudden, unexpected, and often untimely nature of such deaths in tragic circumstances, the absence or destruction of the body, and the survivor guilts which may appear. As well, the ego's struggle to deal with the disaster experience and issues of survival may all interfere with adaptive grieving and resolution.

Other problems for the survivors of community disasters may include the loss of a home and dislocation from familiar environment. Research has shown that more than four moves in the postdisaster year is likely to be associated with poorer emotional recovery (5). But particularly important are ongoing chronic stresses related to delays, bureaucratic inefficiencies, broken promises, and the loss of networks and community resources. If there has been any major destruction of the fabric of the community as occurred with Buffalo Creek, then the disruption of the social networks that appear to be so important in facilitating recovery through support and integration of the experience, as well as mutual aid, may mean that morbidity levels become very high.

Intervention to provide counseling and support for disaster victims has been widespread but rarely systematically evaluated. When this has been done, for instance with those bereaved in a major rail disaster and following fire, it has been shown that such support can lessen morbidity, when it is perceived as helpful by those who receive it (42, 73).

The value of social systems of support was also substantiated in this study and another following bushfires (8). It should be noted that people often find counseling helpful when it is provided with other aid. Other studies (46) have shown that there are some problems when relief workers are not able to identify and refer major mental health problems after a disaster, through either lack of knowledge or stereotyped views of psychiatry. Thus illnesses such as post-traumatic stress disorder and depression may go untreated, leading to entrenched and chronic disability. There is obviously a need for more systematic evaluations of the most effective preventive and therapeutic regimes. It is important to avoid convergence of interventions, which may do more harm than good, yet at the same time to develop skilled preventive and therapy regimes for those at risk.

THE PERSONAL DISASTER OF WAR

In perhaps no other field of human experience are entire populations likely to be subjected to prolonged death and destruction as is frequently commonplace in war. Stresses of war relate to combat soldiers as well as to civilians subjected to bombing, artillery, and so forth, and to those exposed to concentration camp experiences.

Hammond (22) described psychological reactions to combat based on clinical observations during the Civil War, while DaCosta in 1871 published his article "On Irritable Heart" (10), a "cardiac malady common among soldiers" characterized by palpitations, chest pain or heaviness, shortness of breath, sweating, and gastrointestinal disturbances.

In a period of unprecedented peace in Europe, Kraepelin, Jaspers, and others made the observation that in the absence of a constitutional predisposition, any individual would recover from the emotional effects of severe psychological and physical traumas within two years. Pavlov held a similar view until an accidental flooding of his animal laboratory drew him to the conclusion that at least in the case of dogs, each individual will develop neurotic symptoms if subjected to sufficient stress (25).

However, peace did not last, and to date more people have been killed in war in the 20th century than in all the wars in recorded history prior to 1900.

At the end of World War I there were many bitter complaints about the harsh or even cruel way in which Austrian military doctors had treated the war neurotics (30). Although Freud stated his intention of not making a special study of the subject, he implied that if the external threat was great enough, any individual would develop neurotic symptoms (15). He also noted the "fixation to the moment of trauma" that was manifest in the dreams of sufferers.

Early theories relating "shell shock" to physical lesions in the brain were largely abandoned by the time that Kardiner and Spiegel (31) suggested that war created only one stress-related syndrome, which was essentially no different from traumatic neuroses in peacetime.

The immense and often chronic stress of combat is illustrated by numerous personal accounts, e.g., the following observation made by Ernst Udet, quoted in Winter (80), of a fellow World War I fighter pilot:

> Gontermann halted and picked up a leaf, a handful of pebbles. Placing the leaf on the table, he opened the palm of his hand and slowly released the stones. As each fell, there was a sharp metallic sound as the pebbles hit the tabletop. "It's like this Udet," he said. "The bullets fall all round us" — he pointed to the leaf — "and gradually they get nearer and nearer. Eventually they hit us. We're bound to get hit in time." With an impatient movement of the hand he swept his playthings from the table. I was watching him from the side. Obviously he was in a highly emotional state and my desire to get away from the place increased a hundredfold. . . . Gontermann died three months later. (p. 165)

World War II was responsible for the deaths of 51.7 million people. Wartime destruction and killing had reached a new scale.

A close correlation between the degree of combat stress and the number of psychological casualties was demonstrated by such studies as that of Reid (69), who found that within Bomber Command "flying stress" was directly related to the number of losses sustained in flying operations. Studies of the psychological effects of war were bedeviled by the same sort of interpretation problems that are seen with disaster studies; i.e., not all war-related stresses studied were equivalent in either magnitude or duration. Studies showed, however, that when the combat stresses were high, the breakdown rate was directly related to the degree of stress to which a soldier was subjected (25, 26). By the end of the war Grinker and Spiegel (21) were able to state that "the stresses of combat tend(ed) to reduce all individuals to a common denominator — the combat personality."

A classic study by Archibald and Tuddenham (2) showed that 70% of soldiers diagnosed as having an acute traumatic reaction during World War II still had their symptoms 17 years later. Some symptoms had worsened with time.

Only 1 in 600 concentration camp victims survived. By the mid-1950s reports on the longer-term symptoms of the survivors of the holocaust appeared. Clinical features of the so-called K-Z syndrome included persistent insomnia, depression, anxiety, difficulty in thinking, and startle reactions. Guilt over survival was common (34).

One sustaining hope for many survivors had been the thought of reunion with families. With liberation came the knowledge that most family members and friends had perished. Marriages on short acquaintance were common, and many women in displaced-persons camps gave birth as soon as was possible, naming the baby after someone lost (11). A conspiracy of silence surrounded the survivors' stories. Their new society was uncomfortable or disbelieving in its response or compounded the survivors' guilt by somehow implying that they had been partly responsible for their fate.

Guilt was also a central theme for the survivors of the atomic bombing of Hiroshima, which left 60% of the city's population killed or injured. As had been the case in the bombing of British and German cities, despite catastrophic destruction there had been no disintegration of the social order; e.g., the day after the bombing, survivors from the 12 banks got together and resumed banking services.

In Japan the Hiroshima survivors became members of a new caste called Hibakusha, a group that were disfigured, frequently suffered chronic diarrhea, etc., due to radiation or who were later to give birth to babies with hideous deformities, which in turn fueled their guilt and ostracization (17).

Lifton (40) documented the survivor guilt and other persisting emotional disturbances of Hiroshima survivors.

In 1977, one Hibakusha, Kaz Tanaka, arranged for a Japanese medical team to make yearly visits to the United States in order to review the problems of Hiroshima survivors living there, an initiative she took over 30 years after her own personal disaster (17). One is reminded of Victor Frankl, who, having survived the holocaust, posited the need for meaning as a fundamental human motivation (14).

With Vietnam veterans, it has become more and more apparent that a significant proportion have had or are having problems in readjusting to civilian life (13). Chief among their many problems is combat-related post-traumatic stress disorder. Its exact incidence among Vietnam veterans is not known, but estimates range from 15% to 35% (32). Indeed, many feel that Vietnam veterans are as a group more seriously disturbed than combatants from other wars, and reasons given for this include the nature of the war, in which the enemy was frequently undefined and in which there was a high incidence of atrocities, the unpopularity of the war on the home front, the rapidity with which combatants could leave a combat zone and be back in America, the one-year tour of duty, and the lack of any significant homecoming. (It was not until 1985 that 25,000 Vietnam veterans were to march as a welcomed body through New York [38].)

Of course, it is not only the combatants who are vulnerable to the traumatic stresses of war. Janis (29) found that the psychological casualties among civilians in areas that are bombed are proportionate to the deaths and mutilating casualties in the neighborhood. And the millions of refugees moved from home and homeland by war suffer many traumatic stresses which must induce a state of personal disaster for them. Home and family are lost, and even when a new country offers sanctuary, the evidence suggests that more than 50% of people will still be suffering psychological disturbance up to two years later (51).

The individual's disastrous experience in war seems to become submerged in the mass response of his society, and in the needs and cause for which the war is fought. Nevertheless, the same themes are relevant for him: shock, helplessness, fear, denial, numbing, anxiety, helplessness, anger, sadness, guilt, despair. The stressors, too, are the same life threat and encounter with the massive deaths of others, loss, dislocation, moral conflict, the degree of effect on the overall community, and so forth. We know little about the psychological coping processes except that they seem to be similar to those in other personal-disaster situations. Powerful attachment bonds, hope, catharsis, support, review, and integration of experiences are important. The individual may be bolstered by the need for courage and endurance in the face of threat and hardship.

Catharsis, support, and bonds to fellow soldiers are valuable in resolving combat stress, but less is known of the recovery of noncombatant populations exposed to war stressors, except that refugees may suffer considerable psychiatric morbidity. Studies of civil war as in Belfast and Lebanon show some remarkable adjustments in civilian populations during the time of stress, but subsequent outcomes do not appear to be known, except to suggest that people may become conditioned to violence.

MORBID PATTERNS OF PERSONAL DISASTER

The common themes that have been discussed here can be drawn together as a conceptual framework in which to view intensely stressful experiences that overwhelm the individual through the confrontation with death, loss, and the changes they bring.

The patterns of morbidity that follow may include post-traumatic stress disorder, now well delineated by DSM-III-R (1) presenting in many situations from the victims of rape and abuse, the fighters of forest fires, to the veterans of the Vietnam War. The phenomenology of repetitive intrusions and avoidant processes, startle, phobic reactions, nightmares, irritability, guilt, and depression may occur immediately, or after a latent period, and may run an acute, chronic, or fluctuating course (27, 65). Psychic numbing may appear in association with this, or withdrawal and social isolation may make it difficult for those affected to return to the previous lifestyle. Treatment of entrenched disorder is notoriously difficult.

Survivor syndromes, as they are called, vary from psychic numbing and loss of capacity to feel; to chronic guilt preoccupation; to the "death imprint" described by Lifton in the survivors of Hiroshima (40). More subtle survivor guilts may appear for many who survive the death of another, especially if there is any sense of responsibility for the death.

Generalized anxiety syndromes may persist for some who experience such personal catastrophes and may be triggered by any subsequent stressors that are threatening, particularly if they are reminders of the original experience.

Major depressive illness or dysthymic symptoms may follow personal disasters of loss or dislocation and are likely if there are ongoing chronic stresses that make adaptation difficult. Bereavement pathology is often in the form of inhibited or delayed grief — or chronic unremitting sorrow that cannot be relinquished.

It is also possible for pathology following personal disaster to take less specific forms, with a general increase in psychological symptomatology in the form of tiredness, fatigue, sleep disturbance, and so forth. Changes in interpersonal relationships are fueled by irritability and anxiety. Acting out may also be a consequence, especially among adolescents, where delinquency and teenage pregnancy have been described, and among adults, where alcohol problems may develop. As noted earlier, physical problems of health may occur.

Despite such potential for morbid outcomes, people, for the most part, respond with great altruism and courage and are often resilient in the face of such stresses and indeed may ultimately grow in personal strength. But the experience of personal disaster is not forgotten and is always a point of great significance in the individual's life, perhaps even leading him to reevaluate his priorities and to live his life differently thereafter.

While much of this description has referred to the individual, he must also be seen in the context of his family. So often the circumstances of personal disaster are such as to damage or destroy part of the family unit, to place stresses on it. The members of this group need each other's support, yet may all be severely affected by what has happened. Thus each faces this additional harassment of stress—the need to be both comforted and comforter.

THE MANAGEMENT OF PERSONAL DISASTER

In the situations of acute and overwhelming stress that may constitute many personal disasters, several principles apply.

The need for a compassionate, concerned human response is primary. Touch, comforting, and consoling as well as general caring support will assist the individual to come to a more stable state of ensured survival and reality. This framework is one from which a range of preventive and therapeutic interventions may subsequently develop. Opportunities to talk through, review, and make meaning of what has happened, cathartic release, and active mastery within a psychotherapeutic framework will be sufficient for many. As well there is a need to facilitate supportive interpersonal interactions with family, friends, and perhaps others who have shared or been through the same experience. Specific bereavement counseling (58, 67) in the model described elsewhere may be necessary for those who have suffered losses. The management of post-traumatic stress reactions and disorder (PTSD) may involve psychotherapeutic techniques that facilitate review and release, if inhibitory processes predominate, or more controlling processes limiting affect, if intrusive aspects are more pronounced (27). Desensitization may be useful. If depression or panic phenomena are prominent, appropriate medication may be necessary. Medication use largely relates to anxiety, panic attacks, and depression, which are frequent findings in patients with PTSD, and acute psychosis which is an infrequent finding.

Interventions with patients suffering from chronic or delayed PTSD also need to take account of associated symptomatology or maladaptive coping styles that have evolved over time and represent the victim's attempt to cope with or avoid unresolved PTSD symptomatology. Scurfield (71) identifies five key principles in the treatment of such disorders: (1) establishment of a therapeutic trust relationship; (2) education regarding the stress recovery process; (3) stress management/reduction; (4) regression back to or reexperiencing of the trauma; and (5) integration of the trauma experience, including both positive and negative aspects. Lindy et al. (42) report on short-term (6 to 12 sessions) psychodynamic psychotherapy conducted with 30 survivors a year after the Beverly Hills Club fire. The therapies were rated by independent judges in terms of completion: five non-engaged, 15 interrupted, and 10 completed. Survivors with completed treatments showed considerable improvement at three months; the interrupted group showed no change. Group therapy, particularly with Vietnam veterans, is seen as offering several advantages. While family therapy in a number of instances offers theoretical advantages, e.g., with rape victims whose spouses become psychologically incapable of providing the necessary support/acceptance, clinical reports are few.

It is likely, although not established, that early and rapid treatment or preventive intervention, probably in the crisis intervention mode, may do much to lessen the level of chronic disorder and disability.

For the person who provides help at this time there may be difficulties. The nature of the circumstances and the lowered defenses of the sufferer often lead to particular empathy and identification which may help understanding, but may also produce an additional emotional burden for the worker. This may be more pronounced if the disaster is one personally feared, or if there are many such experiences to be shared. Nevertheless, the compassionate concern of one human being for another is a powerful and healing emotion.

REFERENCES

1. American Psychiatric Association (1987). *Diagnostic and statistical manual of mental disorders* (3rd ed., rev.). Washington, DC: APA.
1a. ANDERSON, H., LEWIS, D., LIV, M., TSURUOKA, D., & LUBIC, W. (1985). What went wrong? *Newsweek* (Australian ed.), Aug. 27, 102–107.
2. ARCHIBALD, H., & TUDDENHAM, R. (1965). Persistent stress reactions after combat. *Arch. Gen. Psychiatry, 12*, 475–481.
3. BAILEY, P., & WYNHAUSEN, E. (1985). Like living in a disaster movie. *Sydney Morning Herald Magazine*, Oct. 26, 6–10.
4. BARCS, E. (1985). The year of cruel terror and natural disasters. *The Bulletin*, Dec. 24/31, 42–51.
5. BOLIN, R. C. (1982). *Long-term family recovery from disaster*. Monograph no. 36. Boulder: University of Colorado, Institute of Behavioural Science.
6. BORDOW, S., & PORRIT, D. (1979). An experimental evaluation of crisis intervention. *Social Sci. Med., 13A*, 251–256.
7. BROMET, E. J., SHULBERG, H. C., & DUNN, L. O. (1982). Reactions of psychiatric patients to the Three Mile Island nuclear accident. *Arch. Gen. Psychiatry, 39*, 725–730.
8. CLAYER, J. (1984). *Evaluation of the outcome of disaster*. Report. Adelaide, Australia: Health Commission of South Australia.

9. COHEN, R. E., & AHEARN, F. L. (1980). *Handbook for mental health care of disaster victims*. Baltimore: Johns Hopkins University Press.
10. DACOSTA, J. M. (1871). On irritable heart: A clinical study of a form of functional cardiac disorder and its consequences. *Am. J. Med. Sci., 61*, 2–53.
11. DANIELI, Y. (1985). The treatment and prevention of long-term effects and intergenerational transmission of victimization: A lesson from holocaust survivors and their children. In C. R. Figley (Ed.), *Trauma and its wake*. New York: Brunner/ Mazel.
12. DIMSDALE, J. E. (1974). The coping behaviour of Nazi concentration camp survivors. *Am. J. Psychiatry, 131*, 792–797.
13. EGENDORF, A., KAOUSHIN, C., LAUFER, R. S., ROTHBART, G., & SLOAN, L. (Eds). (1981). *Legacies of Vietnam: Comparative adjustment of veterans and their peers*. New York: Centre for Policy Research.
14. FRANKL, V. (1971). *Man's search for meaning: An introduction to logotherapy*. New York: Pocket Books.
15. FREUD, S. (1959). Psycho-analysis and war neuroses. In J. Strachey (Ed.), *Collected Papers*, Vol. 5. New York: Basic Books.
16. GLESER, G. C., GREEN, B. L., & WINGET, C. N. (1981). *Prolonged psychological effects of disaster: A study of Buffalo Creek*. New York: Academic Press.
17. GOLDMAN, P. (1985). Forty years on — Confronting the long shadows of the bomb. *The Bulletin* with *Newsweek*, July 30, pp. 128–144.
18. GREEN, A. H. (1983). Child abuse: Dimensions of psychological trauma in abused children. *J. Am. Acad. Child Psychiatry, 22*(3), 231–237.
19. GREEN, B. L., GRACE, M. C., & GLESER, G. C. (1985). Identifying survivors at risk: Long-term impairment following the Beverly Hills Supper Club fire. *J. Consult. Clin. Psychol., 53*, 672–678.
20. GREEN, B. L. (1982). Assessing levels of psychological impairment following disaster. *J. Nerv. Ment. Dis., 170*(9), 544–552.
21. GRINKER, R., & SPIEGEL, J. (1945). *Men under stress*. New York: Blakiston.
22. HAMMOND, W. A. (1883). *A treatise on insanity in its medical relations*. London: H. K. Lewis.
23. HARSHBARGER, D. (1976). An ecologic perspective on disaster intervention. In H. J. Parad, H. L. P. Resnick, & L. G. Parad (Eds.), *Emergency and disaster management: A mental health sourcebook*. Bowie, MD: Charles Press.
24. HENDERSON, S., & BOSTOCK, T. (1977). Coping behaviour after shipwreck. *Br. J. Psychiatry, 131*, 15–20.
25. HOCKING, F. (1965). Human reactions to extreme environmental stress. *Med. J. Aust.*, Sept. 18, *II*, 477–483.
26. HOCKING, F. (1970). Psychiatric aspects of extreme environmental stress. *Dis. Nerv. Syst., 31*(8), 542–545.
27. HOROWITZ, M. J. (1976). *Stress response syndromes*. New York: Jason Aronson.
28. JANERICH, D. T., STARK, A. D., GREENWALD, P., BURNETT, W. S., JACOBSON, H. I., & McCUSKER, J. (1981). Increased leukaemia, lymphoma and spontaneous abortion in western New York following a flood disaster. *Public Health Rep., 96*, 350–354.
29. JANIS, I. L. (1951). *Air war and emotional stress: Psychological studies of bombing and civilian defense*. Westport, CT: Greenwood Press.
30. JONES, E. (1961). *Sigmund Freud: Life and work*. New York: Basic Books.
31. KARDINER, A., & SPIEGEL, H. (1947). *War, stress and neurotic illness*. New York: Paul B. Hoeber.
32. KEANE, T. M., FAIRBANK, J. A., CAODEIL, J. M., ZIMERING, R. T., & BENOER, M. E. (1985). A behavioural approach to assessing and treating post-traumatic stress disorder in Vietnam veterans. In C. R. Figley (Ed.), *Trauma and its wake*. New York: Brunner/Mazel.
33. KRIM, A. (1978). Urban disaster: Victims of fire. In H. P. Parad, H. L. P. Resnick, & L. P.

Parad (Eds.), *Emergency and disaster management: A mental health sourcebook.* Bowie, MD: Charles Press.
34. KRYSTAL, H., & NIEVERLAND, W. G. (1968). Clinical observations on the survivor syndrome. In H. Krystal (Ed.), *Massive psychic trauma.* New York: International Universities Press.
35. LIE, P. L. (1971). Suffering. *Philippine J. Ment. Health, 2,* 43–51.
36. The wreck of the "Petragen One" (1985). *LIFE,* July, 46–47.
37. Mourning a lost community (1985). *LIFE,* July, 40–41.
38. A parade long overdue (1985). *LIFE,* July, 57–58.
39. LIFTON, R. J., & OLSON, E. (1976). The human meaning of total disaster. *Psychiatry, 39,* February, 1–18.
40. LIFTON, R. J. (1967). *Death in life: Survivors of Hiroshima.* New York: Random House.
41. LINDEMANN, E. (1944). Symptomatology and management of acute grief. *Am. J. Psychiatry, 101,* 141–148.
42. LINDY, G. D., GREENE, B. L., GRACE, M., & TITCHENER, J. (1983). Psychotherapy with survivors of the Beverly Hills Supper Club fire. *Am. J. Psychother., 37,* 593–610.
43. LUNDIN, T. (1984). Disaster reactions: A study of survivors' reactions following a major fire disaster. University of Uppsala, Sweden. Unpublished paper.
44. LUCHTERHAND, E. G. (1971). Sociological approaches to massive stress in natural and man-made disasters. *Int. Psychiatric Clin., 8,* 29–53.
45. McCALMAN, J. (1986). Lessons from the Bradford disaster. *Aust. Doctor,* p. 12, April.
46. McFARLANE, A. C., & RAPHAEL, B. (1984). Ash Wednesday: The effects of a fire. *Aust. NZ J. Psychiatry, 18,* 341–351.
47. McFARLANE, A. C. (in press). Posttraumatic phenomena in a longitudinal study of children following a natural disaster. *Am. J. Child Psychiatry.*
48. McFARLANE, A. C. (1985). The etiology of post-traumatic stress disorders following a natural disaster. Department of Psychiatry, The Flinders University of South Australia. Unpublished paper.
49. MAGNUSSON, M. (Ed.) (1985). *Readers Digest Book of Facts.* London: The Readers Digest Association Ltd.
50. MALT, U. (1983). *Studies in the effects of accidents.* Oslo: University of Oslo, Norway.
51. MASUDA, M., LIN, K., & TAZUMA, L. (1982). Life changes among Vietnamese refugees. In Richard C. Nann (Ed.), *Uprooting and surviving.* London: D. Reidel.
52. MILNE, G. (1977). Cyclone Tracey: 1. Some consequences of the evacuation for adult victims. *Aust. Psychologist, 12,* 39–54.
53. NADELSON, C. N., NOTMAN, M. T., ZACKSON, H., & GORNICK, J. (1982). A follow-up study of rape victims. *Am. J. Psychiatry, 139,* 1266–1270.
54. The death of a star (1985). *Newsweek,* pp. 14–15, Dec. 31.
55. OCHBERG, F. (1978). The victim of terrorism: Psychiatric considerations. *Terrorism, 1,* 147–167.
56. PARKER, G. (1977). Cyclone Tracy and Darwin evacuees: On the restoration of the species. *Br. J. Psychiatry, 130,* 548–555.
57. PARKES, C. M. (1972). The components of reaction to loss of a limb, spouse or home. *J. Psychosom. Res., 16,* 343–349.
58. PARKES, C. M. (1980). Bereavement counseling: Does it work? *Br. Med. J., 281,* 3–6.
59. POPOVIC, M., & PETROVICK, D. (1964). After the earthquake. *Lancet, 2,* 1169–1171.
60. QUARANTELLI, E. L. (1985). An assessment of conflicting views on mental health: The consequences of traumatic events. In C. R. Figley (Ed.), *Trauma and its wake.* New York: Brunner/Mazel.
61. RAPHAEL, B. (1981). Personal disaster. Squibb Academic Address. *Aust. NZ J. Psychiatry, 15,* 183–198.
62. RAPHAEL, B. (1983). *The anatomy of bereavement.* New York: Basic Books.
63. RAPHAEL, B. (1978). Mourning and the prevention of melancholia. *Br. J. Med. Psychol., 51,* 303–310.

64. RAPHAEL, B. (1977). Preventive intervention with the recently bereaved. *Arch. Gen. Psychiatry, 34*, 1450–1454.
65. RAPHAEL, B. (1986). *When disaster strikes*. New York: Basic Books.
66. RAPHAEL, B., WEISAETH, T., & LUNDIN, T. (1984). *Draft methodology for psychosocial study of disasters*. Newcastle, Australia: International Study Group for Disaster Psychiatry.
67. RAPHAEL, B. (1979). A psychiatric model for bereavement counseling. In B. M. Schoenberg (Ed.), *Bereavement counseling: A multidisciplinary handbook*. Westport, CT: Greenwood Press.
68. RAPPAPORT, E. A. (1968). Beyond traumatic neurosis. *Int. J. Psycho-Anal., 49*, 719–731.
69. REID, D. D. (1944). Neurosis on active services: Experience among aircrew on a bomber station. International Allied Conference on War Medicine. *Neuropsychiatry, 230*, 123.
70. SANDERS, C. M. (1979–1980). A comparison of adult bereavement in the death of a spouse, child and parent. *Omega, 10*(4), 303–321.
71. SCURFIELD, R. M. (1985). Post-trauma stress assessment and treatment: Overview and formulations. In C. R. Figley (Ed.), *Trauma and its wake*. New York: Brunner/Mazel.
72. SHANFIELD, S. B., & SWAIN, B. J. (1984). The death of adult children in traffic accidents. *J. Nerv. Ment. Dis., 172*, 533–538.
73. SINGH, B., & RAPHAEL, B. (1981). Postdisaster morbidity of the bereaved: A possible role for preventive psychiatry. *J. Nerv. Ment. Dis., 169*(4), 203–212.
74. TITCHENER, J. L., & KAPP, F. (1976). Family and character change at Buffalo Creek. *Am. J. Psychiatry, 133*, 295–299.
75. VINEY, L. L., CLARKE, A. M., BUNN, T. A., & BENJAMIN, Y. N. (1985). Crisis intervention counseling: An evaluation of long and short term effects. *J. Counseling Psychol., 32*(1), 29–39.
76. WEISAETH, L. (1983a). Personal communication.
77. WEISAETH, L. (1983b). The study of a factory fire. Doctoral dissertation. University of Oslo, Oslo, Norway.
78. WESTERN, J. S., & MILNE, G. (1979). Some social effects of a natural hazard: Darwin residents and Cyclone Tracy. In R. L. Heathcote & B. G. Thom (Eds.), *Natural hazards in Australia*. Canberra: Australian Academy of Science.
79. WILSON, J. P., SMITH, W. K., & JOHNSON, S. K. (1985). A comparative analysis of PTSO among various survivor groups. In C. R. Figley (Ed.), *Trauma and its wake*. New York: Brunner/Mazel.
80. WINTER, D. (1982). In *The first of the few*. London: Allen Lane, Penguin Books, p. 165.

18

CULTS AND NEW RELIGIOUS MOVEMENTS

MARC GALANTER, M.D.

Professor, Department of Psychiatry,
New York University School of Medicine,
New York, New York

This chapter provides a psychological perspective on the new religious movements, or cults, of recent years. The natural history of membership in these movements will first be examined and relevant explanatory perspectives will be discussed.

Let us first consider the charismatic large-group, a term we shall use for one that contains more than a dozen members, typically many more. Members of large-groups typically: (a) adhere to a consensual belief system; (b) sustain a high level of social cohesiveness; (c) are strongly influenced by group behavioral norms; and (d) impute charismatic (or divine) power to the group or its leadership. This definition includes most of the contemporary new religious movements, but also other nonreligious zealous groups, ranging from Alcoholics Anonymous to radical political organizations.

The concept of a cult, more specifically religious, connotes religious deviancy and, often, transcendental experience. Most cults would fall within our definition of the large-group. The cult has been characterized as a "religious movement which makes a fundamental break with the religious traditions of the culture and which is . . . composed of individuals who had or seek mystical experiences" (1). Troeltsch (2), in his classical discourse on the Christian church, distinguished the established church from church sects. He then characterized a third entity, "spiritual and mystical religion," akin to the cult phenomenon, which conveys "the direct inward and present religious experience." This latter subtype of religious experience has also been described from a sociological perspective, as a "mystic collectivity . . . understood to refer to all people who hold tenets of mystical religion and consequently have a sense of common solidarity and obligation, even though they do not interact" (3). This latter description is also of considerable psychological importance, as it points to the existence of a real or pseudocommunity (4) that serves as a basis for defining reality. Such a community provides consensual validation for its own system of beliefs.

A study of the social origins of cults leads to the observation that their growth is often promoted by a crisis within the culture. Other large-groups may emerge because of focal failings in the culture. But when the plausibility of a society is diminished because of crisis, or fails to meet the needs of a group, its ideological underpinnings cease to be credible (5). Individuals may then become deprived of a meaningful orientation to their lives. This observation bears on the impact of the counterculture and Vietnam protests of the previous decade. These were clearly important to the emergence of such sects among American youth. Since news of social change vis-à-vis the mass media could be disseminated instantaneously to disenchanted youth, the development of alternative groups and ideologies on a national basis was facilitated.

THE NATURAL HISTORY OF MEMBERSHIP

Definitions of the phenomena convey neither the particulars of lifestyle and belief nor the subjective quality of membership. It is important, therefore, to review descriptive findings on contemporary sects in order to understand the psychology of these groups.

Members' Backgrounds

Most reports have characterized subjects as coming from middle- and upper-middle-class social backgrounds (6–9). We studied representative samples of members from two sects through structured self-reports; in both the Divine Light Mission, an Eastern sect, and the Unification Church ("Moonies"), a neo-Christian group, the majority of members had attended college, as had one or both of their parents (10, 11). Similar observations were made on young people who had left charismatic sects (12, 13). Many of the sect members' families have also been reported to be troubled, on the basis of members' self-reports (12, 14). Schwartz and Kaslow (15) also reported patterns of "pseudo-mutuality" and "overly enmeshed families" from studies of the family members themselves.

Psychological distress among potential members is found to be an important antecedent to joining. Based on interviews with members, ex-members, and relatives, a number of clinicians have described members as emotionally disturbed. They have been seen as predominantly "depressed, inadequate, or borderline anti-social youths" (16) or as "lonely, rejected and sad" (8). Inductees are reported to have limited social ties before joining the sect. Their preoccupations with purpose and destiny have been closely associated with a dissatisfaction with interpersonal relations, leading to loneliness and a sense of alienation (14). Some adolescents are thus described as using these sects to reduce a sense of personal incompleteness, often at a time of normative crisis.

Recruitment

Public interest has focused on the role of active recruitment by religious sects. Lofland and Stark (17) proposed a model for this phenomenon based on their observations of a small millenarian Christian group. They emphasize acutely felt tension on the part of a convert, experienced within the context of a religious problem-solving perspective. This lends itself to acquiring the role of a "religious seeker." The encounter with the cult then becomes a turning point in the person's life. Close ties are developed to other members as they shower the convert with affection. The exceptionally friendly and accepting attitude sustained by recruiters has been noted by others (16, 17), and the importance of early contacts with the group in relation to feelings of meaningfulness and deprivation has also been stressed (18–21). This induction through psychological engagement rather than coercion is further underlined by the findings that cult members have not reported overt coercion or physical constraint during the course of their own conversions (11). After the initial involvement, extracult attachments are soon neutralized, as a commitment begins to grow and consolidate.

In a controlled assessment of these issues (22), we undertook a longitudinal study of the induction process and followed a cohort of 106 persons entering a workshop sequence for induction into the Unification Church. Workshop registrants were found to score below the general population on psychological well-being, and those who ultimately joined scored lower than the ones who did not. In addition, the joiners were found to score lower than the nonjoiners on affiliative ties outside the group. Interestingly, the affiliative ties developed toward sect members during the long-term induction workshop were as high for those who elected to leave as for those who chose to join. The latter finding corroborated naturalistic observations on the effectiveness of the group's intense interpersonal input, which complements the alienation among those who ultimately join.

The role of transcendental or mystical experiences in both individual conversion and group induction procedures can be very important. This was, of course, emphasized by both James (23) and Freud (24). The importance of transcendental experiences in conflict resolution has also been noted, even to the point of precipitating acute hallucinatory episodes in nonpsychotics (25, 26) and in psychotics, too (27, 28). In any case, these experiences are integral to conversion and to continuing membership (10, 29) for many charismatic sect members.

Explanatory models for the appearance of "psychotic-like" phenomena in normals within the context of religious experience have not yet been developed. It should be noted, however, that rather striking perceptual phenomena are regularly reported in the religious context. For example, 30 % of members of one sect, the Divine Light Mission, reported hallucinatorylike experiences during their meditation (10). Clearly, such phenomena should carry considerable import for our understanding of pathological as well as normal mental process; they may, perhaps, help us to understand the nature of certain contexts that can precipitate hallucinatory states among those who are designated as mentally ill.

Life in the Sects

An orientation toward communal living is characteristic of many charismatic sects. This is typical both of contemporary sects and of those in previous centuries, such as the Shakers and the original Mormons. Members may live together in an institutional setting or in smaller private residences. For example, among members of the Divine Light Mission, we found that 20 % lived in communal ritual residences with stringent behavioral norms (Ashrams), 50 % with other members in smaller informal private residences, and the remaining 30 % independently. In this sect, the spouses of all married and common-law respondents surveyed were also members. In the Unification Church, on the other hand, fully 94 % of members lived in Church-owned residences.

Some sects, such as the Maher Baba movement, do not have a tight-knit communal structure. This group, studied by Anthony and Robbins (30), consisted of local autonomous groups with members developing independent living arrangements. Nonetheless, most followers of Maher Baba were found to associate primarily with other members of the group and constituted an informal community, based on close friendships and social affiliations.

Measures of social affiliation that we have applied to sect members demonstrate a strong differential between the intensity of ties felt toward nonmembers and members, even members whom respondents did not know personally (10, 11). Sect members frequently refer to each other as "family." This style also emerges in charismatic groups directed primarily toward therapeutic purposes. For example, Ofshe (31) studied patterns of relating in Synanon, a self-help group that was initiated in 1958 for the treatment of drug abusers. Shared residential facilities and economic resources and a "familylike atmosphere" underlay a considerable degree of intimacy within this group. Behaviorally, this was manifest in patterns of social intercourse, in both structured group communication (the "games") and informal socialization.

The behavioral norms of many sects appear to express a reaction to the sexual permissiveness characteristic of the 1960s and 1970s. Harder, Richardson, and Simmonds (32), for example, studied courtship, marriage, and family style in one segment of the Jesus movement. They describe the express avoidance of situations that may be sexually charged and outline specific sect regulations regarding courtship and bodily pleasures. Dating, for example, was considered inappropriate because it might lead to temptations and possible transgression. In our study of engaged Moonies (33), we found similar norms for behavior among these maritally engaged members. Fiancés refrained from physical contact with their future spouses.

Elements of the same behavior were also found (34) among a small Hindu-oriented group, devotees of Baba. Baba encouraged sexual restraint, while not always practicing it himself. Members typically reported that the sexual act brought them down from the "high" they experienced from their religious affiliation. Some, however, continued to practice sexual relations, while the stronger adherents eschewed an interest in sexuality. We observed a similar transformation in attitude among recruits to the Unification Church members, of whom 76% indicated that they should "very much" avoid thinking about sex, although only 11% reported feeling this way prior to joining.

Norms for residence and sexual behavior reflect the profound influence that charismatic groups may bring to bear on the lifestyle of their members. More compelling examples, of course, for the impact of cults on members' behavior have been reported in the popular press in settings where leaders have driven members to participate in deviant behaviors. The impact of psychotic behavior of a charismatic sect leader was undertaken from a psychiatric perspective by Deutsch (35). Because of the grandiose role vested in this charismatic leader, members' reality testing was suspended in the face of the avowals presented them. When necessary, rationalizations emerged so that the leader's bizarre commands might be perceived as reasonable and then be accepted.

Religious Orientation and Consensual Validation

The belief systems that characterize many contemporary sects may seem confusing to the outsider. Many are based on transcendental and mystical experiences. Some are drawn from unfamiliar Eastern traditions, and others embellish on established religions to the point of reconstructing Biblical doctrine. Singer (12) divided the many cult orientations into nine types, although many typologies are possible. In addition, not all types are described in published scholarly reports (or even in the general press), often due to their secretiveness and inaccessibility.

One common orientation is based on neo-Christian ideas, as illustrated by the True World Evangelical Christian Church associated with the Pentecostal movement (36). This group accepts the Bible as the literal word of God, and members have been observed to speak in tongues and believe in personal prophecy and faith healing.

Eastern groups typically emphasize meditation and transcendental experiences. The most common Eastern orientation is based on Hindu concepts, as in the Divine Light Mission and the small Baba group discussed above, as well as the Hare Krishna movement (37). Some groups are based on Zen or other Sino-Japanese practices. Soka Gakkai (38), for example, is a Buddhist sect that originated in Japan and now has headquarters in major American cities; its belief system emphasizes religious chanting and a positive attitude, but does not impose extensive behavioral restrictions on its followers.

Not all charismatic groups are religiously oriented. Some emphasize contemporary psychology as an ideological perspective, to the point of a charismatic commitment. The ideology of groups like these, however, such as Synanon (31) and est (39), may be more palatable to the mental health professional. This supports the consideration that although mystification may enhance the attraction of an ideology for a member, a group is more likely to elicit a positive response in the outsider if its beliefs are comprehensible in terms of the outsider's own world view. Politically oriented or racially based groups, such as the People's Temple or the Italian Red Brigades, are better known through the popular press. Less familiar groups may be subsumed under the headings of witchcraft, Satanism, spiritualism, and outer-space orientation. The term *autism*, typically applied to an individual's cognitive framework, may have its own counterpart on a group's level in this context. It would apply when ideas contrary to those consensually validated by the society become entwined in the members' coping system.

The impact of group influence on members' perception of reality and documented examples of destructive behavior had led many, parents in particular, to fear for the sanity of sect members. In this relation, however, Bromley, Shupe, and Ventimiglia (40) studied the psychological impact of cult "atrocity tales" on the media. They pointed out that examples of presumed deviancy are often used to justify coercive behavior in forcibly removing members from peaceable settings on behalf of the members' families; such atrocity tales may thus serve as a moral legitimation for deprogramming.

Leaving Charismatic Sects

According to Richardson (41), the term *deprogramming* refers to "a set of techniques for removing persons from new religious groups and involving them in a rigorous and even coercive resocialization process in an attempt to get them to renounce their beliefs and accept more traditional ones." Psychiatric options for deprogramming have been discussed by Etemad (8). He suggests that the process be preceded by a physical examination and a comprehensive psychiatric evaluation and recommends that it take place in a "pleasant psychiatric facility"; when possible, the family should be firm but gentle and should accompany and support the patient. Etemad maintains that the therapist should be firm but gentle and should avoid "the adversary techniques of self-styled deprogrammers who attack patients' rights, beliefs, and religion." Based on his own experience, he states that the process takes between 30 and 60 hours, and that the goal is primarily to reorient the subject to think for himself and be independent of the cult member.

There are no survey data nor is there a clear basis for estimating how many sect members leave under coercion and how many voluntarily. There are also no controlled observations of the deprogramming process. Ungerleider and Wellisch (42), however, did contrast a sample of members who left their groups subsequent to deprogramming with another sample who had been "unsuccessfully" deprogrammed and returned. They found that the majority of those who did leave the sects had been members for less than a year. Conversely, the majority of those who returned after deprogramming had been members for more than a year. In addition, a majority of those who were successfully deprogrammed later elected to become involved in conducting deprogramming themselves; sect members who left voluntarily did not choose to pursue this course.

This latter observation, regarding deprogramming, was confirmed in our controlled comparison (13) of 66 persons who had left the Unification Church. After an average of 3.8 years, members had apparently achieved a stable social adjustment. Most had left because they saw themselves at odds with the operating principles of the Church, usually after being frustrated in their work or relationships within the Church. Those who left voluntarily retained a notable fidelity to the sect, in contrast to those who were deprogrammed. Significantly, 36% of the sample reported they had experienced serious emotional problems shortly after leaving. This latter phenomenon is probably reflected in Singer's experience (12) with therapeutically oriented groups for persons who have left, a majority of whom experience deprogramming. She suggests that people who join were troubled to begin with and have difficulty with their subsequent community adjustment. Problems of depression, loneliness, and uncertainty were frequent among ex-members.

EXPLANATORY PERSPECTIVES

Psychopathology and Mental Health

The natural history of membership in these charismatic large-groups raises a number of issues that are qualitatively different from those generally considered by the clinician. These will be discussed below, in relation to both individual and group psychology.

Individual members generally state that joining has a positive effect on their psychological state. Interviewers describe reports of new strength and "spiritual resources," as well as reduced "self-hatred" (14). Increased feelings of calm and happiness and a capability for better relationships are also noted (16, 43).

In our studies, we conducted controlled comparisons to measure the psychological impact of membership in the Divine Light Mission and the Unification Church. Among representative samples of members in the two groups, analysis of structured self-reports indicated considerable amelioration of emotional state over the course of joining, with stability in this improved state maintained over the course of long-term membership (two to three years). Interestingly, however, despite the reported improvement, long-term members' scores on the psychological General Well-Being Schedule were slightly below those of an age- and sex-matched sample from the general population. This was compatible with the finding of a notably low level of psychological well-being measured in a separate sample of nonmembers who had registered for the sects' workshops prior to joining. These studies support the hypothesis that, at least for certain sects, many of those attracted to joining are in a state of significant emotional distress, and do indeed experience an amelioration of their affective status on conversion.

These findings, based on self-report data, should be compared with the impressions of certain observers who report their own assessments of members' status (6, 12, 44). Clark (6), for example, states that, "Converts often seem drab and dreamy outside the group, stereotyped, and somewhat expressionless when discussing anything other than their new experience. They lacked mirth and richness of vocabulary." If such observations do reflect a negative impact of membership in charismatic groups, they should be considered in relation to studies of psychopathology induced within certain groups in more controlled settings. Yalom and Lieberman (45), for example, in a carefully controlled study, noted a 7.5% incidence of psychological casualties in time-limited encounter groups, a setting with much less prolonged, directed interpersonal input. Similarly, casualties have also been reported among members of est (46), a self-help group involving commitments generated in a large-group setting, based on teachings of a charismatic secular leader.

The diagnosis of major psychopathology among converts is difficult to undertake because interviewing of volunteer members does not necessarily reach a more dysfunctional minority, and more widely distributed self-report instruments may not accurately tap more severe symptoms. Nonetheless, certain findings do shed light on this issue. For example, in our studies, emotional problems among Divine Light respondents had led 38% to seek professional help prior to joining and 9% to hospitalization. For the Unification Church, corresponding figures were 30% and 6%, respectively. A number of members to whom we gave clinical interviews were found to have experienced amelioration of symptoms of major psychopathology subsequent to joining.

It appears that certain sects attract members with considerable psychopathology. For example, among the small band of 24 devotees of Baba, "virtually all gave histories of chronic unhappiness and unsatisfactory parent relations" (34). Similar findings were reported with regard to the Subud sect, which appeared to attract individuals in considerable distress. Kiev and Francis (47), who studied the sect, also described members of this group with known psychiatric illness. They observed that although the group appeared to offer temporary remission to such persons, it would probably contribute to later exacerbation of their illness because the pressure for personal change promoted anxiety in those who did not achieve clear-cut progress.

Mystical experiences associated with religious conversion have, conversely, been described as having a salutary effect on psychopathology. Thus, there have been reports of schizophrenic adolescents emerging from transcendental religious experience with a resolution of suicidal impulses (48), bizarre behavior (49), and psychotic decompensation (10).

Another area to be considered is substance abuse. Remission in patterns of abuse is frequently reported, along with rapid changes in attitudes toward drugs on conversion (10, 11, 16, 50–52). These changes occur among young people who were acculturated into patterns of rather heavy drug use during the "counterculture" period of the 1960s and 1970s. The apparent potential of charismatic groups to enforce new behavioral norms is well illustrated by their impact on intoxicant use.

Thought Control

The issue of thought control, or "brainwashing," in sects has been raised in both the popular press and the scientific literature (18, 42, 53, 54). Lifton (55) originally studied this process as applied by Chinese Communists to Western prisoners of war during the Korean conflict. Richardson and Stewart (56) drew on a number of these traits in their own study of the Jesus movement.

Milieu control, for example, entails establishing constraints over all facets of communication; the degree of such control varies between religious sects, usually contingent on the proximity of residential and work arrangements. A shared belief that members' work is devoted to some grand plan (whether revealed or not) is the basis for the mystical manipulation of members' activities; all planned and observed events are thereby rationalized on the basis of the group's mystified goals. The sect is presumed to maintain a sacred science, whereby unquestioned dogma can explain all facets of life; this effectively eliminates the difference between the sacred and secular spheres.

This model was found well suited to explain certain aspects of the Jesus movement, although there are some salient differences (57). Among these are the lack of direct physical coercion in the charismatic groups and, in most cases, the absence of aggressive attempts at stripping away the individual's antecedent identity. In fact, Richardson and Stewart had observed that for most converts entry into the sects appeared to be an attempt to try out something new, often lacking the intensity of a genuine religious conversion. They felt that such converts should be differentiated from persons whose conversion experience came as the culmination of a positive and conscious search. Whether these two different routes to conversion lead to different outcomes has yet to be studied.

REFERENCES

1. NELSON, G. K. (1972). The membership of a cult: The Spiritualists National Union. *Rev. Religious Res.*, *13*, 170.
2. TROELTSCH, E. (1931). The social teaching of the Christian churches. London: George Allen and Unwin.
3. CAMPBELL, C. (1977). Clarifying the cult. *Br. J. Sociol.*, *28*, 376.
4. CAMERON, N. A. (1974). Paranoid conditions and paranoia. In S. Arieti and E. B. Brody (Eds.), *American handbook of psychiatry* (Vol. 3:679–693). New York: Basic Books.
5. EISTER, A. W. (1972). An outline of a structural theory of cults. *J. Sci. Study Religion, 11,* 319–333.
6. CLARK, J. G., JR. (1979). *JAMA,* 279–281.
7. COX, H. (1977). *Turning east: The promise and peril of the new orientalism.* New York: Simon & Schuster.
8. ETEMAD, B. (1978). Extrication from cultism. *Current Psychiatric Ther., 18,* 217–223.
9. DAVIS, R., & RICHARDSON, J. T. (1976). The organization of functioning of the Children of God. *Sociol. Anal., 37,* 321–339.
10. GALANTER, M., & BUCKLEY, P. (1978). Evangelical religion and meditation: Psychotherapeutic effects. *J. Nerv. Ment. Dis., 166,* 695–691.
11. GALANTER, M., RABKIN, R., RABKIN, J., & DEUTSCH, A. (1979). The "Moonies": A psychological study of conversion and membership in a contemporary religious sect. *Am. J. Psychiatry, 136,* 165–170.
12. SINGER, M. (1978). Therapy with ex-cult members. *Nat. Assoc. Private Psychiatr. Hosp. J., 9,* 14–18.
13. GALANTER, M. (1983). Engaged "Moonies": The impact of a charismatic group on adaptation and behavior. *Arch. Gen. Psychiatry, 40,* 1197–1201.
14. NICHOLI, A. M. (1974). A new dimension of the youth culture. *Am. J. Psychiatry, 131,* 396–401.
15. SCHWARTZ, L. L., & KASLOW, F. W. (1958). Religious cults, the individual and the family relations of schizophrenics. *Psychiatry, 21,* 205–220.
16. LEVINE, S. V., & SALTER, N. E. (1976). Youth and contemporary religious movements: Psychological findings. *Can. Psychiatr. Assoc. J., 21,* 411–420.
17. LOFLAND, J., & STARK, R. (1965). Becoming a world-saver: A theory of conversion to a deviant perspective. *Am. Sociol. Rev., 30,* 862–875.

18. GLOCK, C. Y., & STARK, R. (1965). *Religion and society in tension.* Chicago: Rand McNally.
19. GORDON, D. (1974). The Jesus people: An identity synthesis. *Urban Life Culture, 3,* 159–178.
20. SIMMONDS, R. B., RICHARDSON, J. T., & HARDER, M. W. (1976). A Jesus movement group: An adjective check list assessment. *J. Sci. Study Religion, 15,* 323–337.
21. ADAMS, R. L., & FOX, R. J. (1972). Maintaining Jesus: The new trip. *Society, 9,* 50–56.
22. GALANTER, M. (1980). Psychological induction into the large-group: Findings from a modern religious sect. *Am. J. Psychiatry, 137,* 1574–1579.
23. JAMES, W. (1926). *The varieties of religious experience.* New York: Modern Library. (Original work published 1902.)
24. FREUD, S. (1955). Group psychology and the analysis of the ego. In J. Strachey (Ed. and Trans.), *Standard edition of the complete psychological works of Sigmund Freud.* London: Hogarth Press. (Original work published 1921.)
25. STERBA, R. (1968). Remarks on mystic states. *Am. Imago, 25,* 77–85.
26. JACOBSEN, E. (1964). *The self and the object world.* New York: International Universities Press.
27. SEDMAN, G., & HOPKINSON, G. (1966). The psychopathology of mystical and religious conversion experiences in psychiatric patients, I. *Confina Psychiatr., 9,* 65–77.
28. SEDMAN, G., & HOPKINSON, G. (1966). The psychopathology of mystical and religious conversion experiences in psychiatric patients, II. *Confina Psychiatr., 9,* 65–77.
29. BUCKLEY, P., & GALANTER, M. (1979). Mystical experience, spiritual knowledge and a contemporary ecstatic religion. *Br. J. Med. Psychol., 52,* 281–289.
30. ANTHONY, D., & ROBBINS, T. (1974). The Meher Baba movement: Its effects on post-adolescent social alienation. In I. I. Zaretsky and M. P. Leone (Eds.), *Religious movements in contemporary America* (pp. 479–571). Princeton, NJ: Princeton University Press.
31. OFSHE, R. (1976). Synanon: The people business. In C. Y. Glock and R. N. Bellah (Eds.), *The new religious consciousness* (pp. 116–137). Berkeley, CA: University of California Press.
32. HARDER, M. W., RICHARDSON, J. T., & SIMMONDS, R. (1976). Lifestyle: Courtship, marriage and family in a changing Jesus movement organization. *Int. Rev. Modern Sociol., 6,* 155–172.
33. GALANTER, M. (1983). Unification Church ("Moonie") drop-outs: Psychological readjustment after membership in a charismatic religious group. *Am. J. Psychiatry, 140,* 98–99.
34. DEUTSCH, A. (1975). Observations on a sidewalk Ashram. *Arch. Gen. Psychiatry, 32,* 166–175.
35. DEUTSCH, A. (1980). Tenacity of attachment to a cult leader: A psychiatric perspective. *Am. J. Psychiatry, 137,* 1569–1573.
36. HARDYCK, J. A., & BRADEN, M. (1962). Prophecy fails again: A report of a failure to replicate. *J. Abnorm. Soc. Psychol., 65,* 136–141.
37. NAGY, I. B., & STARK, G. (1973). *Invisible loyalties.* New York: Harper & Row.
38. KUMASAKA, Y. (1966). Soka Gakkai: Group psychologic study of new religio-political organization. *Am. J. Psychother., 20,* 46–47.
39. SIMON, J. (1978). Observations on 67 patients who took Erhard Seminars Training. *Am. J. Psychiatry, 135,* 686–691.
40. BROMLEY, D. G., SHUPE, A. D., JR., & VENTIMIGLIA, J. C. (1979). Atrocity tales, the Unification Church, and the social construction of evil. *J. Commun., 29,* 42–53.
41. RICHARDSON, J. T. (1980). Conversion careers. *Society, 3,* 47–50.
42. UNGERLEIDER, J. T., & WELLISCH, D. K. (1979). Coercive persuasion (brainwashing), religious cults, and deprogramming. *Am. J. Psychiatry, 136,* 279–282.

43. WILSON, W. P. (1972). Mental health benefits of religious salvation. *Dis. Nerv. Syst.*, *33*, 383–386.
44. SHAPIRO, E. (1977). Destructive cults. *Fam. Physician*, *15*, 80–83.
45. YALOM, I. D., & LIEBERMAN, M. A. (1971). A study of encounter group casualties. *Arch. Gen. Psychiatry*, *25*, 16–30.
46. KIRSCH, M. A., & GLASS, L. L. (1977). Psychiatric disturbances associated with Erhard Seminars Training: II. Additional cases and theoretical consideration. *Am. J. Psychiatry*, *134*, 1254–1258.
47. KIEV, A., & FRANCIS, J. L. (1964). Subud and mental illness: Psychiatric illness in a religious sect. *Am. J. Psychother.*, *18*, 66–78.
48. HORTON, P. C. (1973). The mystical experience as a suicide preventive. *Am. J. Psychiatry*, *130*, 290–296.
49. LEVIN, T. M., & ZEGANS, L. S. (1974). Adolescent identity crisis and religious conversion: Implications for psychotherapy. *Br. J. Psychol.*, *47*, 73–82.
50. SIMMONDS, R. B. (1977). Conversion or addiction. *Am. Behav. Scientist*, *20*, 909–924.
51. ROBBINS, T. (1969). Eastern mysticism and the resocialization of drug users: The Meher Baba cult. *J. Sci. Study Religion*, *8*, 308–317.
52. GALANTER, M. (1981). Sociobiology and informal social controls of drinking. *J. Stud. Alcohol*, *42*, 64–79.
53. CLARK, J. G., JR. (1978). Problems in referral of cult members. *Nat. Assoc. Private Psychiatr. Hosp. J.*, *9*(4), 27–29.
54. RICHARDSON, J. T., HARDER, M., & SIMMONDS, R. B. (1972). Thought reform and the Jesus movement. *Youth Society*, *4*, 185–200.
55. LIFTON, R. J. (1961). *Thought reform and the psychology of totalism*. New York: Norton.
56. RICHARDSON, J. T., & STEWART, M. (1977). Conversion process models and the Jesus movement. *Am. Behav. Scientist*, *20*, 819–838.
57. ZABLOCK, B. D. (1971). *The joyful community*. Baltimore: Penguin.

19

TERRORISM

DAVID A. SOSKIS, M.D.

Research Psychiatrist, Unit for Experimental Psychiatry,
The Institute of Pennsylvania Hospital and the
University of Pennsylvania,
Philadelphia, Pennsylvania

and

JAN R. LINOWITZ, ED.D.

Lecturer, Graduate School of Education,
University of Pennsylvania,
Philadelphia, Pennsylvania

TERRORISM: THE PHENOMENON

Although relatively few individuals have been direct victims of terrorism during the twentieth century, the victim of terrorism could be anybody. Terrorists carefully plan their attacks to communicate this point as widely as possible, and the timing of the television evening news is as important to them as the schedule of sentries. Thus the number of people exposed to terrorism is much greater than the number of people directly affected. What is terrorism, and what can clinicians learn from it that will help them in their work, and in their lives?

Efforts to produce a coherent and generally accepted definition of terrorism have met with only limited success. The problem is easier to understand when we realize that terrorists themselves almost never accept this label, preferring to describe themselves as "freedom fighters" or "guerrillas." The definition offered and explained below will not please everybody, certainly not most terrorists, but we believe that it captures the essentials that are most useful for clinicians trying to make sense out of a constantly changing international phenomenon.

We define terrorism as the use or threat of violence to achieve a social, political, or religious aim in a way that does not obey the traditional rules of war. The three parts of this definition move progressively further from issues that the average citizen encounters in his or her daily life. The threat or use of violence is, unfortunately, a part of life for many citizens. For those in most developed countries this is most often associated with crime, with the victim and perpetrator having a direct or dyadic relationship. For the most deadly crime, murder, this is often an intimate love relationship that has turned to hate and/or been distorted by intoxication. Even in crimes such as mugging or armed robbery, the criminal wants something *directly from the victim*, and that something goes to, and ends with, the criminal. In other words, the goal of the crime is basically personal.

As we move further in our definition of terrorism, it begins to part company with "ordinary" violent crime. Terrorism uses violence to achieve social, political, or religious aims that are fundamentally transpersonal. In the first three-quarters of this century, terrorism was identified almost exclusively with traditional political goals, such as the overthrow of a particular government or the acquisition of a homeland by a displaced group. This identification has recently begun to shift; there is a clear increase in the role of religious motivations, often mixed with political goals, in the terrorist groups of the late twentieth century. The comforting notion among some Westerners that this trend is limited to Islam and confined to Third World countries has been shattered by the appearance of groups like the Aryan Nations in the United States whose ideology is based on their version of Protestant theology.

For most people, the use of violence to achieve transpersonal goals is associated with war. The thing that differentiates a terrorist from a soldier is that the terrorist does not obey the rules of war. These rules, as codified in the various Geneva Conventions, cover many areas, such as permissible weapons, identification standards, and so forth (1). For the purpose of understanding terrorism, two persistent themes in the various versions are crucial: the definition of who is, and who is not, involved in the struggle, and what happens to people who are captured.

Those who call themselves soldiers are, or should be, the basic combatants in a war. One of the great psychological stressors for American soldiers in Vietnam was the significant number of enemy soldiers who were much younger or older than they were, or who were women, i.e., who did not correspond to their American stereotype of a soldier. Despite these demographic differences between forces, both sides knew that they were fighting in a war. The targets of terrorist attacks, on the other hand, typically do not know or accept the definition of themselves as soldiers in the conflict in which the terrorists are involved. The glib assertions by terrorists that all citizens of a certain country, or anyone who is in the wrong place at the wrong time, are or support their enemies do not really speak to this point. To the extent that terrorists persistently and intentionally attack these citizens, their victims are victims of crime rather than losers in a military struggle.

For those seeking an historical perspective, the closest analogy to modern terrorists may be pirates, who regularly mixed the "instrumental" use of victims (e.g., for ransom) with murder and vicious assaults, including rape. This instrumental or triadic aspect of terrorist violence is sometimes difficult to understand. Thus there may indeed be "nothing personal" in the feelings of the terrorist who executes an innocent hostage; the hostage is being used to influence a third party who is the object of the terrorist's hate or simply to draw the attention of a violence-sated public to the terrorist's cause. For this purpose, the more innocent the victim and the more shocking the attack, the better. As has been noted many times, terrorists want a lot of people watching more than they want a lot of people dead. Like pirates, terrorists depend on their image as much as on their reality to create and amplify fear or interest. Indeed, one of the dangers of terrorism, as with piracy, is that the criminal may be romanticized and glamorized while the victim is forgotten. These issues create a large number of ethical and practical dilemmas for the press and broadcast media in a free society: the media must fulfill its responsibility to inform without compromising government efforts to deal with terrorist incidents, invading the privacy of hostages and their families, or, even worse, being manipulated by the terrorists to serve their instrumental ends.

Most careful students of terrorism feel that the rapid availability of worldwide publicity through the broadcast media serves as a potent motivating factor for much of current international terrorism. In closed, totalitarian societies, there is much less to be gained by terrorist incidents since the government effectively controls the press, and the response to incidents is usually swift and harsh. But where the society values individual human lives, where the press is free, and where small, portable, and lethal weapons are available, terrorism may make sense for a variety of groups who for various reasons have rejected nonviolent means of conflict resolution or ongoing struggle. The analogy with piracy may provide a hopeful perspective: in some areas of the world, interference with international commerce and travel did indeed mobilize successful cooperative efforts to stop piracy. But even with the will to and means for such concerted action, we will probably have terrorism (and perhaps piracy) with us for some time.

For the clinician interested in pursuing the general subject of terrorism, the writings of Brian Jenkins of the RAND corporation present a unique combination of in-depth expertise with a broad, intelligent view of the issues involved (12). A creative clinical and psychodynamic approach to the subject by a psychiatrist is presented in *Crusaders, Criminals, Crazies: Terror and Terrorism in Our Time* by Frederick J. Hacker (8). Perspectives related to the work on the Task Force on Terrorism and Its Victims of the American Psychiatric Association are presented in *Terrorism: Interdisciplinary Perspectives*, edited by Burr Eichelman, David Soskis, and William Reid (5).

THE TERRORISTS

Only a small number of clinicians will ever have the experience of treating a person whom they know is a terrorist, and most of these will be working in specialized forensic settings. Thus, the study of individual terrorists or terrorist groups, as opposed to an understanding of the phenomenon itself and of victims' issues, is not crucial for most clinicians. Moreover, although a large number of theories have been advanced to explain who becomes a terrorist and why, these span a wide range; we still lack, and may always lack, a clear set of necessary and/or sufficient demographic or psychological traits associated with terrorists. A number of trends, however, have emerged.

The most important insight into the terrorist mind for the clinician is probably that it is not necessarily a sick one. Many terrorists, sadly, are all too healthy, adaptive, and highly motivated. In fact, the need to classify terrorists into one or another psychopathological pigeonhole may represent, at best, wishful thinking and, at worst, a maladaptive defensive maneuver that leads to serious underestimation of an adversary. Unfortunately, there are always clinicians, many of them sincere and well meaning, who are willing to speculate in public on the detailed psychological makeup of a person they have never met, let alone examined. The smaller number of clinicians who have made sophisticated and careful studies of terrorists are often constrained by security considerations in their public communications.

The tendency to retreat into a position of "you'd have to be crazy to do that!" may, for many people in liberal, developed countries, reflect their inability to make a wholehearted statement that identifies a person as evil or as their enemy. Either category suggests a need for action, or at least for vigilance, that may be troubling enough to make various psychological avoidance techniques tempting.

Although many terrorists, especially terrorist leaders, are quite healthy, psychopathology is not absent from terrorist groups. Broadly speaking, in countries such as Lebanon and Northern Ireland, many people have had their lives sharply influenced and their options limited by terrorist incidents that most of us see only on TV. The chronic levels of stress and the exposure to recurrent violence in these communities do appear to have taken their toll on residents from all age and economic levels. In addition to expected post-traumatic syndromes, the developmental effects may be most severe, however, in children and adolescents; terrorists recruited from and trained in these communities may perceive themselves and their lives in ways that easily play into agendas for self-destruction and revenge. It now appears that similar effects of major social traumas on cohesive groups can appear in the children or even grandchildren of traumatized individuals who have not suffered the traumas directly themselves (e.g., in Armenian and South Moluccan communities). Even within traumatized or revenge-oriented communities, however, the young people who participate actively in terrorist attacks appear more than usually violence-prone.

Individuals with severe psychopathology have participated in a number of terrorist incidents. They have often been recruited by leaders who have used them, with full knowledge of their problems, to carry out suicidal missions that fit in with delusions or other distorted thinking patterns or to perform menial tasks in return for a sense of belonging or mission. In a sense, they are the expendable appendages of a differentiated social organism. Even more common is the symbiotic alliance in many terrorist groups of idealistic and/or ideologically motivated leaders with individuals who have long histories compatible with diagnoses of antisocial or related personality disorders and who have the practical experience with violence, weapons, and the criminal subculture that the idealists often lack.

Members of the latter group have most often been men, but women have made up a large number of the idealistic terrorist leaders; once socialized to the violent terrorist role, they appear fully as capable of murderous behavior as are their male colleagues.

Many terrorist behaviors that seem to reflect individual psychopathology are instead expressions of the dynamics of socially isolated small groups. This social isolation is a product of the need both to create an environment in which terrorist behavior can "make sense" and to minimize the risk of the capture or defection of any single member (the "cell" system).

Discussions of individual terrorists and terrorist groups can be found in several references (5, 8), including Gerald McKnight's *The Terrorist Mind* (13).

TERRORISM: THE INCIDENTS

Terrorist incidents can be broadly categorized into two groups: those that take place rapidly over seconds or minutes, such as shootings or bombings, and those that are more extended over hours or even days, and often involve the taking of hostages. The more rapid incidents produce victims and survivors who share some clinical features with victims of natural and especially man-made accidents or disasters. The longer incidents have produced some adaptations that have come to be considered distinctive.

The best known of these adaptations is called the Stockholm syndrome after a 1973 hostage incident that occurred as part of a bank robbery in Sweden. Since then it has become clear that other instances of seemingly inexplicable behavior during hostage incidents were probably also manifestations of this phenomenon. We define the Stockholm syndrome as the development by a hostage of positive feelings toward the hostage taker coupled with negative feelings toward the authorities or toward others outside the situation (e.g., the hostage's own family). In many hostage situations there is a reciprocal development of positive feelings toward the hostages by the hostage taker. The syndrome can develop after relatively brief contacts if the situation is sufficiently isolated and intense and can persist in diminishing form for weeks or even months after the incident has concluded.

Early attempts to explain the Stockholm syndrome as identification with the aggressor have been modified as the factors associated with its presence or absence in specific incidents have been clarified. The syndrome seems to require some human contact between the parties involved and to be strongest in situations in which terrorists show some real kindness or nurturing behavior, such as feeding, toward the hostages. Law enforcement and military personnel who are called on to deal with terrorist hostage incidents are aware of the syndrome and tend to foster it if they can while simultaneously maintaining an awareness of its possible effects on hostage behavior both during and after the incident. In the long-run, the development of the Stockholm syndrome seems to somewhat lessen the likelihood of a murderous outcome even if it produces some statements that may embarrass authorities and, ultimately, the hostages themselves. Helping former hostages come to terms with incident-related experiences and behaviors is, in fact, one of the major tasks of postincident therapy.

Recognition of the Stockholm syndrome has led to the development of the discipline of hostage negotiation. The negotiator, who is usually a trained, senior law enforcement officer, tries to establish a helping and mediating relationship with the hostage taker or takers to facilitate a non-violent resolution of the incident (18). In this effort, clinicians have often served as consultants on medical or psychological aspects of the situation. Ethical aspects of this area for clinicians are reviewed in a set of guidelines offered by the Task Force on Terrorism and its Victims of the American Psychiatric Association (5, 21).

Hostage negotiation has had a remarkably successful history in the resolution of the most common types of hostage incidents involving disturbed individuals or couples or stemming from interrupted crimes such as bank robberies. It has a more restricted application in incidents carried out by sophisticated terrorist groups, who usually seek publicity of the incident rather than meaningful negotiation.

A number of adaptive techniques have been used effectively by hostages during terrorist incidents. These include efforts to help other hostages (which seem to have positive effects on both parties), solacing imagery (e.g., of family members or scenes from childhood), religious thoughts and practices, and humor.

For most clinicians, the effects of terrorist incidents on their patients will be extremely indirect. At the present time, the most common effect appears to be an increase in both realistic and unrealistic fear and avoidance behavior related to international travel. These fears are often qualitative rather than quantitative; i.e., they are out of proportion to the actual risks involved and may also have important implications in family systems, as when parents agonize over whether to allow a teenage child to go on a long-anticipated study trip abroad.

PSYCHOLOGICAL EFFECTS OF TERRORISM

Effects on Victims

When an incident of terrorism comes to an end, adult survivors face several difficult psychological tasks. First, they must resolve their feelings about their own behavior under stress. Second, they must resume control over their own lives. Third, they must begin to reestablish belief in the predictability of daily life and the trustworthiness of others.

Many survivors are troubled by guilt over actions they took or failed to take during their ordeal. Concern that the incident could have been resolved more quickly or with less violence "if only I had acted differently" is often voiced. Memories of their own helplessness often arouse feelings of shame and an awareness of human mortality. Many survivors suffer a crisis of identity upon return as they attempt to reconcile their new knowledge of human vulnerability with longstanding beliefs in personal dignity and competence (17).

As they struggle to resolve their feelings about the incident, survivors must also reestablish control over their own lives and behavior. The experience of being a victim is a regressive one for adults; release from captivity involves a return to adult responsibility. In order to function as competent adults, survivors must regain a belief in the world as a safe and predictable place.

Short-Term Effects

In the first days and weeks following a terrorist incident, survivors often report specific changes in thoughts, feelings, and behavior (9, 15, 17, 19, 24). Common short-term effects include nightmares about victimization, insomnia, fears and phobias, general anxiety, and physical complaints. Some survivors report preoccupation with the terrorist incident and loss of interest in sex, eating, or other activities. Positive effects include increased intimacy with family members and friends.

Long-Term Effects

Recent follow-up studies of victims of terrorism suggest that many survivors continue to experience some event-related symptoms several years after the traumatic episode. Preliminary data indicate that although most symptoms fade over time, episodic occurrences of some, such as event-related dreams or intrusive thoughts, may persist for 10 years or longer. Long-term effects include sleep disturbances, physical complaints, fears and phobias, preoccupation with the episode, and feelings of being misunderstood or ostracized by others (3, 6, 9, 16, 19).

Survivors employ a variety of coping mechanisms to help them maintain daily routines. Some avoid thinking or talking about the episode. Others develop personal rituals to ensure safety, such as standing or sleeping by a window to allow a rapid escape. Compensatory behaviors or reenactments may also provide reassurance to survivors. For example, Ayalon and Soskis (3) describe the compensatory behavior of a young woman who missed a chance to escape a terrorist incident because she was too frightened to volunteer to be a messenger. Five years later, she reported that she regularly volunteered for errands at the school in which she worked.

Developmental Issues

While being controlled by others is a regressive experience for adults, children are accustomed to living under the authority of parents and teachers. The task of the child who survives a terrorist episode is to reestablish trust in adults as "good parents" after experiencing the violent authority of "bad parents." Recent research suggests the difficulty of accomplishing this task. Terr (22, 23) interviewed 25 American children who were held hostage for 27 hours when kidnappers stopped their school bus. Four to five years after the event, all of the youngsters maintained intense fears of strangers, vehicles, the dark, or of being kidnapped again. All but two of the youngsters expressed "severe philosophical pessimism" in their follow-up interviews. They were unable to visualize a secure and happy future for themselves. Many predicted that they would die young. Their pessimistic responses suggest that their brief kidnapping experience profoundly affected their views of life.

When the victims of terrorism are adolescents, developmental disruption may be manifested in the area of identity formation. Adolescents, who are engaged in the delicate task of separating from their families and defining independent identities, may find it particularly difficult to integrate their experiences as victims in meaningful ways. Ayalon (2) describes two adolescents who clearly had trouble placing their experiences in perspective following a terrorist attack in Israel. One young man signed all correspondence as "survivor of X" (the name of the town where the incident occurred). In contrast, a young woman avoided all reminders of the attack in order to escape being identified as a survivor. Both these adolescents had understandable difficulty integrating their victimization with other aspects of their developing identities.

Children and adolescents thus face special tasks in the aftermath of terrorist victimization. Nevertheless, when victims have been healthy beforehand, and when adequate supports are provided, psychological development continues even after the most severe trauma.

Effects on Family and Community

The victims themselves are not the only ones to be traumatized by an incident of terrorism; the lives of relatives are also interrupted by the news that a loved one is threatened, and the predictability of family life is shattered. During the course of the incident, and in the first days and weeks following its resolution, family members may suffer from a variety of psychological symptoms, including sleep disturbances, anxiety, phobias, somatic complaints, and depression (9). Their distress, and their sudden awareness of the vulnerability of loved ones, is often overlooked as public attention focuses on the traumas of the victims.

The community itself is violated when members are victimized by terrorists. Neighbors, friends, and co-workers may experience both concern over the victims' fates and the recognition that "it could have been me." The response of the local community to the 1985 MOVE confrontation in Philadelphia illustrates the impact of a violent incident on community members. Eleven people were killed and dozens of homes were destroyed by fire when Philadelphia police dropped a bomb on the headquarters of the radical MOVE group after a prolonged gun battle. In the aftermath, neighborhood children reported nightmares of MOVE members tunneling into their homes and hurting them, regressed to sleeping with their parents at night, refused to walk to school alone, and developed fears of stoves, fire, and darkness. Parents described their own anger and confusion about the day's events and questioned their capacity to provide a satisfactory explanation to their children.

The need to make sense of community disruption often results in stigmatization of the survivors of terrorist incidents. In an effort to overcome a sense of personal vulnerability, community members may distance themselves from survivors and may subtly hold victims responsible for the fates they have suffered (3, 17).

Eric Shaw (16) has suggested that one reason that many of the American ex-hostages held in Iran have had few long-term adjustment problems is the unambivalent welcome they received upon their return to the United States. "No matter what they went through or how they behaved in Iran . . . they came back as heroes" (p. 152). Societal acceptance of and compassion for the ex-hostages facilitated the resolution of their own guilt and shame and allowed them to put their victimization behind them.

When the community fails to provide support for survivors, the victims may have difficulty resolving their own feelings. Survivors may employ denial to avoid thinking about their experiences and may repress feelings of guilt and shame. These unresolved feelings may later surface in nightmares or flashbacks. Support for Shaw's argument comes from Dutch researchers, who report that ex-hostages who are encouraged to talk about their ordeals in the days and weeks after their release suffer fewer long-term symptoms of psychological distress than do victims who are not given an opportunity to discuss their experiences (19).

THE CLINICIAN'S ROLE

Caplan's (4) model of primary, secondary, and tertiary prevention provides a useful framework for exploring the clinician's role in helping survivors, families, and communities cope with terrorist victimization. Primary intervention includes the psychological preparation of high-risk populations and the larger community for incidents of terrorism. Secondary intervention includes crisis intervention with victims, family members, and the affected community during and after an incident. The clinician's role in tertiary intervention involves the long-term treatment of post-traumatic stress disorders and other psychological aftereffects.

Primary Intervention

Primary intervention begins with the assumption that terrorist incidents will occur. Individuals who may be particularly vulnerable to terrorist attacks include people living or working in high-risk areas or other citizens in positions of high visibility. Extensive information about the political and cultural orientation of terrorist groups should be provided for these individuals. Preparation of vulnerable groups should include education about normal responses to danger and victimization, introduction to and practice of relevant coping skills, and the discussion of philosophical and religious contexts for experiences of stress and suffering. Political scientists, military personnel, and clinicians can all be helpful in preparing high-risk populations; the best sources of information and support are the former victims of terrorism. They should be included in the preparation and presentation of all primary-intervention programs.

Primary interventions for the general population should be less focused and less intensive. The community should be prepared for the possibility of terrorist activities, and the vulnerability and disruption that such events cause in individual lives should be acknowledged. General education should include information about public response to victims and about the important role that the community can play in welcoming them back. Efforts should also be made to assist citizens in making rational decisions concerning travel.

Secondary Intervention

Secondary intervention should be initiated as soon as a terrorist action has begun. Clinicians should be available to families of victims, to offer support and listen to relatives' concerns. Victims of former terrorist incidents and their families can be a source of strength and support during this waiting period (14). Clinicians with expertise in the area of crisis intervention and victims' services should plan the activities to follow the survivors' return.

When survivors are released, they should be debriefed before meeting the press or returning to their homes. Debriefing should occur in two phases. In the first, the survivor should be interviewed individually and encouraged to air his thoughts and feelings. Symonds (20) notes the importance of allowing the survivor to assume control of his own life; the clinician can indicate this by requesting permission to sit down, to ask questions, and so forth. The clinician should be particularly attentive to indications of doubt or guilt about the victim's own behavior. Survivors should be reassured that "as long as they are alive, they did the right thing" (p. 102) and that they will not be judged or blamed for what they did. It is often useful to follow the individual interviews with a group debriefing session, in which the survivors can share their experiences and describe their current thoughts and feelings. Clinicians and former victims can play a helpful role by discussing with the survivors the kinds of psychological aftereffects they are likely to experience in the short term.

Crisis intervention should continue beyond the initial debriefing. The clinician should assume an active role in encouraging the survivor and family members to attend regular meetings in the aftermath of the incident (3, 9). Survivors should be encouraged to talk freely about their experiences and to explore the impact that the sudden return to freedom has had on their lives. Clinicians should be aware that relatives may also feel in great need of attention and support during this period.

Regular meetings of survivors may be particularly effective in the days and weeks after they return home. When geographical distance makes this difficult, "reunions" should be arranged, to allow group resolution of the experience.

Victims and their families often feel uncomfortable with the idea of mental health intervention. Stöfsel (19) reports that Dutch survivors felt stigmatized as psychiatric patients. Clinicians should reframe survivors' understandings of their own symptoms; short-term psychological aftereffects should be discussed as understandable responses to extreme stress rather than as indications of psychopathology.

Secondary intervention should extend beyond the victims and their families into the affected community. Neighborhood schools are an excellent setting for mental health efforts; classroom interventions should include careful explanation of the facts of the incident and discussion of students' responses to the news. Parents should be provided the opportunity to talk to mental health experts first about their own reactions and questions and, second, about their children's responses and behaviors. Parents should be reassured that temporary changes in their children's behavior (i.e., nightmares, bed wetting, irritability, reluctance to go to school, and so forth) are normal, but should also be encouraged to consult professionals if symptoms do not subside within several weeks.

Tertiary Intervention

For victims who experience continuing problems in readjustment to work and family life, or for those whose symptoms surface weeks or months after their return, extended psychotherapy may be required (7, 10, 11). Whenever possible, continuity between secondary and tertiary treatment should be maintained, in order to build on the trust established in initial clinical contacts. Clinicians should familiarize themselves with the prior history and mental status of the victim. Golan (7) has discussed the necessity of exploring the developmental issues of particular relevance to the survivor at the time of the incident, in order to understand the "special meaning" of the incident to the patient. She has also pointed out that the stress of post-traumatic adjustment may provide patients with a unique opportunity for resolving difficult dilemmas.

Treatment of patients who have been victims of terrorism requires some special adjustments on the part of the clinician. Their stories are hard to listen to. They often maintain a distrust of others and a reluctance to risk intimate contact. Sometimes this is based on previous exploitation by journalists or researchers who got their stories and then left them with their symptoms. Thus, clinicians who can assume an active, ongoing, direct therapeutic role with survivors are especially valuable, even if they are not "experts" in the field. Therapists must be careful not to undermine idiosyncratic positive coping mechanisms that help survivors participate in daily life (e.g., a former hostage who had been rescued through a window subsequently felt most comfortable when near one). Occasional intrusive thoughts or dreams concerning the incident may be extremely difficult to eliminate; minimizing their negative consequences may be a more realistic goal for treatment.

REFERENCES

1. AXINN, S. (1978, October). The law of land warfare as minimal government. *The Personalist*, 374.
2. AYALON, O. (1982). Children as hostages. *Practitioner*, *226*, 1773.
3. AYALON, O., & SOSKIS, D. A. (1986). Survivors of terrorist victimization: A follow-up study. In N. Milgram (Ed.), *Stress and coping in time of war: Generalizations from the Israeli experience*. New York: Brunner/Mazel.
4. CAPLAN, G. (1964). *Principles of preventive psychiatry*. New York: Basic Books.
5. EICHELMAN, B., SOSKIS, D., & REID, W. (Eds.) (1983). *Terrorism: Interdisciplinary perspectives*. Washington, DC: American Psychiatric Association.
6. FIELDS, R. M. (1981). Psychological sequelae of terrorization. In Y. Alexander, & J. M. Gleason (Eds.), *Behavioral and quantitative perspectives on terrorism*. New York: Pergamon Press.
7. GOLAN, N. (1982). The influence of developmental and transitional crises on victims of disasters. In C. D. Spielberger, I. G. Sarason, & N. A. Milgram (Eds.), *Stress and anxiety, Vol. 8*. Washington, DC: Hemisphere.
8. HACKER, F. J. (1976). *Crusaders, criminals, crazies: Terror and terrorism in our time*. New York: Norton.
9. HAUBEN, R. (1983). Hostage taking: The Dutch experience. In L. Z. Freedman, & Y. Alexander (Eds.), *Perspectives on terrorism*. Wilmington, DE: Scholarly Resources.
10. HELLEKSON-EMERY, C. (1981). Posttraumatic stress disorder of a former hostage. *Am. J. Psychiatry*, *138*, 991.
11. HOROWITZ, M. J. (1986). Stress-response syndromes: A review of posttraumatic and adjustment disorders. *Hosp. Commun. Psychiatry*, *37*, 241.
12. JENKINS, B. M. (1985). *International terrorism: The other world war*. Santa Monica, CA: Rand Corp.
13. McKNIGHT, G. (1984). *The terrorist mind*. Indianapolis, IN: Bobbs-Merrill.
14. OCHBERG, F. M. (1982). A case study: Gerard Vaders. In F. M. Ochberg, & D. A. Soskis (Eds.) *Victims of terrorism*. Boulder, CO: Westview Press.
15. SANK, L. I., & SHAFFER, C. S. (1979). Clinical findings while treating the B'nai B'rith hostages. *Psychiatr. Forum*, *8*, 67.
16. SHAW, E. (1983). Political hostages: Sanction and the recovery process. In L. Z. Freedman, & Y. Alexander (Eds.), *Perspectives on terrorism*. Wilmington, DE: Scholarly Resources.
17. SOSKIS, D. A., & OCHBERG, F. M. (1982). Concepts of terrorist victimization. In F. M. Ochberg, & D. A. Soskis (Eds.), *Victims of terrorism*. Boulder, CO: Westview Press.
18. SOSKIS, D. A., & VAN ZANDT, C. R. (1986). Hostage negotiation: Law enforcement's most effective nonlethal weapon. *Behav. Sci. Law*, *4*(4), 423–435.
19. STÖFSEL, W. (1980). Psychological sequelae in hostages and the aftercare. *Dan. Med. Bull.*, *27*, 239.
20. SYMONDS, M. (1982). Victim responses to terror: Understanding and treatment. In F. M. Ochberg, & D. A. Soskis (Eds.), *Victims of terrorism*. Boulder, CO: Westview Press.
21. Task Force on Terrorism and Its Victims, American Psychiatric Association (1982). Ethical dimensions of psychiatric intervention in terrorist and hostage situations: A report of the APA Task Force on Terrorism and Its Victims. *Am. J. Psychiatry*, *139*, 1529.
22. TERR, L. C. (1981). Psychic trauma in children: Observations following the Chowchilla school-bus kidnapping. *Am. J. Psychiatry*, *138*, 14.
23. TERR, L. C. (1983). Chowchilla revisited: The effects of psychic trauma four years after a school-bus kidnapping. *Am. J. Psychiatry*, *140*, 1543.
24. ZAFRIR, A. (1982). Community therapeutic intervention in treatment of civilian victims after a major terrorist attack. In C. D. Spielberger, I. G. Sarason, & N. A. Milgram (Eds.), *Stress and anxiety, Vol. 8*. Washington, DC: Hemisphere.

20

SOCIAL DISASTER

JAMES H. SHORE, M.D.

Professor and Chairman, Department of Psychiatry,
University of Colorado Health Sciences Center,
Denver, Colorado

ELLIE L. TATUM, M.S.W.

Instructor, Department of Psychiatry,
Oregon Health Sciences University,
Portland, Oregon

and WILLIAM M. VOLLMER, PH.D.

Assistant Professor, Department of Psychiatry,
Oregon Health Sciences University,
Portland, Oregon

With instant news reports we are living in a time of increased awareness of social disasters and the physical health and emotional consequences of catastrophic stress. Social disasters include many types of massive stress experiences that are the result of natural or human-induced violence and affect entire communities or groups of people. These events may be caused by floods, earthquakes, volcanic eruptions, airline crashes, industrial explosions, nuclear accidents, or acts of terrorism. In the United States, for example, the extent of morbidity and mortality from natural disasters has been significant. Between 1971 and 1979 the federal disaster declarations and reported casualties included 108 total disasters, 866 deaths, and 29,713 injuries (24). Throughout history disasters have taken their toll on human life. In A.D. 526 a quarter of a million people died in an earth-

---

The authors wish to thank Elaine Steffen for preparation of the manuscript.

quake in Syria. In China in the 1500s over 800,000 were killed in another massive earthquake, and in that same country 3.7 million lost their lives in a devastating flood of the Huang River in 1931, the largest recorded death toll from any single disaster. More recently, in 1985 thousands died in floods and mudflows from the volcanic eruption of Nevado del Ruiz in Colombia. This is only a small percentage of the world-wide casualties and greatly underestimates the number of social disasters and the subsequent suffering from physical injury and psychiatric morbidity.

Several comprehensive literature reviews focus on the psychological consequences of natural disasters. Logue, Melick, and Hansen (24) reviewed the research on the epidemiology of both physical and mental health effects of natural disasters. In 1984 the National Institute of Mental Health Center for Mental Health Studies of Emergencies published an annotated bibliography (7) covering 20 years of mental health research with disasters in the United States. Kinston and Rosser (16) also reviewed the psychiatric outcomes of disaster-related stress. However, interpreting this literature can be difficult and confusing. Leivesley (21) identified several major inconsistencies in the body of disaster research including: (1) a wide variety in sampling, observation, and nomenclature; (2) significant variation in disaster types occurring in many cultures; and (3) different interpretations applied to the same data.

THEORETICAL ISSUES

These literature reviews identify a number of major variables that may influence the duration and significance of behavioral and emotional response to social disaster. These variables include:

1. nature of the disaster response, whether natural or man-made;
2. premorbid physical and mental health; mediating influences of perception and interpersonal networks; and
3. preexisting psychosocial and economic conditions, and susceptible high-risk subgroups.

Frederick (11) has discussed the different effects of natural versus human-induced violence on victims. The nature and timing of any predisaster warning along with individual, family, and community readiness may prevent undesirable postdisaster stress. The presence of predisaster physical or emotional health problems can significantly impair an individual's adaptive capabilities. Other high-risk groups include those suffering the loss of a loved one or major property damage, children, and the elderly. Interpersonal relationships, social networks, and cultural influences may also be strong determinants of emotional reaction to disaster stress.

Berren, Beigel, and Ghertner (1) suggest a model to predict the variable influence on emotional response of various disaster types. They ask five questions to determine the disaster characteristics:

1. Is the event an act of nature or a purposeful event?
2. Is the disaster of long or short duration?
3. Is the personal impact of the disaster high or low?
4. Is the potential for recurrence high or low?
5. Is the control over similar future events high or low?

For example, an act of nature that is predictable, of short duration, with variable degrees of personal impact, and a low potential for recurrence might predict a more favorable outcome. On the other hand, a terrorist act, of long duration, with a high degree of personal impact, a high potential for recurrence, and with little control over similar events in the future, might predict more serious consequences.

Many researchers have reported the "disaster syndrome," a dazed condition of postdisaster adjustment. The phases of the disaster syndrome often overlap and are seldom discrete. They also vary in both intensity and duration. The range of response in symptom manifestations has been attributed to characteristics of the individual, community, and the specific disaster event. Two main interpretations of these variations have dominated the field of research in social disasters. One interpretation emphasizes the disruption of interpersonal and social linkages and the importance of social support systems in determining disaster response and recovery. This viewpoint has been called "the social fabric view" and represents a sociological perspective. This sociological view has focused on the emotional response to disaster as a group process and has assumed minimal negative mental health consequences to individual victims. The second major view has been classified as a psychiatric approach, which defines the extent to which disaster victims have suffered from significant mental disorder as a result of the specific stress. This position has been called "the individual trauma view." While most psychiatric studies of disaster have drawn conclusions supporting a biomedical perspective, these conclusions often have been criticized for utilizing unreliable diagnostic methods based on loosely defined symptom states and subjective measures of unhappiness. Some of these studies have also been complicated by litigation.

A comprehensive theoretical model of the mental health consequences of natural disaster has been proposed by Perry and Lindell (25). This model integrates both the social fabric and individual trauma views and includes three critical areas that influence the psychological consequences of social disaster. These critical areas are the characteristics of the individual victim, the characteristics of the social system, and the disaster's impact on the individual.

INFLUENCE OF PERCEPTION

Perception is a major factor relating to both the nature of the trauma and the nature of the response. Lazarus (19) has pointed out the importance of cognitive assessment of the stressor as a determinant of anxiety response. Kates (15) identifies perception of threat as a significant variable in his conceptual model of natural hazards in human ecology. Spielberger's (38) state-trait model of anxiety also emphasizes that stressors are linked to anxiety by perception of the threat. In his person-situation interactional model of anxiety, Endler (9) sees perception of threat as the mediator of stress response. It is useful to consider both the stressor and the stress response through the filter of an individual's perception.

A number of disaster studies have focused on the perception of danger. Golant and Burton (12) found considerable variation in individual's perceptions of dimensions of danger associated with a range of types of natural, man-made, and quasinatural disasters. In the Love Canal chemical hazard, younger residents and those with dependent children reported perceptions of more widespread contamination than older residents and those with no dependents (10). Studies of Washington State residents living near Mt. St. Helens revealed that awareness of the hazard potential increased as the tremors became more frequent. Prior to the major eruption, those living in the area also had difficulty identifying the specific nature of the threat (e.g., mudflows, ashfall) although they felt adequately informed (13, 26). Perception of threat was not found to be related to distance from the volcano.

Other researchers have focused on individuals' perception of their response to disaster. Another study of people living near Mt. St. Helens examined perceived stress in families. Perceived stress, measured retrospectively by a stress graph, was found to be directly related to geographical proximity to the mountain and to peak at the time of the major eruption (20). Dunal et al. (8) also utilized a retrospective measure of perceived disruption among Argentine flood victims. Higher levels of perceived disruption were associated with the presence of children in the home, greater perceived danger, high property loss, early evacuation, and lack of assistance in the evacuation process.

Two recent disaster studies have examined the relationship of perceived danger and symptomatic measures of stress response. In studying suspected high-risk groups in the Three Mile Island (TMI) nuclear plant accident, Bromet et al. (2, 3) found perception of danger to be directly related to higher anxiety scores among psychiatric patients. Nuclear plant workers who acknowledged danger were also considerably more symptomatic than the majority who viewed TMI as safe. Tatum et al. (39) found significant correlations between high levels of perceived danger from the Mt. St. Helens volcano and diagnosable stress disorders. Perceived distress and objective symptomatic measures of stress were highly correlated among these subjects.

Perception of control has also been investigated in several disaster studies. Sims and Baumann (36) found geocultural differences between those from northern and southern states in perception of control, perception of tornado threat, and coping styles. They associated the more fatalistic, maladaptive responses of southerners with higher death rates from tornadoes. Simpson-Housely (35) also reported that people with less fatalistic, more internally centered locus of control were more likely to take precautionary measures in response to the threat of earthquakes. In a study of communities exposed to ash fallout from Mt. St. Helens, Roberts and his colleagues (27, 28) found that although most people perceived the disaster events to be out of their realm of control, they did feel in control of their response to those events.

SELECTED SOCIAL DISASTER STUDIES

In 1956 Wallace (42) completed a careful review of victim response following a devastating tornado that touched down in Worcester, Massachusetts. This review resulted in the publication of one of the first systematic descriptions of the stages of the "disaster syndrome." Wallace stated that "one can describe the overt behavior of the disaster syndrome as displaying three stages, corresponding roughly to isolation, rescue, and early rehabilitation periods" (p. 125). In the isolation period the tornado victims were dazed, ineffective in coping, stunned, and apathetic. During the rescue phase they behaved with grateful dependence. In the rehabilitation period they were mildly euphoric, with improved coping capacity and a sense of altruism.

The technique of staging behavioral response to social disasters has characterized the research approach in this field for the past three decades. This staging of the disaster syndrome has undergone considerable revision since Wallace's original description of the tornado victims. Frederick (11) emphasized the contrast between the effects of natural versus human-induced violence. His description of the disaster syndrome resembled Wallace's earlier classification. Frederick's phases are: initial impact, heroic, honeymoon, disillusionment, and reorganization. Each phase is associated with its own specific psychological symptoms. Victims of human-induced violence often feel guilty over their inability to prevent their victimization, whereas victims of natural disasters do not. Aberrant behaviors such as looting or alcohol abuse may occur with victims of some major disasters and riots, but not among victims of other forms of human-induced violence, who may identify with the aggressor. Clearly, the type of collective stress situation and the sociocultural fabric of the community interact to determine the ultimate outcome.

Three of the most frequently cited studies in the disaster literature are Lifton's study of the victims of Hiroshima, Lindemann's work with the survivors of the Coconut Grove night club fire in Boston, and Titchener's study of the victims of the Buffalo Creek flood in West Virginia. Lifton (22) interviewed more than 30 survivors of Hiroshima who were picked at random plus additional victims who were unusually articulate or personally prominent. His book on these interviews, *Death in Life—The Survivors of Hiroshima*, was a winner of the National Book Award. In this book Lifton described the internal worlds of the disaster survivors, emphasizing their personal experience from an existential perspective. He described their personal encounter with death, their subsequent psychic numbing, and their guilt over surviving. Psychosomatic symptoms and physical illness were prevalent and long lasting, although formal psychiatric disorder was not common.

Eric Lindemann (23) is often credited with the description of the stages of normal grief that has contributed significantly to our understanding of disaster response. His study was the outcome of working with survivors from the Coconut Grove night club fire in Boston, Massachusetts. Through these interviews he produced a detailed description of the phenomenology of acute grief, concepts that have been widely used to explain the reaction of disaster victims. In another disaster study Titchener and Kapp (41) directed an evaluation of the victims of a West Virginia slag dam collapse on Buffalo Creek. The destructive flash flood killed 125 victims and left hundreds homeless. Using an evaluation that consisted of psychoanalytically oriented family interviews, the investigators demonstrated widespread psychiatric impairment which persisted for at least two years after the disaster. The reaction, which they described as "the Buffalo Creek syndrome," was characterized by anxious and depressed mood, despair, survivor shame, sleep disturbance, and nightmares. One important outcome of the study was the observation that many victims underwent character adjustments that actually were found to preserve and perpetuate the symptoms.

In his book *Stress Response Syndromes* Horowitz (14) emphasizes that significant and disruptive symptoms may persist long after the actual stress, even in conditions of relative safety. Normal and abnormal disaster responses usually involve both logical and irrational beliefs about the personal meaning of the disaster. Horowitz demonstrates that the fears of the disaster may return at later times when the recall experiences of the threat are triggered. The victim experiences the recall as though a repetition were possible, and even likely. At times it is possible that the victim will use the disaster in an attempt to solve an unrelated life experience. With this dynamic perspective Horowitz focuses on the symbolic significance of the disruptive symptoms and their tendency to persist or recur after the actual stressor has passed. This process becomes an important consideration in treatment planning for disaster victims. Horowitz describes five phases after a stressful event: outcry, denial, intrusiveness, working through, and completion. In parallel to the symptomatology of mourning and grief after the death of a family member, he concludes that the resolution of a major stress response is often a process of one or two years.

The extensive research with military veterans of the Vietnam War also has contributed significantly to our understanding of the psychological response to severe trauma, just as "battle fatigue" taught us about stress response to earlier wars. From the American war veterans' reactions to this experience, clinicians defined a disorder of post-traumatic stress (PTSD), which has been incorporated in the psychiatric diagnostic classification of the American Psychiatric Association (6). The diagnostic criteria for PTSD emphasize the potential for delayed onset and prolonged duration. The criteria must include:

A. Existence of a recognizable stressor that would evoke significant symptoms of distress in almost anyone.
B. Reexperiencing of the trauma as evidenced by at least one of the following:
   1. recurrent and intrusive recollections of the event
   2. recurrent dreams of the event

3. sudden acting or feeling as if the traumatic event were recurring, because of an association with an environmental or ideational stimulus

C. Numbing of responsiveness to or reduced involvement with the external world, beginning sometime after the trauma, as shown by at least one of the following:
   1. markedly diminished interest in one or more significant activities
   2. feeling detachment or estrangement from others
   3. constricted affect

D. At least two of the following symptoms that were not present before the trauma:
   1. hyperalertness or exaggerated startle response
   2. sleep disturbance
   3. guilt about surviving when others have not or about behavior required for survival
   4. memory impairment or trouble concentrating
   5. avoidance of activities that arouse recollection of the traumatic event
   6. intensification of symptoms by exposure to events that symbolize or resemble the traumatic event*

Recent studies of the symptom patterns among Vietnam veterans have suggested that the DSM-III criteria for PTSD may underestimate the prevalence of stress-induced impairment (34). Laufler et al. (18) investigated relationships between PTSD and other types of traumatic stress. The DSM-III approach of aggregating symptoms was compared to an approach that differentiated symptoms into subtypes of denial and reexperiencing. The latter approach of distinguishing responses of denial and reexperiencing was felt to be more useful for evaluating PTSD and its meaning. Laufler et al. suggested that the current PTSD model underestimates the prevalence of stress response disorders and points to the limited applicability of PTSD and to its origins as a combat-induced stress disorder. It is unlikely that the diagnostic criteria for PTSD in DSM-III-R will significantly affect this underestimation.

Terr (40) studied the reactions of 26 children who were kidnapped and buried alive in Chowchilla, California, in 1976. The children, who ranged in age from 5 to 14 years, were kidnapped when their school bus was hijacked. They were locked in an abandoned truck that had been buried

---

*Reprinted with permission from the *Diagnostic and Statistical Manual of Mental Disorders, Third Edition*. Copyright 1980 American Psychiatric Association.

underground. They escaped after 16 hours of imprisonment. Terr began interviewing these children five months after this social disaster. She discovered an absence of denial and flashbacks, two of the most common symptoms of PTSD that had been described from studies of combat soldiers suffering from PTSD. Terr discovered that the children engaged in post-traumatic play in a reenactment of the traumatic events. She described the play as sometimes being dangerous, repetitive, grim, and monotonous. In a few children the reenactments were so intense that personality changes and physical problems followed. She also observed that the symptoms were sometimes contagious and affected friends and schoolmates. Her findings emphasized an important area where research has been lacking and demonstrated important differences in the reaction of children to a traumatic social disaster.

NEW RESEARCH METHODS AND FINDINGS

In a new book entitled *Disaster Stress Studies: New Methods and Findings*, Shore (32) included four separate studies that investigated psychiatric disorders resulting from the life-threatening stress of social disasters. These studies were a combination of man-made and natural disasters and included: the nuclear accident at Three Mile Island in Pennsylvania; flood and toxic chemical disasters in Time Beach, Missouri; the volcanic eruption of Mt. St. Helens in Washington State; and Indochinese refugees. All of these recent research efforts utilized systematic diagnostic criteria with a community epidemiology method. The Diagnostic Interview Schedule (30) was applied for the first time in social disaster studies in two of the four projects. The outcomes demonstrated a differential response of the stress disorders with varying psychiatric impairments. The level of impairment appeared to be related to the nature and intensity of the social disaster, with significant psychiatric morbidity occurring only in certain of the disaster stress experiences.

Shore, Tatum, and Vollmer (33) studied the psychiatric reactions in a disaster and control community following the 1980 Mt. St. Helens volcanic eruption. They utilized the Diagnostic Interview Schedule for psychiatric epidemiological research and found a significant disaster-related onset pattern of psychiatric disorders following the eruption. These Mt. St. Helens disorders included depression, generalized anxiety, and post-traumatic stress reaction. A progressive dose-response relationship was demonstrated in the comparison of control, low-exposure, and high-exposure groups, with the pattern occurring among both bereaved and property loss victims and among both males and females.

Bromet and colleagues (2) evaluated the mental health effects of the Three Mile Island (TMI) nuclear accident in Pennsylvania, utilizing the Schizophrenic and Affective Disorders Scale, another standardized psychiatric interview. They also selected a control community and assessed social support as a mitigating factor in psychiatric morbidity from the disaster. They evaluated three suspected risk groups: the mothers of preschool children living within 10 miles of the TMI plant, workers at the TMI plant, and psychiatric outpatients in the area. Mothers of preschool children who lived in the area were at greater risk for anxiety and depression than a control group in the unaffected community. The two other potential high-risk groups demonstrated no significant difference in psychiatric symptomatology between exposed and control communities.

Robins et al. (29) reported on the results from a study of health effects of environmental hazards in Missouri in 1982 and 1983. The town of Times Beach experienced serious floods and a discovery that roads in the area had been contaminated by dioxin. Coincidentally some residents in this area had previously been interviewed as part of the NIMH Epidemiologic Catchment Area (ECA) Project (31). The ECA Project had estimated the prevalence of specific psychiatric disorders in the general population utilizing the Diagnostic Interview Schedule (DIS). They concluded that in Times Beach the disasters of 1982 and 1983 had little impact on mental health measured by the DIS. There was substantial job and property loss with associated economic consequences. The victims tolerated the severe stress, temporary dislocation, and financial reverses without showing profound effects on their mental health. The authors concluded that the stable mental health outcomes could be explained by victims' avoidance of other adverse life events and by the support of interpersonal and social networks.

Working with Robins, Smith et al. (37) compared victims who had experienced a single disaster (flood or toxic exposure) with victims who experienced both disasters and with a series of control subjects who were not exposed to either disaster. In a detailed analysis they concluded that the victims who survived the double disaster had more physical and mental health problems than those who were not exposed to either disaster. The apparent impact of the disaster was diminished by considering that those who experienced the disaster may have been at higher risk for physical illness and psychiatric symptoms even if the disaster had not occurred.

The victims were younger, poorer, less educated, and more often separated or divorced. The higher rates of psychiatric symptomatology and disorders could be accounted for by an exacerbation of symptoms among those who had already experienced the onset of these symptoms prior to the disaster. Unlike the Mt. St. Helens research, where there was a significant onset of new disorders, the research at Times Beach demonstrated little evidence that the disaster was responsible for the development of new psychiatric disorders and symptoms. One exception was post-traumatic stress disorder, however, which was experienced by 25% of the disaster victims even though only 5% met diagnostic criteria one year postdisaster.

Kinzie (17) reported his investigations of severe post-traumatic stress syndrome among Indochinese refugees. Kinzie studied adult patients at a refugee clinic and Cambodian high-school students who had previously been in concentration camps for up to four years. He concluded that post-traumatic stress disorder among these patients was a chronic, relapsing illness with a differential pattern of symptoms. The avoidance, shame, and decreased ability to function placed a long-term limitation on improvement and created a continuing vulnerability to regression and symptom recurrence. Kinzie defined a hierarchy of symptoms that fluctuated over the course of the illness and was dependent on the treatment and subsequent stressors. The depressive symptoms were the most effectively treated. Startle reaction, hyperalertness, nightmares, insomnia, and low interest were only moderately well treated. The symptoms most resistant to treatment included: shame, avoidance behaviors, and capacity for work. Even with patients who were successfully treated, there remained a significant vulnerability to repeated stresses or stimuli that reinforced recall and reactivated symptoms. The Cambodian adolescents who were living in this country without a nuclear family member were at increased risk for experiencing a psychiatric disorder and for a poor prognosis for recovery.

The comparison of the research outcomes in social disaster from Mt. St. Helens, TMI, Times Beach, and Indochinese refugees, all utilizing criterion-based diagnostic methods, documented differential patterns of psychiatric impairment. The extent of psychiatric impairment appeared to be related to the type and intensity of the disaster stress, community characteristics, and postdisaster interpersonal and social networks. For the Mt. St. Helens and refugee populations, the findings substantiated psychiatric morbidity from the disaster stress experience, with symptoms lasting two years and beyond.

APPROACHES TO TREATMENT

On the whole, communities often demonstrate a remarkable adaptation to social disasters. Widespread panic is relatively uncommon. Intervention efforts should be directed to suspected high-risk groups, and mental health professionals responding to disasters should take an active rather than passive role in initiating contact. Disaster assistance centers, emergency rooms, and the morgue are all likely places to seek out surviving family members.

Trained mental health professionals may be utilized close to the disaster site to treat acutely disturbed victims and to provide consultation to relief coordinators. They will be needed to train and supervise volunteer workers. Indeed, special attention must be given to the physical and emotional needs of disaster workers themselves. They must be provided with a realistic set of expectations both for themselves as well as for the victims they will encounter. Failure to do so can lead to feelings of frustration, helplessness, and ultimately to premature "burnout" (43).

A number of authors have addressed specific issues relating to postdisaster crisis intervention (4). A common theme throughout is the notion that disaster victims are normal people whose ability to function has been temporarily disrupted because of the presence of a severe stress. Although they may show symptoms of psychological distress, they do not view their condition as pathological. Cohen and Ahearn (5), in describing guidelines for crisis intervention, stress the acute nature of treatment in the immediate postdisaster period. Traditional clinical practices must be modified so that assistance is of immediate value to the victim. Furthermore, mental health professionals need to work cohesively with other disaster officials. As Cohen (4) notes, "Mental health professionals will find opportunities to offer direct help to individuals traumatized by the disaster while simultaneously offering indirect services, such as consultation and education, to caregivers" (p. 13). She emphasizes the importance of establishing and maintaining supportive relationships throughout all levels of the disaster response network.

The effects of disaster can be especially pronounced in children. Most researchers have found that children tend to mirror the reactions of their parents. The most important fear among children is that of separation. Researchers have stressed the importance of reestablishing immediate physical contact in the event that separation does take place. Cohen (4) notes that the family should be viewed as the first line of resource in helping children. They also advocate the entire family as the basic unit of service when treatment is indicated.

An important aspect of disaster treatment includes predisaster planning. To be successful, an intervention program must get people to admit to the possibility that the disaster may occur while still believing in their capability to survive it. As Kinston and Rosser (16) note, "Anticipation is a small scale preliminary exposure on the level of imagination and can have an inoculating effect. By rehearsing and familiarizing oneself with the coming event one may reduce the risk of becoming overwhelmed by the experience" (p. 449).

REFERENCES

1. BERREN, M. R., BEIGEL, A., & GHERTNER, S. (1980). A typology for the classification of disasters. *Commun. Ment. Health J.*, *16*, 103–111.
2. BROMET, E., PARKINSON, D., SCHULBERG, H., ET AL. (1982). Mental health of residents near the Three Mile Island reactor: A comparative study of selected groups. *J. Prev. Psychiatry*, *1*, 225–276.
3. BROMET, E. J., & SCHULBERG, H. C. (1986). The TMI disaster: A search for high risk groups. In J. H. Shore (Ed.), *Disaster stress studies: New methods and findings*. Clinical Insights Monograph Series. Washington, DC: American Psychiatric Press.
4. COHEN, R. E. (1986). Crisis counseling principles and services. In M. Lystad (Ed.), *Innovations in mental health services to disaster victims*. Rockville, MD: DHHS Pub. No. (ADM) 86-1390.
5. COHEN, R. E., & AHEARN, F. L., JR. (1980). *Handbook for mental health care of disaster victims*. Baltimore: Johns Hopkins University Press.
6. *Diagnostic and statistical manual of mental disorders* (DSM-III) (1980). Washington, DC: American Psychiatric Association.
7. *Disasters and mental health: An annotated bibliography* (1984). Rockville, MD: NIMH Center for Mental Health Studies of Emergencies, DHHS Pub. No. (ADM) 84-1311.
8. DUNAL, C., GAVIRA, M., FLAHERTY, J., & BRIZ, S. (1985). Perceived disruption and psychological distress among flood victims. *J. Operational Psychiatry*, *16*(2), 9–16.
9. ENDLER, N. S. (1975). A person-situation interaction model of anxiety. In C. D. Spielberger & I. G. Saranson (Eds.), *Stress and anxiety*, Vol 1. Washington, DC: Hemisphere.
10. FOWLKES, M. R., & MILLER, P. Y. (1982). *Love Canal: The social construction of disaster*. Northampton, MA: Smith College, Department of Sociology and Anthropology.
11. FREDERICK, C. J. (1980). Effects of natural vs. human-induced violence upon victims. *Evaluation Change*, Special Issue, 71–75.
12. GOLANT, S., & BURTON, I. (1969). *The meaning of a hazard application of the semantic differential*. Working paper no. 7. Toronto, Ontario: University of Toronto.
13. GREEN, M., PERRY, R., & LINDELL, M. (1981). The March 1980 eruptions of Mt. St. Helens: Citizens perceptions of volcano threat. *Disasters*, *5*, 49–66.
14. HOROWITZ, M. (1976). *Stress response syndromes*. New York: Jason Aronson.
15. KATES, R. W. (1977). Natural hazard in human ecological perspective: Hypothesis and models. *Economic Geography*, *47*, 438–451.
16. KINSTON, W., & ROSSER, R. (1974). Disaster: Effects on mental and physical state. *J. Psychosom. Res.*, *18*, 437–456.
17. KINZIE, J. D. (1986). Severe post-traumatic stress syndrome among Cambodian refugees: Symptoms, clinical course and treatment approaches. In J. H. Shore (Ed.), *Disaster*

stress studies: New methods and findings. Clinical Insights Monograph Series. Washington, DC: American Psychiatric Press.

18. LAUFLER, R. S., BRETT, E., & GALLOPS, M. S. (1985). Symptom patterns associated with posttraumatic stress disorder among Vietnam veterans exposed to war trauma. *Am. J. Psychiatry, 142*, 1304–1311.

19. LAZARUS, R. S. (1966). *Psychological stress and the coping process.* New York: McGraw-Hill.

20. LEIK, R. K., LEIK, S. A., EKKER, R., & GIFFORD, G. A. (1982). *Under the threat of Mt. St. Helens: A study of chronic family stress.* Minneapolis, MI: Family Study Center, University of Minnesota.

21. LEIVESLEY, S. (1985). Epidemiology of natural disasters. In J. Seaman, S. Leivesley, & C. Hogg (Eds.), *Contributions to Epidemiology and Biostatistics* (pp. 109–139). Basel: Karger.

22. LIFTON, R. J. (1968). *Death in life – The survivors of Hiroshima.* London: Weidenfeld and Nicholson.

23. LINDEMANN, E. (1944). Symptomatology and management of acute grief. *Am. J. Psychiatry, 101*, 141–148.

24. LOGUE, J. N., MELICK, M. E., & HANSEN, H. (1981). Research issues and directions in the epidemiology of health effects of disasters. *Epidemiol. Rev., 3*, 140–162.

25. PERRY, R. W., & LINDELL, M. K. (1978). The psychological consequences of natural disasters: A review of research on American communities. *Mass Emergencies, 2*, 105–115.

26. PERRY, R. W., LINDELL, M. K., & GREEN, M. R. (1982). Threat perception and public response to volcano hazard. *J. Soc. Psychol., 116*, 199–204.

27. ROBERTS, M. L., DILLMAN, J. J., & MITCHELL, D. W. (1981). Social-psychological responses to the May 18th eruption of Mount St. Helens: Attributions of causality and perception of control. Paper presented at the Pacific Sociological Association, Portland, OR.

28. ROBERTS, M. L., & DILLMAN, J. J. (1981). *Summary of results: You and the mountain effects of the May 18th Mount St. Helens eruption: A survey of eastern Washington households.* Pullman, WA: Department of Child and Family Studies, Washington State University.

29. ROBINS, L. N., FISCHBACH, R. L., SMITH, E. M., COTTLER, L. B., & SOLOMON, S. D. (1986). Impact of disaster on previously assessed mental health. In J. H. Shore (Ed.), *Disaster stress studies: New methods and findings.* Clinical Insights Monograph Series. Washington, DC: American Psychiatric Press.

30. ROBINS, L. N., HELZER, J. E., CROUGHAN, J., & RATCLIFF, R. S. (1981). *National Institute of Mental Health diagnostic interview schedule,* Vol. 38 (pp. 381–389). Rockville, MD: NIMH.

31. ROBINS, L. N., HELZER, J. E., WEISSMAN, M. M., et al. (1984). Lifetime prevalence of specific psychiatric disorder in three sites. *Arch. Gen. Psychiatry, 41*, 949–958.

32. SHORE, J. H. (1986). *Disaster stress studies: New methods and findings.* Clinical Insights Monograph Series. Washington, DC: American Psychiatric Press.

33. SHORE, J. H., TATUM, E. L., & VOLLMER, W. M. (1986). Psychiatric reactions to disaster: The Mount St. Helens experience. *Am. J. Psychiatry, 143*, 5.

34. SIERLES, F. S., CHEN, J., McFARLAND, R. E., & TAYLOR, M. A. (1983). Posttraumatic stress disorder and concurrent psychiatric illness: A preliminary report. *Am. J. Psychiatry, 140*, 1177–1179.

35. SIMPSON-HOUSELY, P. (1978). *Locus of control, repression-sensitization and perception of earthquake hazard.* Working paper no. 36. Boulder, CO: Natural Hazards Research and Application Information Center.

36. SIMS, J. H., & BAUMANN, D. O. (1972). The tornado threat: Coping styles of the North and South. *Science, 196*, 1386–1392.

37. SMITH, E. M., ROBINS, L. N., PRZYBECK, T. R., GOLDRING, E., & SOLOMON, S. D. (1986). Psychosocial consequences of a disaster. In J. H. Shore (Ed.), *Disaster stress studies: New methods and findings.* Clinical Insights Monograph Series. Washington, DC: American Psychiatric Press.

38. SPIELBERGER, C. D. (1972). Anxiety as an emotional state. In C. D. Spielberger (Ed.), *Anxiety: Current trends in theory and research,* Vol. 1. New York: Academic Press.

39. TATUM, E. L., VOLLMER, W. M., & SHORE, J. H. (1986). The relationship of perception and mediating variables to the psychiatric consequences of disaster. In J. H. Shore (Ed.), *Disaster stress studies: New methods and findings.* Clinical Insights Monograph Series. Washington, DC: American Psychiatric Press.

40. TERR, L. C. (1983). Chowchilla revisited: The effects of psychic trauma four years after a school-bus kidnapping. *Am. J. Psychiatry, 140,* 12.

41. TITCHENER, J. L., & KAPP, F. (1976). Family and character change at Buffalo Creek. *Am. J. Psychiatry, 133,* 295–299.

42. WALLACE, A. F. C. (1956). *Human behavior in extreme situations: A study of the literature and suggestions for further research,* Disaster Study No. 1, Committee on Disaster Studies. Washington, DC: National Academy of Sciences, National Research Council.

43. WILKINSON, C. B., & VERA, E. (1985). The management and treatment of disaster victims. *Psychiatr. Ann., 15,* 174–184.

NAME INDEX

SUBJECT INDEX